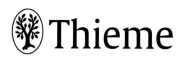

Avoiding Errors in Radiology

Case-Based Analysis of Causes and Preventive Strategies

Klaus-Juergen Lackner, MD
Professor Emeritus
Institute for Diagnostic Radiology
University Hospital
Cologne, Germany

Kathrin Barbara Krug, MD
Professor
Institute for Diagnostic Radiology
University Hospital
Cologne, Germany

956 illustrations

Thieme
Stuttgart · New York

Library of Congress Cataloging-in-Publication Data
is available from the publisher.

This book is an authorized and revised translation of the German edition published and copyrighted 2009 by Georg Thieme Verlag, Stuttgart, Germany.
Title of the German edition: Fehlentscheidungen in der Radiologie: Analyse der Ursachen und Strategien zur Fehlervermeidung.

Translator: Terry Telger, Fort Worth, Texas, USA

Illustrator: Barbara Gay, Stuttgart, Germany

Important note: Medicine is an ever-changing science undergoing continual development. Research and clinical experience are continually expanding our knowledge, in particular our knowledge of proper treatment and drug therapy. Insofar as this book mentions any dosage or application, readers may rest assured that the authors, editors, and publishers have made every effort to ensure that such references are in accordance with **the state of knowledge at the time of production of the book.**

Nevertheless, this does not involve, imply, or express any guarantee or responsibility on the part of the publishers in respect to any dosage instructions and forms of applications stated in the book. **Every user is requested to examine carefully** the manufacturers' leaflets accompanying each drug and to check, if necessary in consultation with a physician or specialist, whether the dosage schedules mentioned therein or the contraindications stated by the manufacturers differ from the statements made in the present book. Such examination is particularly important with drugs that are either rarely used or have been newly released on the market. Every dosage schedule or every form of application used is entirely at the user's own risk and responsibility. The authors and publishers request every user to report to the publishers any discrepancies or inaccuracies noticed. If errors in this work are found after publication, errata will be posted at www.thieme.com on the product description page.

© 2011 Georg Thieme Verlag
Rüdigerstrasse 14, 70469 Stuttgart, Germany
http://www.thieme.de
Thieme New York, 333 Seventh Avenue,
New York, NY 10001, USA
http://www.thieme.com

Cover design: Thieme Publishing Group

Typesetting by Druckhaus Götz GmbH,
   Ludwigsburg, Germany
Printed by L.E.G.O. S.p.A., Vicenza, Italy

ISBN 978-3-13-153881-9   1 2 3 4 5 6

Foreword I

I am pleased to have been asked to write a foreword for this groundbreaking work by Klaus Lackner and Barbara Krug, doing so from a judicial rather than a medical perspective. There have long been conflicts between medicine and law that can be assuaged only if we maintain a dialogue that contributes to mutual understanding. In any event, doctors and lawyers have several characteristics in common: They start their work by making a diagnosis or analyzing the facts of a case, respectively. Then they look for a promising treatment or relevant legal standard, and hopefully they complete their job by finding a cure or reaching a satisfactory resolution.

Sometimes our efforts fail. A judicial decision may be overturned by a higher court and sent back to the lower court for a new ruling. An enviable system! And one that is not often available to doctors who make a mistake. "When you go into a hospital, you never know if you'll come out again," wrote Gottfried Benn, a doctor and author, at the end of his life.

Which brings us to the subject of this book: medical errors. No doctor or patient is safe from them. Some time ago I said to the (now retired) director of a university clinic in Cologne: "A doctor who can say at the end of his career that he has never harmed or killed a patient through negligence may count himself lucky." His reply: "That doctor doesn't exist." Sadly, every honest physician would have to agree.

Yet it is extremely difficult for doctors to admit their mistakes in real-life situations. The exchange quoted above took place during an investigation that I was forced to conduct because medical records were being withheld.

The paths of medicine and law do not separate over malpractice; quite the opposite. But a doctor in this situation must let go of diagnosis and treatment, surrendering them to a legal system that will start by investigating the facts of the case. Legal standards are applied: the doctor is the guarantor of the life and physical well-being of his patient. On the face of it, every intervention meets the criteria of a bodily injury and is therefore unlawful without the consent of the patient. A doctor may also be culpable by failing to perform a necessary intervention. No wonder doctors view their work as a hazardous activity while placing the legal system in the enemy camp.

It all comes down to the patients, however. The physician works for them. Medical malpractice law works for them as well.

Aside from the few cases in which offenders commit criminal acts under the guise of the medical profession, the essential goal of the justice system is special and general prevention. The sheer tenacity of the justice system reflects its efforts to prevent the future endangerment of patients, but this can work only if physicians admit their errors and are prepared to draw conclusions.

This book, too, serves the goal of prevention. I hope that it enjoys a wide readership and will have the greatest possible impact on all medical specialties.

Leonie Kaufmann-Fund
Senior District Attorney,
District Attorney's Office, Cologne

Foreword II

Mistakes happen. Constantly. Some mistakes result from human nature and occur whenever people are involved in the decision-making process. Making mistakes is one of the prime requisites for advancing human understanding and capabilities. It helps us learn how to recognize errors and how to talk about them.

The German Institute for Standardization (DIN) defines a mistake as a "characteristic value that does not meet designated requirements." A mistake can also be defined as a deviation of the results of goal-directed human actions from the goals of that action, thus bringing us quickly to the fine and lofty goals of medical actions. It is clear that errors must be viewed differently in different contexts. The consequences of a broken wire in a CD player are very different from those of a broken wire in a cardiac pacemaker.

Given their potential to cause suffering, disability, and in rare cases even death, medical errors should not happen. But despite the best intentions, they cannot be entirely avoided. Doctors are people, and as such they are affected by moods, by character traits, and by latent and acute influences in their increasingly complex work environments. Doctors are expected to tolerate punishing stress levels almost as a matter of course. It is also taken for granted that we never make mistakes under any circumstances. But we doctors do make mistakes.

The medical profession has long been silent on the subject of medical errors. Who likes to admit mistakes? In grade school we learn that a mistake is a defect, and that a defect is a blemish. But there are many other fields in which quality- and risk-management systems have been implemented with almost perfect success. We see this clearly in commercial airlines, which have dealt with the sobering fact that even a tiny error can result in the deaths of hundreds of people.

In essence, there are two core questions that must be addressed: (1) How can we avoid making a mistake? and (2) How can we avoid repeating a mistake once it has occurred?

If we are to avoid mistakes, we must first analyze working processes, discuss protocols, and make sure that all colleagues receive good basic and advanced training. Even these measures cannot eliminate mistakes (known euphemistically as "adverse events" in modern quality-management systems). When an error occurs, it is imperative that it be discussed. The primary goal is not to unmask and punish the guilty party but to foster a result-oriented approach to problem solving. Repeating the same mistake may suggest stupidity or an ignorance of the problem, neither of which has any place in medicine.

Even among doctors, mistakes must be discussed openly. Traditionally the medical profession has been very reluctant to disclose errors. The reasons for this are diverse and cannot always be rationally explained. Inflated egos are certainly a factor, along with the fear of the potential consequences of admitting a mistake. It is only when we doctors talk openly about our mistakes that the general public will also learn to accept that medical actions are human actions. Medical institutions must foster a culture of awareness that will encourage a solution-oriented analysis of mistakes without finger-pointing.

This book is wonderfully suited for that purpose.

Markus A. Rotschild
Department of Forensic Medicine
Cologne University Hospital

Preface

No one likes to make mistakes. And while constant efforts are being made to reach competent and technically sound decisions in both office and hospital settings, mistakes do happen. There are bound to be differences in individual skills and proficiencies. External factors can adversely affect the quality of decisions as well; current pressures to reduce costs are increasing the risk of medical errors. As a result of staff cutbacks and shift work, experienced physicians are not always available when needed. The advanced training and supervision of young doctors is becoming an increasingly difficult task. The policy intent, of course, is to reduce costs while maintaining a stable quality of care. Quality-management structures in hospitals are developing and implementing key projects aimed at quality assurance. But they are too far removed from the point of care to catch routine errors and generally lack the technical training necessary to evaluate errors and provide didactic feedback. They serve mainly as talking points in the competition among hospitals.

Mistakes are unavoidable. As health-care professionals, we must see to it that they happen rarely and, once discovered, are not repeated. According to a publication by Kohn et al., medical errors account for as many as 40 000 to 100 000 hospital deaths in the United States each year. Individual case reviews are not always easy—a fact that we also experience in insurance claims examinations. But the very magnitude of the problem, which has not been refuted, is definitely cause for alarm.

What can we do with our mistakes?
- Recognize them.
- Discuss them openly.
- Learn from them.
- Develop prevention strategies.
- Implement the strategies developed.
- Test the efficacy of the strategies.

It can be difficult to detect errors in large radiology departments. There is a natural tendency to conceal mistakes. Sometimes the clinician or chief happens to catch the error, and sometimes the initial error comes to light when a patient is sent repeatedly to radiology or develops delayed complications. Some errors are reported by patients or their attorneys.

The detection of errors depends critically on the attentiveness of trained colleagues and their willingness to deal with the incident responsibly and without fear. We must foster a willingness to talk about errors and their prevention. Colleagues should become keen, critical observers at their own initiative rather than in response to external controls. They must be motivated by the need to improve their own quality of work and that of their department. It does no good to look the other way. Respect for the affected patient and regret over the service failure should be reflected in an open discussion of errors among colleagues. The goal of this process is not to assign blame but to establish open communication, convey information, further continuing education, and develop strategies for error prevention. Patients expect dependability. This includes attentiveness to irregularities. As much as we regret them, mistakes provide an opportunity and an obligation to learn and to increase our knowledge of patient safety.

The present collection of case studies summarizes observations made over a period of approximately 10 years. Most of the cases are drawn from our own institution. Some originate from other radiology departments, and the imaging results were interpreted after the patients were transferred. This case collection is intended to alert the reader to potential errors in radiological services and help to ensure that they are not repeated.

Klaus Lackner, Barbara Krug

Abbreviations

AAA	abdominal aortic aneurysm	ICA	internal carotid artery
ACE	angiotensin-converting enzyme	ICH	intracerebral hemorrhage
ACL	anterior cruciate ligament	ICU	intensive care unit
ADC	apparent diffusion coefficient	IDT	intradermal test
AFP	alpha-fetoprotein	IgE	immunoglobulin E
AP	anteroposterior	IgG	immunoglobulin G
ARDS	adult respiratory distress syndrome	IL	interleukin
ASD	atrial septal defect	IRDS	infant respiratory distress syndrome
ASIF	Association for the Study of Internal Fixation	IV	intravenous
AV	arteriovenous	IVP	intravenous pyelogram
AVM	arteriovenous malformation		
		LAO	left anterior oblique
β-HCG	beta human chorionic gonadotropin	LDH	lactate dehydrogenase
BI-RADS	Breast Imaging Reporting and Data System	LHD	left hepatic duct
BPD	bronchopulmonary dysplasia	LLD	left lateral decubitus
b.w.	body weight		
		MALT	mucosa-associated lymphatic tissue
CBC	complete blood count	MCA	middle cerebral artery
CC	craniocaudal	MIBG	$meta$-[^{131}I]iodobenzylguanidine
CCT	cranial computed tomography	MLO	mediolateral oblique
CDU	color duplex ultrasound	MRI	magnetic resonance imaging
CHD	common hepatic duct		
CLL	chronic lymphocytic leukemia	NHL	non-Hodgkin lymphoma
CMV	cytomegalovirus	NSCLC	non–small-cell lung cancer
COPD	chronic obstructive pulmonary disease	NSE	neuron-specific enolase
CRP	C-reactive protein	PA	posteroanterior
CSF	cerebrospinal fluid	PAOD	peripheral arterial occlusive disease
CT	computed tomography	PEEP	positive end-expiratory pressure
CUP	carcinoma of unknown primary	PET	positron emission tomography
CVC	central venous catheter	PML	progressive multifocal leukoencephalopathy
		PSA	prostate-specific antigen
DCIS	ductal carcinoma in situ	PTA	percutaneous transluminal angioplasty
DSA	digital subtraction angiography	PTCD	percutaneous transhepatic cholangio-drainage
DWI	diffusion-weighted imaging	PTT	partial thromboplastin time
ECG	electrocardiogram		
EEG	electroencephalogram	RAO	right anterior oblique
ERC	endoscopic retrograde cholangiography	R-CHOP	chemotherapy regimen involving rituximab, cyclophosphamide, doxorubicin, vincristine, and prednisolone
ER	emergency room		
ESR	erythrocyte sedimentation rate	REE	transesophageal echocardiography
ESWL	extracorporeal shock-wave lithotripsy	RHD	right hepatic duct
		RIS	radiology information system
FDG	2-deoxy-2-(^{18}F)fluoro-D-glucose	ROI	region of interest
		RSNA	Radiological Society of North America
GOT	glutamate-oxalate transaminase	RSV	respiratory syncytial virus
GPT	glutamate-pyruvate transaminase	RT	radiology technician
γGT	gamma-glutamyl transferase		
		SAH	subarachnoid hemorrhage
Hb	hemoglobin	SCLC	small-cell lung cancer
HCC	hepatocellular carcinoma	SEP	somatic evoked potential
IA	intra-arterial		

SSM	superficial spreading melanoma	**TSE**	turbo-spin-echo sequence
STIR	short T1 inversion recovery	**TUR P**	transurethral resection of the prostate (TURP)
SUV	standard uptake value		
TACE	transarterial chemoembolization	**UOQ**	upper outer quadrant
TB	tuberculosis		
TFE	turbo field echo	**VSD**	ventricular septal defect
TIA	transient ischemic attack		
TIPS	transjugular intrahepatic portosystemic shunt	**WBC**	white blood (cell) count
		WHO	World Health Organization
TL	target lesion		

Interdisciplinary Topics for Further Study

Many of the case presentations in this book include an in-depth look at a particular topic for readers who want to know more. The interdisciplinary topics range from the technical aspects and protocols of imaging procedures to issues of differential diagnosis, applied anatomy, pathology, pathophysiology, and treatment options for various diseases.

Contents

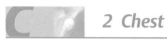

Contents

3 Breast

4 Abdomen

Urogenital Tract ——————————— 223

5 Spinal Column

6 Musculoskeletal System

Contents

7 Vascular System

1

Cranium

Cranium

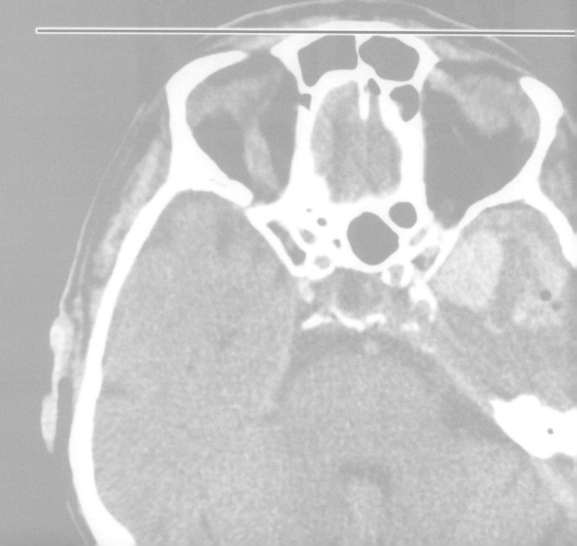

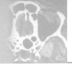

Normal Findings/AV Malformation/Aneurysm/Subarachnoid Hemorrhage (SAH)

History and Clinical Findings

A 39-year-old man was hospitalized with a severe headache of sudden onset. He was experiencing this complaint for the first time. The diagnostic work-up included a lumbar puncture and noncontrast cranial CT scans. The CSF was blood-tinged, and CT scans were interpreted as normal (**Fig. 1.1**). Due to the severity of the headaches, the patient was hospitalized for observation.

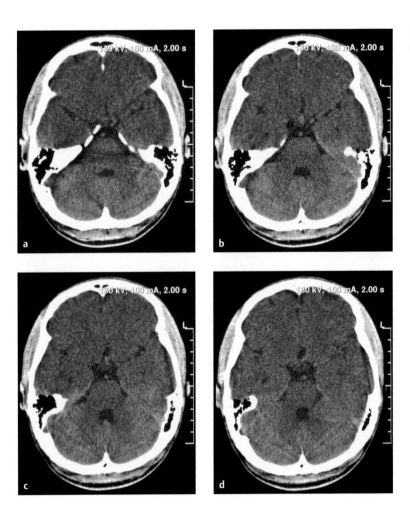

Fig. 1.1 a–d Noncontrast cranial CT scans, interpreted as normal.

Further Case Summary

The patient had no complaints during the night, but his headache returned the next morning. When CT was repeated, scans showed fresh blood in the subarachnoid space, predominantly in the frontal region, in addition to brain edema (**Fig. 1.2**). The patient was transferred to neurosurgery with a suspected ruptured aneurysm of the anterior communicating artery.

CT angiography identified an anterior communicating artery aneurysm as the cause of the SAH (**Fig. 1.3**). Interventional radiology was performed the same day, at which time the aneurysm was occluded by coil embolization (**Fig. 1.4**). There were no complications of treatment.

Error Analysis and Strategy for Error Prevention

The clinical presentation and blood-tinged CSF were consistent with an acute SAH. The most frequent cause of SAH in younger patients is a ruptured arterial aneurysm in the circle of Willis. The anterior communicating artery is most commonly affected (30–40%), followed by the terminal segment of the internal carotid artery (20–30%), the bifurcation of the middle cerebral artery (10–20%), the basilar artery (5–10%), and the vertebral artery (<5%). Less commonly, an SAH is referable to a bleeding AV malformation. A review of the present case shows that the aneurysm was already detectable as a hyperdense "mass" on the initial CT scans (**Fig. 1.5**). However, the finding was so subtle that it was missed.

Peracute subarachnoid hemorrhages only a few hours old may elude CT detection because the blood is still liquid and is isodense to normal brain parenchyma. Because blood in the subarachnoid space directly overlies the cerebral cortex, often there is no attenuation difference at this stage that would cause appreciable CT contrast between the liquid blood and cerebral cortex. It is only in the acute stage (1–3 days) that the density of the hemorrhage rises to 80–100 HU due to the high iron content of the clotted blood, which then becomes distinguishable from surrounding brain parenchyma (which has unenhanced attenuation values of 40–50 HU) (see **Table 1.5**, p. 18 and the interdisciplinary excursion on p. 20).

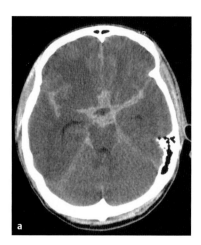 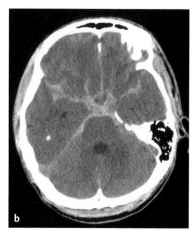

Fig. 1.2 a, b Noncontrast CT scans the following day show a definite subarachnoid hemorrhage, now accompanied by brain edema.

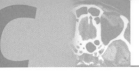
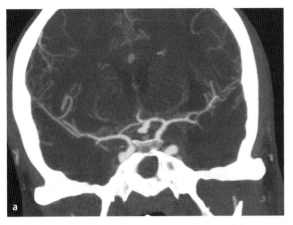 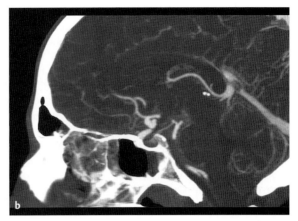

Fig. 1.3 a, b CT angiography confirms an aneurysm of the anterior communicating artery.
a Coronal reformatted image.　　　　　　　　　　**b** Sagittal reformatted image.

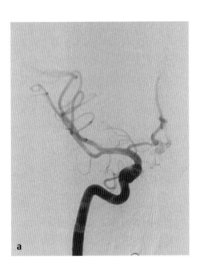 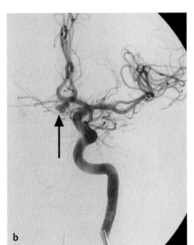

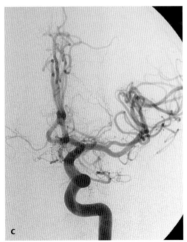 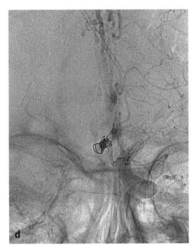

Fig. 1.4 a–d The aneurysm was occluded with coils at interventional radiology.
a Preinterventional DSA shows slight opacification of the aneurysm via the right anterior cerebral artery.
b Preinterventional DSA shows intense opacification of the aneurysm via the left anterior cerebral artery (arrow).
c Postinterventional DSA confirms occlusion of the aneurysm.
d Postinterventional DSA shows coils in the aneurysm lumen.

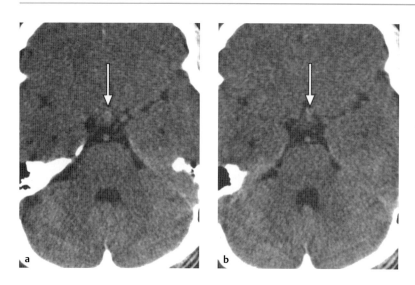

Fig. 1.5 a, b The anterior communicating artery aneurysm was visible on initial CT scans (arrow) but was missed.

References and Further Reading

Bradley Jr WG. Hemorrhag. In: Stark DD, Bradley Jr WG, eds. Magnetic Resonance Imaging. 3rd ed. St. Louis: Mosby; 1999: 1329–1346

Osborn AG. Diagnostic Cerebral Angiography. 2nd ed. Philadelphia: Lippincott Williams & Wilkins; 1999

Osborn AG, Blaser SI, Salzmann KL, Katzman GL, Provenzale J, Castillo M. Diagnostic Imaging Brain. Salt Lake City: Amyrsis; 2004

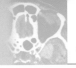

CT Section of a Cerebral Fissure/ Cerebral Infarction

History and Clinical Findings

A 66-year-old man underwent an elective aortocoronary bypass for coronary heart disease. Surgery was repeated on the second postoperative day due to occlusion of the bypass. Shortly thereafter the patient developed hemiparesis on the right side of the body. EEG showed signs of ischemia. Noncontrast cranial CT scans were interpreted as normal. A well-circumscribed hypodensity in the left parietal area was interpreted as a cerebral fissure that had been cut by the scan plane (**Fig. 1.6**).

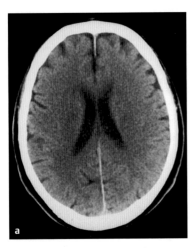 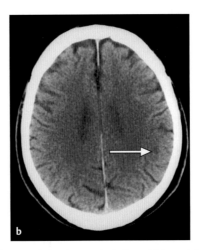 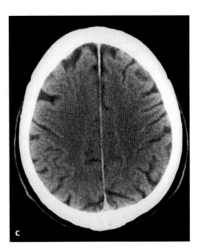

Fig. 1.6a–c   Noncontrast cranial CT scans. The arrow in **b** points to the lesion, which was initially interpreted as a cerebral fissure cut by the scan.

Diffusion and Perfusion Imaging

Diffusion imaging (MRI). Diffusion-weighted imaging shortly after a cerebral ischemic event shows a decrease in the diffusion (motion) of hydrogen protons in the intercellular space caused by the cytotoxic, hydropic swelling of brain cells in the infarcted area.

Perfusion imaging (MRI, CT). Perfusion imaging provides a semiquantitative assessment of cerebral blood flow by documenting the passage of an IV contrast bolus through the brain parenchyma in multiple consecutive data acquisitions.

Perfusion–diffusion mismatch. A mismatch between dying tissue (diffusion) and underperfused tissue (perfusion) correlates with the pathophysiologic concept of the penumbra, or brain tissue bordering an infarction that can potentially be saved. If the hypoperfused area matches the area showing a diffusion deficit, this means that virtually no salvageable tissue is present. If the volume of the perfusion deficit is larger than that of the diffusion deficit, it may be possible to preserve brain tissue by lytic therapy.

Further Case Summary

When cranial CT was repeated the next day, it showed increased volume of the hypodensity in the left parietal white matter and cerebral cortex, which now had ill-defined margins. In addition, a new wedge-shaped hypodensity was found in the left white matter rostral to the first lesion, and effacement of sulci was noted in the parietal left hemisphere (**Fig. 1.7**). The findings were interpreted as fresh infarctions in the territory of the left middle cerebral artery (MCA) with toxic perifocal edema. The hemiparesis responded well to conservative treatment during the next few months.

Error Analysis and Strategy for Error Prevention

In retrospect, the hypodensity indicated by an arrow in **Fig. 1.6b** must be interpreted as a direct, early sign of ischemia due to parenchymal destruction. Indirect early signs caused by toxic postinfarction edema are relative unsharpness of the gray–white matter junction compared with healthy brain and narrowing of the adjacent cerebral fissures.

Given the history and EEG findings and the therapeutic implications, it would have been better to perform MR diffusion and perfusion imaging or CT perfusion imaging to allow for early detection of any ischemic areas not disclosed by plain CT. The cerclage wires in the sternum following coronary surgery would not have contraindicated MRI. CT examination after IV contrast administration was not indicated, because plain scans are better for showing a possible loss of gray–white matter contrast a few hours after an ischemic event. Disruption of the blood–brain barrier is not apparent until 6 hours after the event.

References and Further Reading

Sator K. Diagnostic and Interventional Neuroradiology. A Multimodality Approach. Stuttgart: Thieme; 2001

Osborn AG, Blaser SI, Salzmann KL, Katzman GL, Provenzale J, Castillo M. Diagnostic Imaging: Brain. Salt Lake City: Amyrsis; 2004

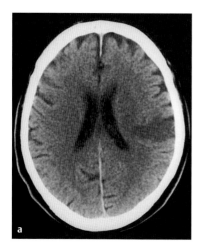 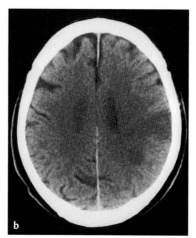 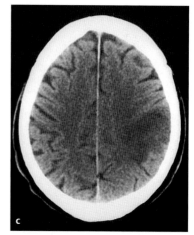

Fig. 1.7 a–c Noncontrast cranial CT scans taken the following day show increased volume and ill-defined margins of the hypodensity in the left white matter, decreased gray–white matter contrast, and effacement of cerebral sulci in the affected area.

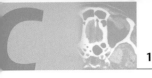

Age-Normal Findings/ Fresh Cerebral Ischemia/ Old Infarction

History and Clinical Findings

A 61-year-old man was found in an unconscious state. The emergency physician noted anisocoria. Noncontrast cranial CT scans prior to ICU admission showed an old postischemic lacunar defect in the right frontal white matter, small microangiopathic white-matter defects in both hemispheres, and a cavum septi pellucidi as a normal variant (**Fig. 1.8**). There was no evidence of intracranial hemorrhage, impaired CSF circulation, or a skull fracture.

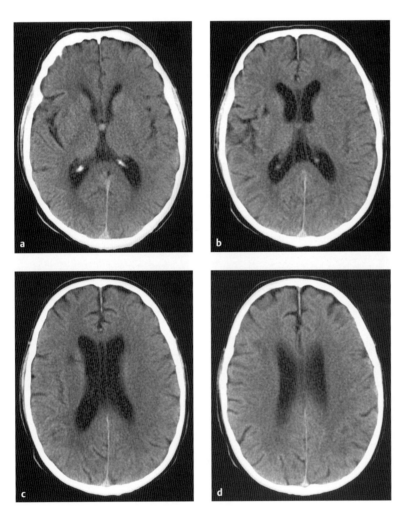

Fig. 1.8 a–d Noncontrast cranial CT scans on admission show a lacunar defect in the right white matter and bilateral areas of microangiopathic white matter degeneration. A cavum septi pellucidi is present as a normal variant.

Further Case Summary

The patient was found to have an extensive left hemispheric infarction, which was confirmed by further CT follow-up (**Figs. 1.9, 1.10**). The patient died 10 days later from complications relating to increased intracranial pressure.

Error Analysis and Strategy for Error Prevention

The asymmetry of the outer CSF spaces (smaller on the left side), the effacement of cerebral sulci relative to the opposite side, the loss of gray–white matter differentiation in the left parieto-occipital area, hypodensity of the left white matter, and poor delineation of the left basal ganglia had all been missed as early signs of cerebral ischemia during interpretation of the initial CT scans (**Fig. 1.11, Table 1.1**).

Table 1.1 CT features of acute cerebral ischemia

Pathophysiology	CT morphology
Mass caused by cytotoxic brain edema	Narrowing of inner and/or outer CSF spaces in the affected region Narrowing or effacement of cerebral sulci (compared with the opposite side)
Parenchymal destruction, cytotoxic edema	Hypodensity of ischemic parenchyma (compared with the opposite side) Poor delineation of affected basal ganglia Incipient loss of gray–white matter differentiation
Acute thrombosis of arterial vascular lumen	Plain scans show increased density of the occluded vascular segment (**Fig. 1.12**)

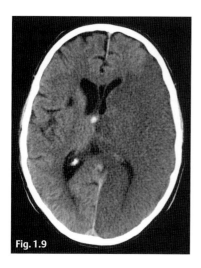

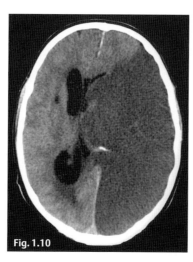

Fig. 1.9

Fig. 1.10

Fig. 1.9 CT scan 1 day after admission shows hypodensity of the left middle and posterior cerebral artery territory with a shift of the midline.

Fig. 1.10 Noncontrast CT scan 3 days after admission shows global cerebral edema with an increasing midline shift toward the right side.

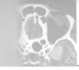
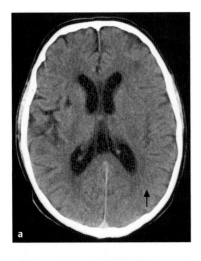

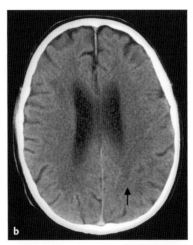

Fig. 1.11 a, b Noncontrast CT scans on admission (**Fig. 1.8**). Initial reading of the scans missed early signs of cerebral ischemia (arrows): narrowing of the outer CSF spaces in the left parieto-occipital region (**a, b**) with loss of gray–white matter contrast (**a, b**) and poor delineation of the left basal ganglia (**a**).

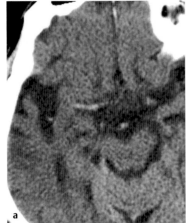

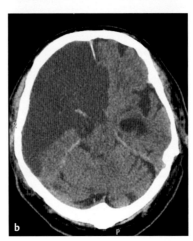

Fig. 1.12 a, b Noncontrast CT of an acute right middle cerebral artery infarction shows increased intraluminal density of the right MCA (in a different 62-year-old patient with clinical manifestations of right cerebral ischemia).
a Initial findings.
b Scan 2 days later documents the development of a large MCA infarction.

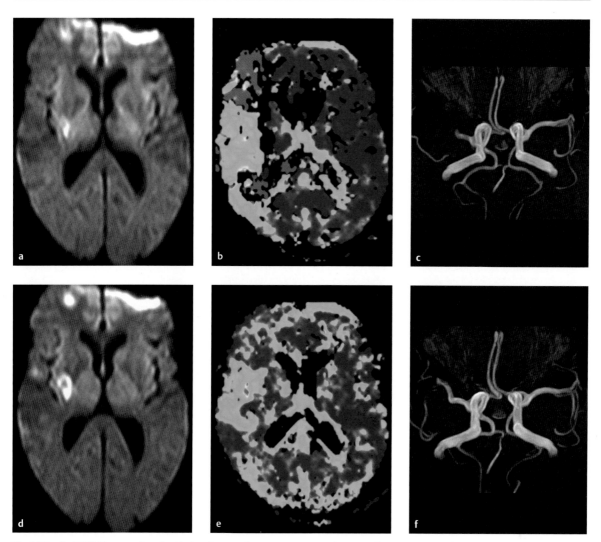

Fig. 1.13 a–f   MRI follow-up of cerebral ischemia secondary to occlusion of the right middle cerebral artery (different patient). Examination 2 hours after onset of symptoms shows a mismatch between a circumscribed diffusion abnormality in the right paraventricular white matter (**a**) and a perfusion deficit throughout the MCA territory (**b**). The changes were caused by thromboembolic occlusion of the main trunk of the right MCA (**c**). The right MCA was reopened by local lytic therapy (**f**), leading to regression of the perfusion deficit (**e**). The diffusion abnormality shows no significant change, indicating circumscribed irreversible damage to the brain tissue (**d**).

a Diffusion-weighted image 2 hours after the event.
b Perfusion image 2 hours after the event.
c MR angiography 2 hours after the event.
d Diffusion-weighted image 24 hours after the event.
e Perfusion image 24 hours after the event.
f MR angiography 24 hours after the event.

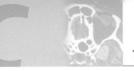
Ischemic Brain Diseases

Pathophysiology

Several stages are recognized in the natural history of a brain infarction: the necrotic stage (days 0–3 after the event), the absorption stage (day 4 to <week 6), and the organization stage (week 6 and after). The normal blood flow rate in the gray matter is 80 mL/100 g brain tissue/min. Brain function is reversibly compromised at flow rates between 15 and 25 mL/100 g tissue/min (penumbra, **Fig. 1.13**). An infarction exists when perfusion falls below 15 mL/100 g tissue/min.

During the *necrotic stage*, failure of the Na^+/K^+ pump in the cell membrane, which normally controls the exchange of fluids and electrolytes between the intra- and extracellular spaces, leads to the development of cytotoxic brain edema, which is manifested by the swelling of perivascular astrocytes and endothelial cells. As the volume of the intracellular space increases, the extracellular space becomes smaller. This compromises the brownian motion of hydrogen protons in the infarcted tissue. Disruption of the blood–brain barrier occurs approximately 6 hours after the ischemic event, allowing macromolecules to enter the extracellular space of the ischemic tissue. Following the osmotic pressure gradient, this results in an influx of water from the blood vessels into the extracellular space. The cytotoxic edema is accompanied by *vasogenic edema*. Leukocytes begin to infiltrate the margins of the infarcted area by approximately 24 hours, followed by the necrosis of ganglion cells and glial cells and damage to the myelin sheaths.

The dominant process in the *absorption stage* is phagocytosis of the necrotic tissue. Neutral fat-laden macrophages leave the infarcted area through newly formed capillaries. Postinfarction edema is greatest between days 3 and 5 and clears during the second week after the event.

Necrosis and absorption are largely complete by the *organization stage*. The principal findings at this stage are colliquation cysts and gliosis.

Imaging and Treatment Planning

Diffusion-weighted MRI sequences are used to evaluate the free mobility of hydrogen protons. A decrease in the apparent diffusion coefficient (ADC) is detectable by MRI (**Fig. 1.13**; see also p. 23). The increased water content of ischemic brain parenchyma due to cytotoxic and vasogenic edema is mainly responsible for the changes on CT (hypodensity of the infarcted area) and T2-weighted MRI (increased signal intensity) that are seen at least 2–3 hours after the ischemic event.

The treatment options for acute arterial cerebral ischemia range from anticoagulation, neuroprotection (glutamate antagonists, free-radical scavengers), anticytokines, calcium channel blockers, etc.), systemic transvenous and local transarterial thrombolysis, to hypothermia and decompressive craniotomy. The maximum time window for local lytic therapies is the first 6 hours after the onset of symptoms; otherwise there would be a disproportionately high risk of bleeding complications in the infarcted area. The imaging work-up should answer the following questions as an aid to treatment planning:

1. Stroke: Does the patient have cerebral ischemia or a primary cerebral hemorrhage?
2. Acute ischemia: How much brain tissue has already been irreversibly damaged?
3. Acute ischemia: How much brain tissue is reversibly damaged and therefore potentially salvageable?
4. Acute ischemia: Is there an occlusion of major cerebral supply arteries?

Question 1: CT is the most sensitive and specific imaging modality for the detection or exclusion of cerebral hemorrhage. CT can detect cerebral ischemia as early as 2–3 hours after the event on the basis of regional narrowing of the cerebral sulci, a circumscribed loss of gray–white matter differentiation, and circumscribed hypodensity of the affected brain area (**Table 1.1**, p. 9). Diffusion-weighted MRI sequences can show initial changes during the first hour after the event based on a focal increase in the ADC. T2- and T1-weighted MR sequences, like CT, can detect acute ischemia no earlier than 2–3 hours after the event on the basis of ischemic cerebral sulci, loss of gray–white matter differentiation, ill-defined increase in T2-weighted signal intensity, or decrease in T1-weighted signal intensity).

Question 2: Irreversibly damaged brain tissue is characterized by a diffusion abnormality (increased ADC in diffusion-weighted MR sequences) and also by a perfusion defect (MR perfusion imaging).

Question 3: Reversibly damaged brain tissue is characterized by a perfusion deficit in the absence of a diffusion abnormality, known as a "perfusion–diffusion mismatch."

Question 4: A high-grade stenosis or occlusion of the cerebral supply arteries can be detected or excluded noninvasively by CT or MR angiography.

Thus, the radiological work-up of acute stroke should include noncontrast CT scans and MRI with diffusion-weighted, perfusion-weighted, and angiographic sequences, depending on available equipment and individual treatment options (availability of a stroke unit, neuroradiology, and neurosurgery).

References and Further Reading

Sator K. Diagnostic and Interventional Neuroradiology. A Multimodality Approach. Stuttgart: Thieme; 2001

Osborn AG, Blaser SI, Salzmann KL, Katzman GL, Provenzale J, Castillo M. Diagnostic Imaging Brain. Salt Lake City: Amyrsis; 2004

Traumatic Intraparenchymal Hemorrhage/ Cavernoma/Tumor

History and Clinical Findings

A 32-year-old man drove his bicycle into a post while under the influence of alcohol, sustaining multiple midfacial fractures. CT scans of the facial skeleton taken in the emergency room confirmed the presence of complex Le Fort III midfacial fractures (**Fig. 1.14**). Cranial CT showed enlarged third and lateral ventricles with no hypodense subependymal caps near the ventricular horns and no evidence of blood in the CSF. The findings were interpreted as normal-pressure hydrocephalus unrelated to the injury (**Fig. 1.15**). CT also demonstrated an approximately 2-cm rounded hyperdensity in the left frontoparietal region that was interpreted as a possible intraparenchymal hemorrhage or, less likely, an intracerebral tumor.

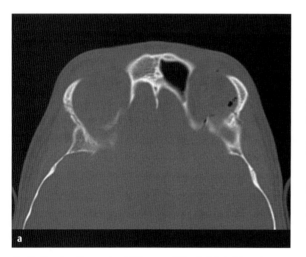
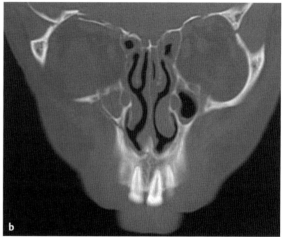

Fig. 1.14 a, b Noncontrast CT scans of the facial skeleton show a Le Fort III midfacial fracture with involvement of the anterior skull base (see **Fig. 1.16**).

a Axial scan.
b Coronal scan.

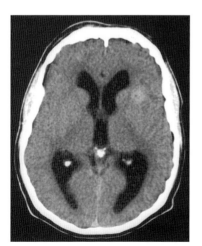

Fig. 1.15 Noncontrast CT scan of the skull shows triventricular internal hydrocephalus with an approximately 2-cm rounded hyperdensity in the left frontoparietal white matter.

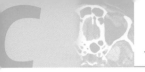

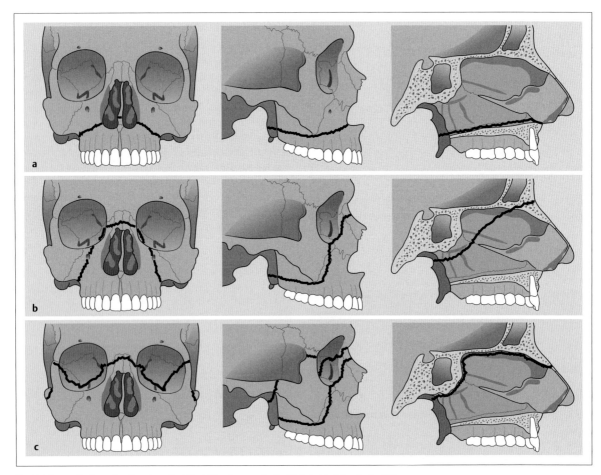

Fig. 1.16a–c   Le Fort classification of midfacial fractures. **a** Le Fort I. **b** Le Fort II. **c** Le Fort III.

Further Case Summary

MRI one week later revealed a cavernoma in the anterior external capsule with:

- A nodular mass, predominantly hyperintense in all sequences, whose signal intensity was influenced by slow blood flow and thrombi in lacunar venous cavities.
- A rim of low T2-weighted signal intensity caused by hemosiderin deposits due to chronic recurrent petechial hemorrhages.
- Slight homogeneous enhancement after IV contrast administration (**Fig. 1.17**).

CT confirmed finely dispersed calcifications within the cavernoma, which appeared iso- to hypointense to normal brain on MRI. The calcifications were displayed less clearly on MRI than CT due to limitations of spatial and contrast resolution.

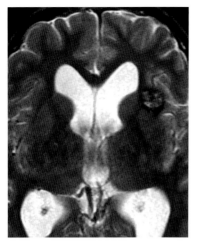 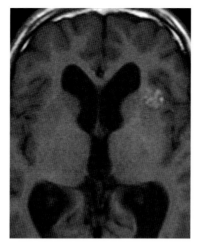 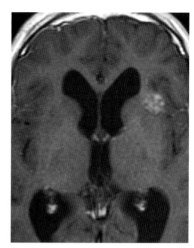

Fig. 1.17 a–c   MR images of a cavernoma.
a T2-weighted TSE sequence.
b T1-weighted TSE sequence without contrast medium.

c T1-weighted TSE sequence after IV contrast administration.

Error Analysis and Strategy for Error Prevention

The hyperdense intraparenchymal lesion visible on non-contrast CT suggested a chronic, inactive process based on its location, symmetry, and the absence of perifocal edema. The most likely diagnosis was a cavernoma, which typically contains finely dispersed calcifications, or a calcified postinflammatory or postinfectious focus (**Table 1.2**). The absence of soft-tissue signal intensity and/or perifocal edema was inconsistent with a fresh posttraumatic hemorrhage, acute intratumoral hemorrhage, or a calcified primary brain tumor or calcified metastasis (from colon cancer, osteosarcoma, or lung cancer). A meningioma with stromal calcifications, a giant aneurysm with a calcified thrombus, and calcifications in the basal ganglia were unlikely because the lesion was located in the external capsule and was not closely related to the meninges.

Table 1.2   Morphologic imaging findings in 2000 asymptomatic patients who underwent cranial MRI for enrollment in the Rotterdam Study

Findings	Number of patients (n)	Percentage of patients (%)
Asymptomatic cerebral infarction	145	7.2
▪ Lacunar infarction	112	5.6
▪ Cortical infarction	41	0.2
Primary brain tumors, benign	31	1.6
▪ Meningioma	18	0.8
▪ Vestibular schwannoma	4	0.2
▪ Intracranial lipoma	2	0.1
▪ Trigeminal schwannoma	1	<0.1
▪ Pituitary adenoma	6	0.3
Primary brain tumors, malignant	1	<0.1
Other findings		
▪ Aneurysm	35	1.8
▪ Cavernous angioma	7	0.4
▪ Metastases	1	<0.1
▪ Subdural hematoma	1	<0.1
▪ Arachnoid cyst	22	1.1
▪ Chiari malformation type I	18	0.9
▪ Stenosis of large cerebral arteries	9	0.5
▪ Dermoid cyst	1	<0.1
▪ Fibrous dysplasia	1	<0.1
Total	**456**	**22.8**

* Source: Vernooij MW, Ikram MA, Tanghe HL, et al. Incidental findings on brain MRI in the general population. N Eng J Med 2007; 357 (18): 1821–1828. Reprinted with permission.

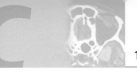

Hydrocephalus

Obstructive (Noncommunicating) Hydrocephalus

- Mechanical obstruction of CSF flow in the aqueduct, in the foramina of Luschka or Magendi of the fourth ventricle, or in the foramen of Monro at the junction of the lateral ventricles and third ventricle.
- Ventricular dilatation upstream of the obstruction (particularly, enlargement of the temporal horns and ballooning of the third ventricle).
- Narrowing of the outer CSF spaces and sulci.
- Hypodense caps around the horns of the lateral ventricles caused by pressure-induced diapedesis of CSF into the subependymal parenchyma.

Malabsorptive (Communicating) Hydrocephalus

- Impairment of CSF absorption due to inflammatory or infectious meningitis, carcinomatous meningitis, subarachnoid hemorrhage, venous sinus thrombosis, trauma, or a neurosurgical procedure.
- Ventricular dilatation.
- Relatively late narrowing of the outer CSF spaces and sulcal effacement.
- Otherwise, same imaging features as obstructive hydrocephalus

Normal-Pressure Hydrocephalus (Special Form of Communicating Hydrocephalus)

- Ventricular dilatation. Various portions of the inner CSF spaces may be affected, but dilatation is usually limited to the lateral ventricles and third ventricle.
- Normal caliber of outer CSF spaces.
- Normal appearance of periventricular parenchyma

References and Further Reading

Litt AW, Maltin EP. Cerebrovascular abnormalities. In: Stark DD, Bradley WG, eds. Magnetic Resonance Imaging. Volume III. 3rd ed. St. Louis: Mosby; 1999: 1317–1327

Ott A, Breteler MM, van Harskamp F, Stijnen T, Hofman A. Incidence and risk of dementia: the Rotterdam Study. Am J Epidemiol 1998; 147: 574–580

Vernooij MW, Ikram MA, Tanghe HL, et al. Incidental findings on brain MRI in the general population. N Engl J Med 2007; 357: 1821–1828

Normal Variant/ AV Malformation/ Aneurysm/ Subarachnoid Hemorrhage

History and Clinical Findings

A 22-year-old woman was struck by an automobile while under the influence of alcohol, sustaining anterior dental injuries, a left paramedian fracture of the mandible, bilateral fractures of the mandibular neck and condyles, a fracture of the right radius, chest contusions, and grade 1 head trauma (**Table 1.3**). Noncontrast cranial CT scans obtained during critical care were interpreted as normal (**Fig. 1.18**). The patient was transferred the next day to the oral and maxillofacial surgery clinic for treatment of her complex mandibular fractures. Another noncontrast cranial CT examination was performed 2 days later (**Fig. 1.19**). The report described "marked density of the tentorium" as a normal variant with no change relative to the previous examination. Subarachnoid hemorrhage (SAH) and intracerebral hemorrhage (ICH) were excluded.

Table 1.3 Hunt and Hess scale for grading the clinical severity of head trauma (after Hunt and Hess 1968)

Grade	Symptoms
1	Asymptomatic or minimal headache and slight nuchal rigidity
2	Moderate to severe headache; nuchal rigidity; no neurologic deficit except cranial nerve palsy
3	Drowsy; minimal neurologic deficit
4	Stuporous; moderate to severe hemiparesis; possibly early decerebrate rigidity and vegetative disturbances
5	Deep coma; decerebrate rigidity; moribund

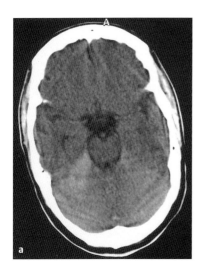
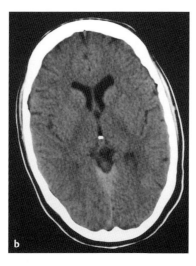

Fig. 1.18 a, b Noncontrast cranial CT on the day of the injury.

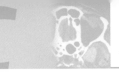

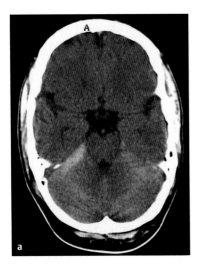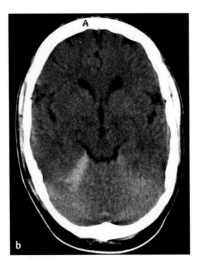

Fig. 1.19 a, b CT scans 2 days later.

Further Case Summary

The patient first complained of diplopia one week after the injury. Right abducens nerve palsy was diagnosed on day 13. Another CT examination yielded the diagnosis of a SAH in the absorption stage (**Fig. 1.20**). The next day this diagnosis was confirmed by a pathognomonic set of MRI findings (patchy tentorial deposits with high T1- and T2-weighted signal intensity and low T2*-weighted signal intensity; meningeal enhancement after IV contrast administration; **Fig. 1.21**). The findings indicated a subarachnoid hemorrhage classified as grade 2 on the Hunt and Hess scale and grade 3 on the Fisher scale (**Tables 1.4, 1.5**).

Table 1.4 Fisher scale for grading the CT appearance of sub-arachnoid hemorrhage (after Fisher et al. 1980)

Grade	Findings
1	SAH is present pathoanatomically, but no blood is evident at CT
2	Diffuse hemorrhage or subarachnoid hemorrhage less than 1 mm thick
3	Subarachnoid clot or hemorrhage more than 1 mm thick
4	SAH of any thickness with intraventricular or parenchymal extension

Table 1.5 Effect of the denaturation of hemoglobin in a subarachnoid hemorrhage on MRI and CT findings

Stage of hemorrhage	Hemoglobin (Hb) and its breakdown products	Patho-physiology	MRI				CT
			Location of Hb products (red cells)	Magnetic properties	T1 relation to brain parenchyma	T2 relation to brain parenchyma	Density relative to brain parenchyma
Peracute (hours)	Oxyhemoglobin	Serum and red cells in clot	Intracellular	Diamagnetic	Isointense	Hyperintense	Isodense
Acute (days 1 + 2)	Deoxyhemoglobin	Deoxygenation	Intracellular	Paramagnetic	Isointense	Hypointense	Hyperdense
Early subacute (days 3–7)	Methemoglobin	Absence of iron reduction (oxygenation) and denaturation of Hb	Intracellular	Paramagnetic	Hyperintense	Hypointense	Hyper- to isodense (fogging)
Late subacute (weeks 2–4)	Methemoglobin	Breakdown of red cells	Extracellular	Paramagnetic	Hyperintense	Hyperintense	Hypodense
Chronic (months to years)	Hemosiderin, ferritin	Iron deposition and storage	Extracellular	Para- and ferro-magnetic	Iso- to hypo-intense	Hyperintense with a hypo-intense rim	Hypodense

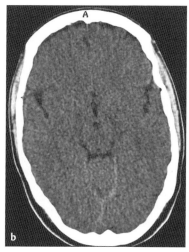
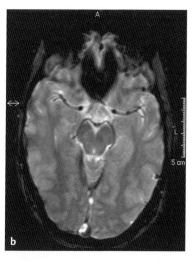

Fig. 1.20 a, b Noncontrast cranial CT scans on day 13 post injury show decreased density of the hemorrhagic deposits on the tentorium compared with **Fig. 1.18**.

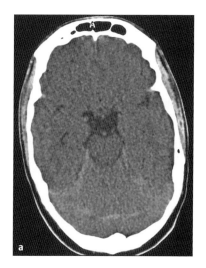
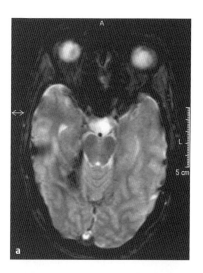
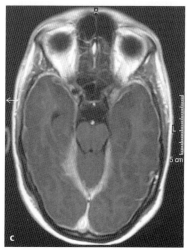
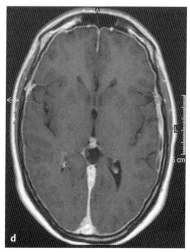

Fig. 1.21 a–d Cranial MRI on day 14 post injury. The T2*-weighted sequence shows pathognomonic signal voids in the subarachnoid space due to susceptibility changes caused by extracellular iron deposits from blood breakdown products (**a, b**). Meningeal enhancement in the T1-weighted sequence after IV contrast administration (**c, d**) results from inflammation of the meninges caused by the hemorrhagic deposits.

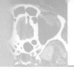

Error Analysis and Strategy for Error Prevention

Confinement of the subarachnoid hemorrhage to the tentorium was unusual and led to misinterpretation of the initial CT scans. This pattern arose because the traumatizing force was directed posteriorly from the mandible toward the brainstem, causing a local shearing action between the firmly attached tentorium and the more mobile meningeal and parenchymal soft tissues. This led to the rupture of meningeal veins.

A subarachnoid hemorrhage at an atypical location could have been diagnosed in the initial CT examinations because the attenuation values of the hemorrhage, at 85–93 HU, were significantly higher than the attenuation values of normal brain (43–48 HU).

References and Further Reading

Bradley Jr. W. Hemorrhage. In: Stark DD, Bradley Jr. WG, eds. Magnetic Resonance Imaging. Volume III, 3rd ed. St. Louis: Mosby; 1999: 1329–1346

Fisher CM, Kistler JP, Davis JM. Relation of cerebral vasospasm to subarachnoid hemorrhage visualized by computerized tomographic scanning. Neurosurgery 1980; 6: 1–9

Hunt WE, Hess RM. Surgical risk as related to time of intervention in the repair of intracranial aneurysms. J Neurosurg 1968; 28: 14–20

Sator K. Diagnostic and Interventional Neuroradiology. A Multimodality Approach. Stuttgart: Thieme; 2001

Subarachnoid Hemorrhage

CT

Acute subarachnoid hemorrhage is detected most reliably by CT. Hemoglobin detection in the CSF after lumbar puncture is also available as an adjunct. The CT detection of hemorrhage depends on the hemoglobin concentration and age of the hemorrhage. Pathophysiologically, the initially liquid blood that extravasates into the subarachnoid space (*peracute stage*) coagulates over a period of minutes to several hours. The subarachnoid blood is completely coagulated by the first to third day after the injury (*acute stage*). The blood clots break down during the next two weeks (*subacute stage*), generally leaving only a few residual iron particles in the subarachnoid space after that period (*chronic stage*).

A *peracute* hemorrhage may elude CT detection because the blood is still liquid and is therefore isodense to brain parenchyma. Due to the high iron content of clotted blood, an *acute* hemorrhage is hyperdense to the brain parenchyma. Attenuation values at this stage are in the range of 80–100 HU, compared with 40–50 HU for normal brain parenchyma on unenhanced scans. The density of the hemorrhage declines steadily during the *subacute* and *chronic* stages, initially becoming isodense ("fogging") and then hypodense to the parenchyma. In anemic patients with a hemoglobin content below 5 mmol/L (8 g/dL), even acute hemorrhages may appear iso- or hypodense.

MRI

The MRI signal intensity of a hemorrhage depends on the selected pulse sequence and the age of the collection, i.e., the pathophysiologic and magnetic properties of the hemoglobin breakdown products (**Table 1.5**, p. 18). Oxygen exchange causes intravascular hemoglobin to change from oxyhemoglobin to deoxyhemoglobin through iron reduction. The hemoglobin denatures to methemoglobin. Initially (days 3–7) the methemoglobin is still contained within red cells, but later (weeks 2–4) it is extracellular. The ferromagnetic and paramagnetic breakdown products hemosiderin and ferritin are deposited at the periphery of the hemorrhage.

Acute hemorrhages are isointense to brain tissue in T1-weighted spin-echo sequences and hyperintense in T2-weighted spin-echo sequences. Occasionally they are difficult to detect because of their low contrast with healthy tissue. It is not until day 3 that enough intracellular paramagnetic methemoglobin has formed to cause increased signal intensity in T1-weighted spin-echo sequences. By day 7 the hematoma is hyperintense on T2-weighted spin-echo images due to breakdown of the red cells and the release of methemoglobin. Gradient-echo sequences are sensitive to susceptibility differences, allowing the early detection of hemorrhage based on signal losses due to the paramagnetic properties of the blood breakdown products, regardless of the age of the hemorrhage.

$T2^*$-weighted MR sequences are the most sensitive for detecting small hemorrhages. Even small extracellular iron deposits will produce signal voids ("susceptibility effect") by slightly altering the main magnetic field strength. In some cases, hypointense hemosiderin and iron deposits can still be detected at the margins of a hemorrhagic area even years after the hemorrhage occurred.

Pharmacologic Effect/ Primary Brain Tumor/ Multiple Sclerosis

History and Clinical Findings

A 25-year-old man with a psychotic disorder had taken a carbamazepine product commonly used in antiepileptic therapy as part of a clinical study. His psychotic symptoms increased during the following two weeks, and the drug was discontinued. Cranial MRI was ordered to exclude a somatic cause of the clinical deterioration (**Fig. 1.22**). The images revealed an approximately 2-cm rounded lesion in the splenium of the corpus callosum with an associated diffusion abnormality. The lesion had low T1-weighted signal intensity and high T2-weighted signal intensity. Lumbar puncture revealed oligoclonal bands in the CSF. Multiple sclerosis was diagnosed on the strength of the MRI and CSF findings. A primary brain tumor was excluded on the basis of the atypical location in the posterior corpus callosum and the absence of perifocal edema.

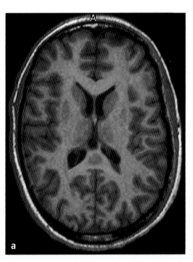
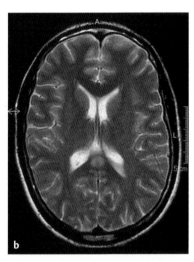
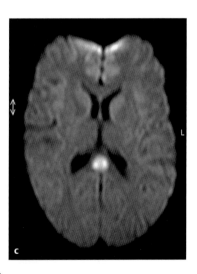

Fig. 1.22 a–c MRI demonstrates an elliptical lesion with abnormal diffusion in the posterior corpus callosum. The lesion, which has low T1-weighted signal intensity and high T2-weighted signal intensity, was attributed to multiple sclerosis.

a T1-weighted image.
b T2-weighted image.
c Diffusion-weighted image.

Further Case Summary

When MRI was repeated 4 weeks later, the lesion was no longer visible (**Fig. 1.23**). Follow-up examination 6 months later yielded normal neurologic and MRI findings, and multiple sclerosis was excluded.

Drawing on case observations published in 1999 and 2003, the initial MRI findings could be explained as follows. Carbamazepine affects the hormone arginine vasopressin, which regulates regional blood flow and fluid balance in the brain. The prolonged use of carbamazepine tends to lower arginine vasopressin levels, and the regional blood flow and fluid balance adapt to this change. Abrupt discontinuation of the drug leads to a temporary, reactive rise in the arginine vasopressin level, resulting in transient ischemia and transient cytotoxic edema in the splenium of the corpus callosum. This produced the signal pattern seen in **Fig. 1.22**. The pathognomonic location in the splenium is attributable to special aspects of local vascular anatomy.

Error Analysis and Strategy for Error Prevention

The local diffusion abnormality showing low T1-weighted and high T2-weighted signal intensity represents a brain area affected by intracellular cytotoxic edema. The differential diagnosis is broad and includes ischemic, inflammatory, immunologic, neurodegenerative, and neoplastic changes. Since the first MRI examination was done without IV contrast, it could not detect an associated disruption of the blood–brain barrier signifying increased permeability of the arteriolar and capillary walls to macrophages, contrast molecules, and serum.

Multiple sclerosis typically presents with multiple lesions distributed chiefly in the white matter but also appearing in the gray matter of the brain and spinal cord. Occurrence in the corpus callosum and an elliptical lesion shape are common due to the perivascular location. Contrast enhancement results from the inflammatory component of multiple sclerosis. Parenchymal defects and brain atrophy reflect the neurodegenerative component of the disease.

The detection of monoclonal bands in the CSF steered the MRI diagnosis toward multiple sclerosis. But this failed to take into account that the detection or exclusion of monoclonal bands or an elevated IgG index in the CSF has a negative predictive value of $<95\%$ but a positive predictive value of only about 70%. Like MRI, then, negative CSF findings are useful for excluding an inflammatory and/or neurodegenerative disease like multiple sclerosis, but a positive finding still leaves a broad differential diagnosis.

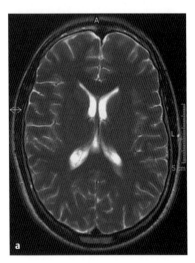
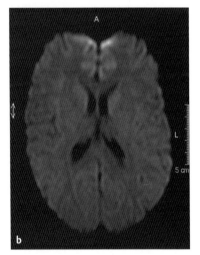
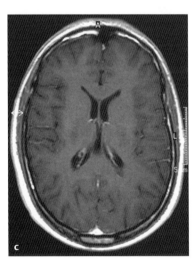

Fig. 1.23 a–c   MRI 4 weeks later shows no abnormalities. The area no longer enhances after IV contrast administration.

a T2-weighted image.
b Diffusion-weighted image.
c T1-weighted image after IV contrast administration.

Diffusion-Weighted MRI (Diffusion-Weighted Imaging)

Diffusion-weighted imaging (DWI) records molecular motion. This phenomenon is based on the fact that all gases, liquids, and tissues contain kinetic energy that causes molecules to move at a particular average speed. Collisions with other molecules constantly alter the direction of this molecular motion. The higher the molecular density, the more frequent the collisions and the shorter the distance traveled by a molecule in any given direction. DWI relies critically on the motion of water molecules in the extracellular space. The diffusion of molecules inside the cell is so limited by the nucleus, organelles, and cell membrane that it cannot contribute to imaging. When the molecules are free to move in an extracellular space of normal dimensions, all of the molecules lose signal intensity. The greater the limitation of molecular motion, the smaller the signal loss.

Diffusion-weighted images are produced with special T2-weighted MRI sequences that include the application of two equal but opposite diffusion gradients (one for dephasing and one for rephasing). The measured signal intensity corresponds to the signal intensity of a T2-weighted image minus the signal loss caused by the diffusion of mobile water molecules. Because the vectors of molecular motion cancel out under normal circumstances, a comparison of diffusion-weighted images with normal T2-weighted images shows a reduction of signal intensity in healthy tissue. Abnormal tissues have a smaller extracellular space in which a greater number of hydrogen protons undergo rephasing. This results in less signal reduction compared with healthy tissue.

Cytotoxic edema (inflammation, ischemia) and primary brain tumors increase the overall volume of the intracellular space, with a correspondingly smaller extracellular space. The result is increased signal intensity in the diffusion-weighted image. In the case of cytotoxic edema, failure of the Na^+/K^+ pump causes a shift of extracellular water molecules into the intracellular space. In the case of brain tumors, cellular proliferation causes the intracellular space to expand at the expense of the extracellular space. On the other hand, perifocal edema, which is characterized by an increase in extracellular water content, promotes the diffusion of hydrogen atoms in the extracellular space, causing decreased signal intensity in the diffusion-weighted image.

Multiple Sclerosis

Multiple sclerosis is an inflammatory, neurodegenerative immune disorder whose pathogenesis is not yet fully understood. The inflammation is believed to be incited by the activation of myelin-specific $CD4^+$ T lymphocytes in the peripheral immune system. Viral infections and viral antigens presumably initiate the process. Proinflammatory factors help to enable activated $CD4^+$ T lymphocytes, macrophages/monocytes, and B lymphocytes to cross the blood–brain barrier. Once inside the CNS, the T lymphocytes form cytokines and chemokines that amplify the inflammatory process and recruit additional inflammatory cells. The degenerative component of the disease arises from a cellular and humoral immune response to the inflammatory process, resulting in damage to oligodendrocytes, myelin sheaths, and axons. This is accompanied by an activation of local antigen-presenting cells that perpetuate the inflammatory process. It has also been suggested that some forms of multiple sclerosis may arise from primary damage to oligodendrocytes rather than the activation of peripheral $CD4^+$ T lymphocytes and that this mechanism may trigger an inflammatory–immunologic-degenerative cycle.

References and Further Reading

Davies G, Keir G, Thompson EJ, Giovannoni G. The clinical significance of an intrathecal monoclonal immunglobulin band: a follow-up study. Neurology 2003; 60: 1163–1166

Fortini AS, Sanders EL, Weinshenker BG, Katzmann JA. Cerebrospinal fluid oligoclonal bands in the diagnosis of multiple sclerosis. Isoelectric focusing with IgG immunoblotting compared with high-resolution agarose gel electrophoresis and cerebrospinal IgG index. Immunopathology 2003; 120: 672–675

Kim SS, Chang KH, Kim ST, et al. Focal lesion in the splenium of the corpus callosum in epileptic patients: antiepileptic drug toxity. AJNR 1999; 20: 125–129

Link H, Huang Y-M. Oligoclonal bands in multiple sclerosis cerebrospinal fluid: an update on morphology and clinical usefulness. J Neuroimmunol 2006; 180: 17–28

Mirsattari SM, Lee DH, Jones MW, Blume WT. Transient lesion in the splenium of the corpus callosum in an epileptic patient. Neurology 2003; 60: 1838–1841

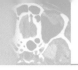

Cause of Intracerebral Hemorrhage: Arterial Hypertension/ AV Malformation/ Aneurysm/Glioblastoma

History and Clinical Findings

An 81-year-old woman was hospitalized with an initial occurrence of severe headaches and speech impairment. She had a prior history of arterial hypertension. CT demonstrated a left temporal intracerebral hemorrhage (ICH) as the cause of her symptoms. Because of increasing obtundation, the patient was intubated and taken to neurosurgery, and the ICH was decompressed by craniotomy the same day.

Postoperative CT scans (**Fig. 1.24**) revealed postoperative air inclusions in the left temporal region and a large, hyperdense residual hematoma. According to the surgical report, blood clots had been left in the medial portion of the operative site because the hypertension and hemorrhage location suggested a middle cerebral artery aneurysm as the cause of the ICH, and the surgeon did not want to damage the aneurysm.

Due to the atypical location of the ICH, cerebral angiography was performed 3 days later. The angiograms displayed normal vascular anatomy (**Fig. 1.25**). In particular, they showed no evidence of a vascular malformation or aneurysm of the left middle cerebral artery. Angiography also showed no pathologic vessels or vascular cutoffs.

The further postoperative course was uneventful, and the patient was discharged home without complaint.

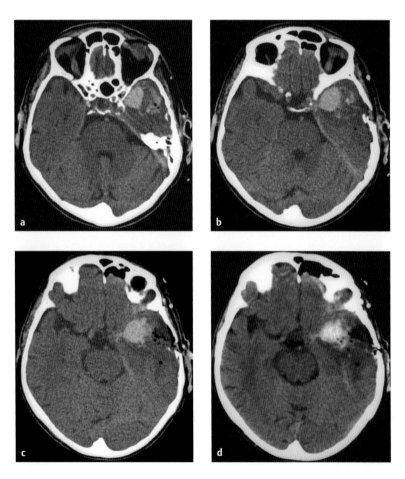

Fig. 1.24 a–d Cranial CT scans following a left temporal craniotomy. Air inclusions are visible at the operative site. The hyperdense area in the left temporal region was interpreted as an intracerebral hemorrhage, possibly originating from an aneurysm of the middle cerebral artery (**c, d**).

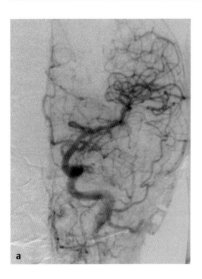
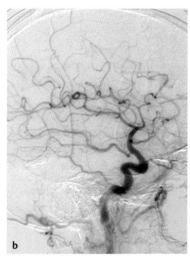

Fig. 1.25 a, b   Intra-arterial DSA of the left internal carotid artery shows no abnormalities.
a Sagittal series.
b Lateral series.

Further Case Summary

The patient was readmitted 4 months later with increasing obtundation, aphasia, and right spastic hemiparesis. Noncontrast cranial CT scans taken on admission and scans taken the following day after IV contrast administration showed a solid, intensely enhancing mass in the left temporal region bordered posteriorly by a larger cystic component showing peripheral enhancement (**Fig. 1.26**). Faint perifocal edema surrounded the mass. A ventricular drain was placed for relief of new internal hydrocephalus. The patient's condition deteriorated during her hospital stay. Respiratory failure and sepsis ensued, and the patient

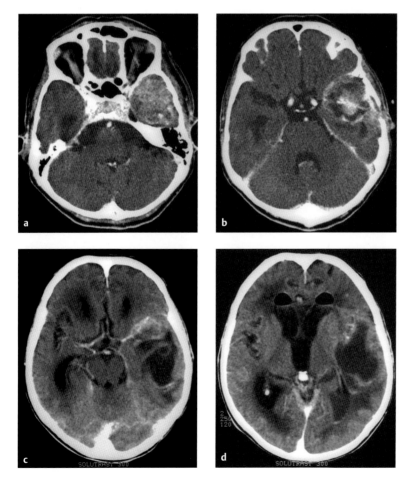

Fig. 1.26 a–d   Cranial CT scans after IV contrast administration, 4 months after **Fig. 1.24**, show an enlarging solid left temporal mass with a new posterior cystic component and nonhomogeneous enhancement. Mild perifocal edema is present along with triventricular internal hydrocephalus. Air–fluid levels are present in both anterior horns following placement of a ventricular drain.

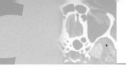

died a short time later due to failure of central regulatory functions. Autopsy revealed a mixed solid–cystic glioblastoma multiforme in the left temporobasal area that had infiltrated the dura of the middle cranial fossa.

Error Analysis and Strategy for Error Prevention

The proximity of the ICH to the middle cerebral artery (**Fig. 1.27 b**) suggested a perforated aneurysm of that vessel. The differential diagnosis also included a bleeding vascular malformation and a cerebral tumor. A hypertensive hemorrhage was unlikely because it most commonly involves the basal ganglia, centrum semiovale, or thalamus. A perforated aneurysm and AV malformation were excluded by angiography. While grade IV astrocytomas (glioblastomas) are generally hypervascular, a small glioblastoma could not definitely be excluded by angiography due to the projection nature of the study and the spatial and contrast resolution, which are too low for defining capillary vessels.

The glioblastoma was initially missed for the following reasons:

- The tumor component extending toward the suprasellar cistern and dorsum sellae was not recognized (**Fig. 1.27 a**). It could not be clotted blood, because clots do not transgress the dura.
- The tumor was masked by the high density of the fresh hemorrhage. Extravasated blood is hyperdense during the first 3 days due to the iron content of the hemoglobin component of the clot (fresh blood has unenhanced attenuation values of 80–100 HU, compared with 40–50 HU for brain tissue). Afterward the density fades as the hemoglobin is denatured, and hemorrhages more than 2 weeks old are generally hypodense. The correct procedure, then, would have been to schedule follow-up CT scans (or preferably MRI) at 3 weeks so that a tumor could be detected while still at an operable stage.

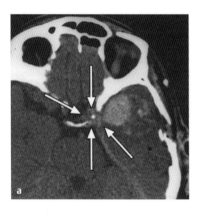
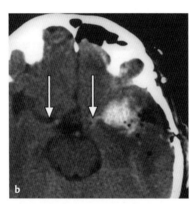

Fig. 1.27 a, b Initial findings.
a Noncontrast CT. Magnified view of the lesion in **Fig. 1.24 b**. The medial portion of the middle cranial fossa, which was not inspected during decompressive surgery, contains a mass that has infiltrated the dura, suprasellar cistern, and dorsum sellae (arrows).
b CT after IV contrast administration. Magnified view of the lesion in **Fig. 1.24 d**. Arrows indicate the right and left middle cerebral arteries. Note the close relationship of the left middle cerebral artery to the tumor and its associated hemorrhage.

Postoperative: Cerebellar Infarction/ Residual Tumor/ Hematoma/Abscess

History and Clinical Findings

A 62-year-old man underwent surgical removal of a left acoustic neuroma. Routine cranial CT scans the following day documented status post craniectomy through an occipitolateral presigmoid approach (**Fig. 1.28**). The CT report described an approximately 1-cm×2-cm hypodense area located posterior to the left petrous apex. The hypodensity contained hyperdense elements and was inter-preted as edema due to bloody imbibition. Enhancing residual tumor tissue was not found. Other postoperative findings were left-sided brain edema and air inclusions in the outer CSF spaces.

Another routine postoperative CT examination without contrast medium was performed one week later (**Fig. 1.29**). Scans now showed an inhomogeneous hy-podensity measuring 2 cm×3 cm in the area of the left cerebellar peduncle with extension to the dorsolateral pons, interpreted as a zone of acute ischemia. Hemor-rhagic areas at the surgical site were undergoing absorp-tion and appeared less dense. The findings were otherwise unchanged.

CT was repeated 13 days postoperatively (**Fig. 1.30**) for investigation of left abducens nerve palsy, meningism, and fever. The CT report described a new, patchy, inhomo-geneous but nonenhancing hypodensity with a small central gas inclusion located at the surgical access site. The differential diagnosis included a fading hematoseroma or a CSF pocket with bloody imbibition. The report cited no evidence of meningitis or abnormal enhancement after IV contrast administration. The hypodensity in the area of the left cerebellar peduncle and dorsal pons was still interpreted as acute ischemia and was described as unchanged from the previous examination.

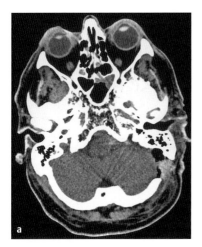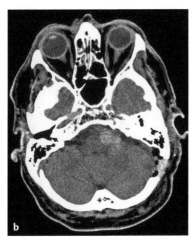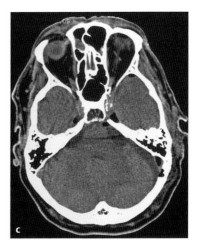

Fig. 1.28 a–c Noncontrast cranial CT scans after surgical removal of a left acoustic neuroma show patchy hyperdensities and postoperative air inclusions.

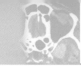

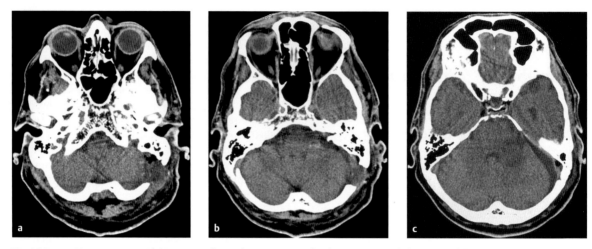

Fig. 1.29 a–c   Noncontrast cranial CT scans on the ninth postoperative day document normal absorption of the hematoma. The decreased density of the left cerebellar peduncle was interpreted as ischemia.

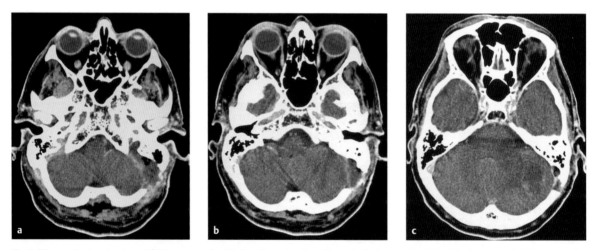

Fig. 1.30 a–c   Postcontrast cranial CT scans on day 13 show hypodensity with gas inclusions and peripheral enhancement at the surgical access site.

Further Case Summary

The surgical site was reopened on day 15 because of a wound infection and clinical signs of inflammation. This disclosed an abscess arising from the mastoid cells, which had been opened during the initial operation and had been inadequately sealed with bone wax. The abscess was drained and triple antibiotic therapy was instituted. The patient's condition improved in response to this therapy, and he was discharged for follow-up care.

Error Analysis and Strategy for Error Prevention

The fact that mastoid cells had been opened during the first operation and sealed secondarily with bone wax was not known during interpretation of the CT scans. Even so, the scans acquired 9 days after the first operation (**Fig. 1.29**) still detected air at the posterior border of the petrous bone, as in the initial scans (**Fig. 1.28**). This should have raised the possibility of an infectious complication and prompted a CT examination after IV contrast administration. When additional scans were taken on day 13 (**Fig. 1.30**), the radiologist did not notice that the air inclusions were progressive or that the cerebellar, meningeal, and extracranial soft tissues showed a new, scalloped pattern of contrast enhancement. The abscess contents produced the patchy hypodensity described in the CT report.

References and Further Reading

Osborn AG, Blaser SI, Salzmann KL, Katzman GL, Provenzale J, Castillo M. Diagnostic Imaging: Brain. Salt Lake City: Amyrsis; 2004

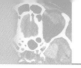
Cranial CT: Exclusion of Metastases

History and Clinical Findings

A 58-year-old woman underwent a cranial CT examination 2½ years after having a superficial spreading melanoma (SSM, Clark level IV, tumor thickness 1.4 mm) removed from her back. She had no neurologic symptoms. One month earlier she had undergone a left axillary lymphadectomy for lymph node metastasis. Current thoracic and abdominal CT scans revealed pulmonary, hepatic, splenic and skeletal metastases. Cranial CT scans were interpreted as normal (**Fig. 1.31**).

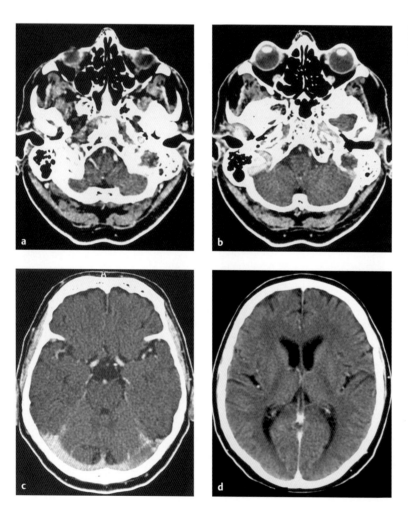

Fig. 1.31 a–d   Cranial CT. Axial scans after IV contrast administration were interpreted as normal.

Further Case Summary

Three weeks later the patient was again referred for CT due to left facial paralysis. These scans demonstrated osteolytic metastasis in the left petrous bone (**Fig. 1.32**), which had already been present and detectable in the previous examination. Destruction of the posterior border of the left petrous bone and left mastoid bone had progressed during the interval between examinations. Invasion of the clivus and left sigmoid sinus had also occurred.

Error Analysis and Strategy for Error Prevention

When the first CT examination was interpreted, all attention was focused on the exclusion of cerebral metastases. Despite the positive thoracic and abdominal scans, the possibility of skeletal metastases was not considered.

Cranial Computed Tomography (CCT)

A **systematic review** of all image information contained in the CCT data set should include the scrutiny of:
- Image data sets acquired with a **soft-tissue window** before *and* after IV contrast administration
- Image data sets acquired with a **bone window** without contrast medium *or* after IV contrast administration

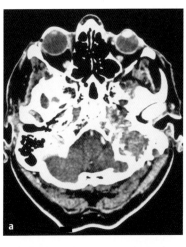
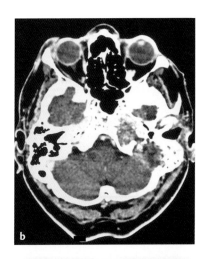
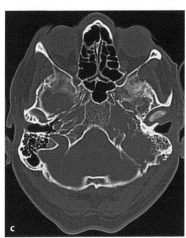
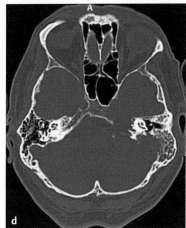

Fig. 1.32 a–d Cranial CT scans 3 weeks later document the progression of osteolytic metastasis in the left skull base.

Carcinoma of the Oral Floor/Soft-Tissue Abscess/Osteomyelitis

History and Clinical Findings

A 70-year-old man was referred to the oral and maxillofacial surgery clinic with clinical suspicion of a malignant tumor in the left side of the mandible. CT scans were obtained for preoperative planning (**Fig. 1.33**). Consistent with clinical findings, CT showed an approximately 3-cm mass with a hypodense center located in the subcutaneous fat and bordering the posterior mandibular segment. The mass was surrounded by streaky densities in the subcutaneous fat. The mandible showed no osteolysis in proximity to the tumor. Enlarged lymph nodes up to 1 cm in diameter were found in the submental region on both sides, at both mandibular angles, and posterior to the left sternocleidomastoid muscle. The findings were interpreted as a carcinoma that had invaded the oral floor muscles and mandible, accompanied by perifocal carcinomatous lymphadenitis and lymph node metastases.

MRI was performed 5 days later and confirmed the CT findings (**Fig. 1.34a, b**). The mass had a hyperintense center on T2-weighted images and showed peripheral enhancement after IV contrast administration. Portions of the mandible bordering on the mass were eroded. The bone marrow in the same area showed increased T2-weighted signal intensity and abnormal enhancement in a T1-weighted sequence after IV contrast administration.

CT, MRI, and radionuclide bone scans showed no evidence of hematogenous metastasis.

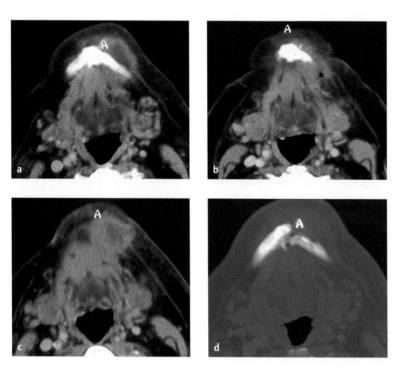

Fig. 1.33a–d   CT shows a left submental density with an enhancing rim, initially interpreted as carcinoma.

Further Case Summary

An excisional biopsy of the suspected carcinoma was performed under general endotracheal anesthesia. Blunt dissection of the subcutaneous fibrofatty tissue revealed an encapsulated mass. Pus was released by incision of the capsule. Smears and tissue samples were taken from the capsule. The cavity was irrigated with 5% iodine solution, and a drain was inserted. Histology showed no evidence of malignancy. Although microbiology did not reveal a causative organism, the abscess resolved in response to drainage and broad-spectrum antibiotic therapy. CT follow-up at 2 weeks showed only residual postinflammatory changes and the known circumscribed bone defect in the mandible. It was finally concluded that the soft-tissue abscess was secondary to dentogenic osteomyelitis.

Error Analysis and Strategy for Error Prevention

The history and clinical findings, as well as the frequency of hypopharyngeal malignancies in patients referred for oral and maxillofacial surgery, biased the initial interpretation toward cancer. The following aspects suggested the inflammatory etiology of the mass (**Fig. 1.34c**):

- The mass was not in contact with the tongue base, which is the most frequent starting point for hypopharyngeal cancers.
- The bulk of the lesion was located in the subcutaneous tissue and not in the floor of the mouth.
- Thickening of a long portion of the left anterior platysma, fluid collections in the subcutaneous fibrofatty tissue of the submental region, and skin thickening in the same region were consistent with inflammatory spread and were not typical of carcinoma.

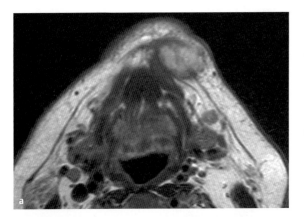

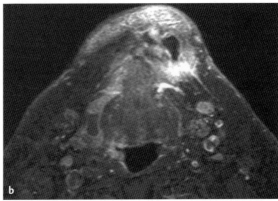

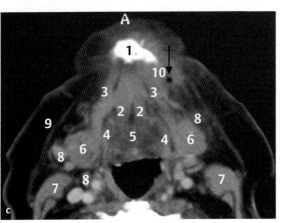

Fig. 1.34 a–c MRI confirms the CT findings and raises suspicion of lymph node metastases.
a T2-weighted turbo spin-echo sequence.
b T1-weighted fat-suppressed STIR sequence after IV contrast administration.
c Topographic anatomy (CT).
   1 Mandible
   2 Geniohyoid muscle
   3 Mylohyoid muscle
   4 Hyoglossus muscle
   5 Tongue base
   6 Sublingual gland
   7 Sternocleidomastoid muscle
   8 Lymph nodes
   9 Platysma
 10 Tumor
 ↓ Air

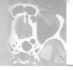
The gas inclusion in the thickened subcutaneous tissue was caused by air in a fistulous tract.

Lymph node enlargement was a result of lymphadenitis and, as is often the case, was indistinguishable from early metastasis.

The images in **Fig. 1.35 a–c**, acquired in an 87-year-old woman, raised premature suspicion of carcinoma due to an incomplete history and physical examination. The patient had lost considerable weight during the previous months. A CT tumor screening examination revealed concentric wall thickening of the ascending colon, which was interpreted as typical of carcinoma. The patient's husband

stated that on the day before the CT examination, the patient had undergone a colonoscopy with biopsies. The colon wall was thickened as a result of biopsy-related intramural hemorrhage. The patchy increased density of the colon wall on plain CT (**Fig. 1.35 a**) is typical of intramural hemorrhage and was initially disregarded during image interpretation.

In a different woman, aged 57 years, with CT findings of a polypoid mass in the gastric fundus, the history and repeat endoscopy identified the lesions as postbiopsy blood clots rather than carcinoma (**Fig. 1.35 d**).

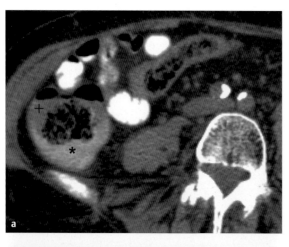

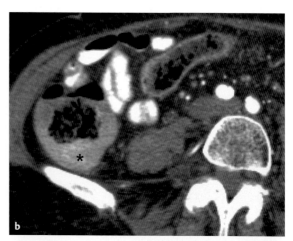

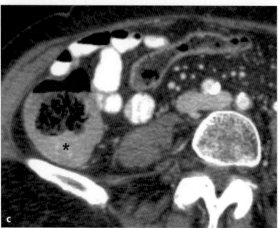

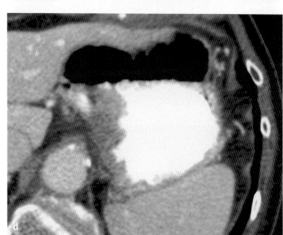

Fig. 1.35 a–d Other misinterpretations based on a failure to consider the history and clinical findings.

a–c Concentric wall thickening of the ascending colon due to intramural hemorrhage was misinterpreted as carcinoma. The increased density of the affected wall segment on noncontrast spiral CT is typical of intramural hemorrhage (**a**). Perfusion analysis shows no density changes in the hematoma (asterisk) compared with healthy colon segments (cross).

d CT after gastroscopy in a different patient shows polypoid wall thickening of the gastric fundus, which was initially interpreted as carcinoma. Repeat gastroscopy identified the polypoid lesions as clots.

2

Chest

Chest

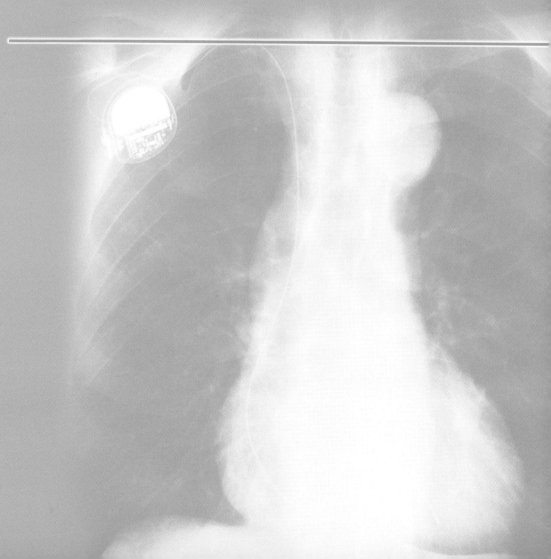

Normal Postoperative Findings?

History and Clinical Findings

A 52-year-old woman underwent a segmental colon resection for pT3 N1 M1 colon carcinoma with hepatic metastases. The next day, a routine postoperative chest radiograph taken in the ICU was described as showing normal heart and lungs, a normal position of the endotracheal tube, superimposed ECG leads and ventilation hose, and a plate of metallic density superimposed on the upper abdomen (**Fig. 2.1**).

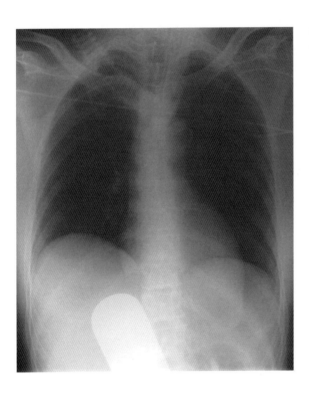

Fig. 2.1 Chest radiograph. The radiography report described normal-appearing heart and lungs, correct position of the endotracheal tube, ECG leads, ventilation hose, and an external metal plate projected over the upper abdomen.

Further Case Summary

Laparotomy was repeated the same day and disclosed a retractor left from the previous operation.

Error Analysis and Strategy for Error Prevention

The radiologist who read the chest radiograph had not considered the possibility of an iatrogenic foreign body due to the patient's history and the rarity of the finding.

A foreign body was also missed in a different, 43-year-old patient who had undergone a vaginal hysterectomy for cervical cancer. A bleeding complication was caused by injury to a large pelvic vessel. A critical fall in blood pressure occurred after the surgery. Suspected recurrent hemorrhage was investigated by CT (**Fig. 2.2**).

CT scans showed a fresh retrovesicular hematoma spreading toward the left side and a hypodense foreign body that contained a metallic string, indicating a foreign body at the operative site. Re-laparotomy was performed to secure hemostasis and extract the foreign body.

Injury to the left uterine artery and the resulting hematoma were confirmed at operation. No sponges or lap pads were found at the operative site, but sponges had been packed into the rectum for tamponade during the initial operation. The foreign material was initially forgotten and was later removed after CT imaging and reoperation.

The CT diagnosis of injury to a branch of the left internal iliac artery, the associated hematoma, and a retained sponge in the lesser pelvis was correct. Localization of the sponge was incorrect, as the possibility of an intrarectal location had not been considered and so a detailed anatomical analysis had not been performed.

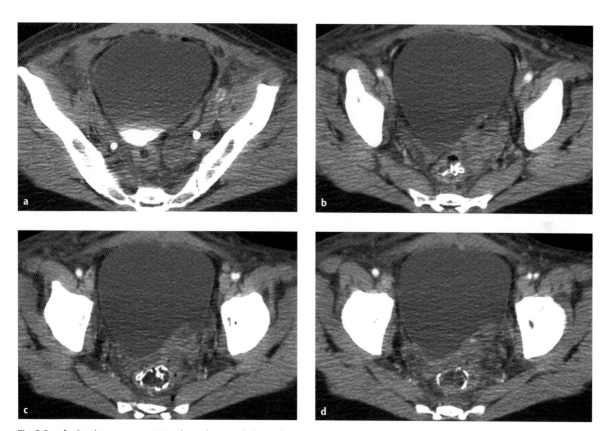

Fig. 2.2 a–d Posthysterectomy CT in the early arterial phase after IV contrast administration shows a hematoma at the site of the resected uterus. The metallic markers are typical of surgical sponges or lap pads.

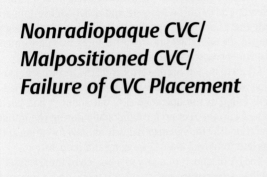

Nonradiopaque CVC/ Malpositioned CVC/ Failure of CVC Placement

History and Clinical Findings

A radiology technician obtained a frontal chest radiograph in a 66-year-old man at 10:24 and sent it to the attending radiologist for interpretation (**Fig. 2.3**). The clinical question on the surgical request form was "CVC position?" The chest radiograph showed dystelectasis of the right lower lobe and aortic elongation. A central venous catheter (CVC) was not visible.

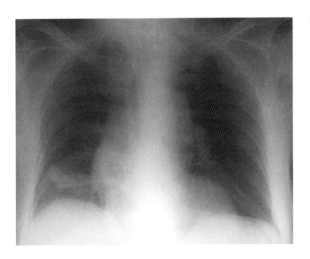

Fig. 2.3 Chest radiograph taken at 10:24 shows dystelectasis of the right lower lobe and aortic elongation. There is no indication of a CVC.

Further Case Summary

Physical inspection of the somnolent patient revealed that no attempt had been made to place a CVC. Because the ward physicians were operating and the ward nurse could not explain the situation, the patient was returned to the ward. Approximately 1 hour later an anesthesiologist in the emergency department again requested a chest radiograph for the same patient to check for CVC placement.

A subsequent telephone call showed that, consistent with standard protocols, an anesthesia consult form (placement of the CVC) and radiology request form (check the CVC position) had been sent with the patient to the emergency department. The department staff failed to note the logical sequence of the two referrals and sent the patient to radiology first. The radiology technician "automatically" exposed a chest radiograph without reviewing the information on the request form.

Finally, a chest radiograph taken at 12:58 documented the correct placement of a CVC.

Error Analysis and Strategy for Error Prevention

The RT should have noticed that the patient did not have a central venous line before taking the radiograph.

Since it is common practice at maximum-care hospitals to obtain a chest radiograph after CVC placement to verify a correct catheter position and exclude pneumothorax, the indication for the chest radiograph went unquestioned.

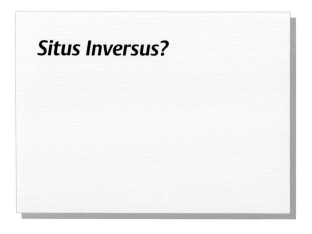

Situs Inversus?

History and Clinical Findings

A 61-year-old man was scheduled to have a squamous cell carcinoma of the skin removed from his right shoulder. The preoperative work-up included a frontal chest radiograph (**Fig. 2.4**), which showed kyphoscoliosis secondary to ankylosing spondylitis in addition to apparent situs inversus (cardiac shadow and gastric bubble on the right side).

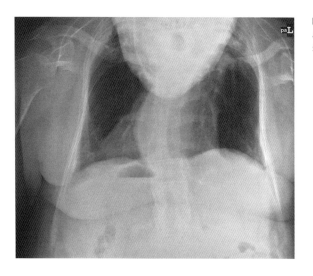

Fig. 2.4 Chest radiograph shows kyphoscoliosis secondary to ankylosing spondylitis. The film initially prompted a diagnosis of situs inversus.

Further Case Summary

When the RT was questioned, it was learned that a PA radiograph could not be taken due to the patient's kyphoscoliosis, and therefore an AP view had been obtained. The RT forgot to change the side marker (which indicates left PA in **Fig. 2.4**). Another technical deficiency was that the beam had not been collimated.

Error Analysis and Strategy for Error Prevention

The examination conditions were made difficult by significant kyphoscoliosis. The RT did not collimate the beam to improve visualization of all relevant anatomic structures and also forgot to change the side label or communicate the special circumstances to the radiologist. The projection of the chin over the superior thoracic aperture on the frontal chest radiograph is typical in patients with significant kyphosis.

A radiologic examination consists of numerous steps that generally involve various RTs and physicians. To avoid misunderstandings and prevent time lost due to follow-up questions, all special circumstances in an examination should be routinely noted and communicated to the radiologist.

Normal Findings after Pacemaker Implantation/Broken Wire/Insulation Defect

History and Clinical Findings

A pacemaker was implanted in an 82-year-old man for bradyarrhythmia. The postoperative chest radiograph was described as showing enlargement of the left ventricle, bilateral pleural effusions, and chronic obstructive pulmonary disease (COPD) (**Fig. 2.5**).

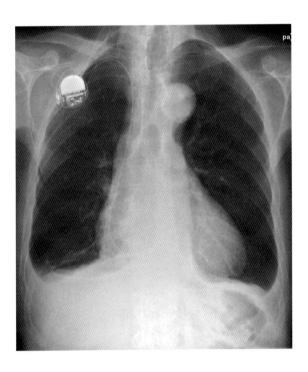

Fig. 2.5   Frontal chest radiograph after pacemaker implantation shows the ventricular lead, enlargement of the left atrium and left ventricle, bilateral pleural effusions due to congestive failure, and signs of COPD.

Further Case Summary

During subsequent months the patient developed fasciculations in his right arm, and the pacing threshold of the pacemaker steadily increased. A chest radiograph taken 4½ months after pacemaker implantation showed a normalization of cardiac size and configuration, regression of the pleural effusions, and a lucent defect in the axillary part of the pacemaker lead, which was already visible in the initial examination (**Figs. 2.6, 2.7, 2.8**). The lucency was interpreted as a break in the pacemaker wire, but surgical reexposure showed no evidence of a broken wire. The pacemaker lead was moved to a subpectoral site and reinsulated. This led to improvement of clinical complaints.

Error Analysis and Strategy for Error Prevention

A suture had fixed the wire too tightly to the pectoralis muscle. Traction on the wire caused its outer covering to split open, damaging the insulation. The thinned portion of the wire created the lucent line visible on radiographs. Fasciculations occurred because some of the pacemaker current leaked through the insulation defect and stimulated the surrounding muscle. This also caused the pacing threshold to increase. Based on clinical experience, from 0.1% to 1% of all implanted pacemakers must be revised because of manufacturing defects or flaws in operating technique.

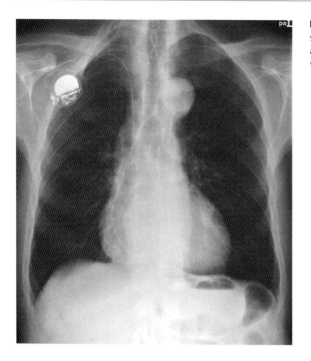

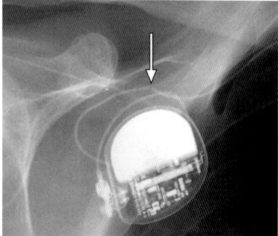

Fig. 2.6   Chest radiograph taken 4½ months after **Fig. 2.5**. Heart size has returned to normal and the pleural effusions have been reabsorbed. The lucent defect in the axillary part of the pacemaker wire has increased in size.

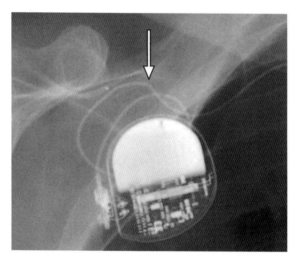

Fig. 2.7   Initial examination shows a faint lucency in the axillary part of the pacemaker lead, which was interpreted as a break in the wire.

Fig. 2.8   Follow-up at 4½ months.

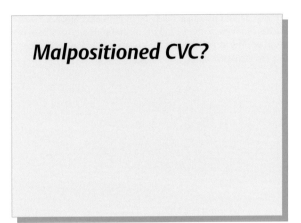

Malpositioned CVC?

History and Clinical Presentation

A 12-year-old girl underwent a chest radiographic examination in the ICU after being resuscitated from an anesthesia incident (**Fig. 2.9**). She was known to have a persistent left superior vena cava. Based on information from her treating physicians, blood could be aspirated from a subclavian catheter that had been introduced from the left side. The radiology technician (RT) performed the examination without a formal order, as the ICU physician had no time to submit a request because of the urgency of the situation. Consequently, the chest radiograph was developed and sent directly to the ICU.

Another chest radiograph was performed by on-call staff approximately 12 hours later (**Fig. 2.10**) after the patient had required a second resuscitation. Again, the RT sent the radiograph directly to ICU because the radiologist on duty was in a different building at the time.

Both examinations were forwarded to pediatric radiology 2 days later. Analysis of the radiographs at that time yielded the following main findings:

- The endotracheal tube and nasogastric tube were correctly positioned.
- The second examination additionally showed a CVC advanced through the left subclavian vein with the catheter tip projected at the T9 level.

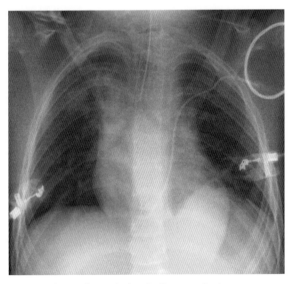

Fig. 2.9   Chest radiograph after the first resuscitation.

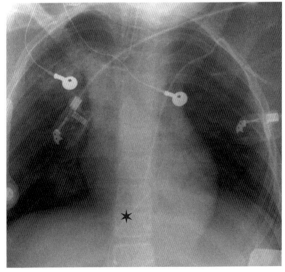

Fig. 2.10   Chest radiograph after the second resuscitation 12 hours later. Asterisk = extracorporeal catheter.

Further Case Summary

Infusion therapy had been administered through the CVC. Pericardial tamponade was diagnosed after the second resuscitation, and pericardiocentesis yielded a clear liquid aspirate that looked like the infusion solution. The CVC was removed that same night. In the days that followed, the heart and mediastinum regained a normal radiographic appearance. However, the circulatory arrest and two resuscitations led to hypoxic brain damage that resulted in the patient's death. Autopsy confirmed a persistent left superior vena cava, which drained into the coronary sinus and thence into the right atrium. A perforation was not grossly visible.

It was reasonable to conclude that the CVC had perforated the persistent left superior vena cava or the junction of the superior vena cava with the coronary sinus, causing the catheter tip to enter the pericardial sac. Infusion therapy administered via the CVC had caused the pericardial tamponade. The inability to find a perforation at autopsy was not considered contradictory: Booth et al. (2001) described a fatal pericardial tamponade that had been caused by the inadvertent intrapericardial infusion of alimentation fluid. In this case as well, blood had been aspirated appropriately from the CVC used for the infusion. The diagnosis of CVC malposition was confirmed by the liquid contents of the pericardial cavity and laboratory data identifying the aspirate as infusion solution. The perforation site was not found, even though the CVC had been removed shortly before autopsy was performed.

Error Analysis and Strategy for Error Prevention

The following errors were made during the diagnostic work-up:

- Radiographic examinations in ICU require prompt interpretation because of their clinical relevance.
- The attending radiologist was unaware of the risk of intrapericardial catheter placement.
- The radiographic signs of pericardial tamponade (loss of normal cardiac borders, decreased pulmonary blood flow) were missed in the second chest radiograph.

A CVC in a persistent left superior vena cava runs parallel to the border of the descending thoracic aorta. The catheter deviates medially because the left superior vena cava drains into the coronary sinus. For anatomic reasons, the bend at this location creates a site of predilection for wall perforation by the catheter tip. Thus the distal end of the catheter should not go past the coronary sinus, which is located at the level of the AV valves. A chest radiograph following the injection of contrast medium through the CVC would have shown the distribution of the contrast bolus, thereby defining the catheter position.

The heart and mediastinum were too wide for a 12-year-old child on both radiographs (**Fig. 2.11**). Given the history and the CVC position, the differential diagnosis included dilated cardiomyopathy, which may have developed during resuscitation, and a pericardial effusion. Mediastinal widening was probably a result of the prior resuscitations.

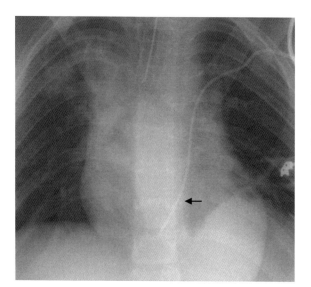

Fig. 2.11 Retrospective interpretation of **Fig. 2.9**. A catheter introduced through the left subclavian vein descends in a left paravertebral course. It runs parallel to the lateral border of the descending aorta at the T4/T5 level, then makes a medial turn at the T6/T7 level. This is suspicious for catheter malposition because the lower portion of the CVC runs unusually far medially and ends below the valve plane (arrow). The heart is too large for a 12-year-old, and the enlargement is not limited to one chamber. The mediastinum is widened. The differential diagnosis of these post-resuscitation findings includes dilated cardiomyopathy, pericardial effusion, hemopericardium, mediastinal hematoma, and hydromediastinum.

Persistent Left Superior Vena Cava

Persistent left superior vena cava is a congenital anomaly in which the left cardinal vein is not obliterated during prenatal development. Generally the persistent vena cava descends to the left of the midline, passing anterior to the aortic arch and draining in approximately 90% of cases into the right atrium by way of the coronary sinus. Leibowitz et al. (1992) reported that in a series of 4000 examinations for CVC localization, only 5 of the patients (0.1%) had a persistent left superior vena cava.

On the basis of published reports, passage of the catheter through the coronary sinus may lead to mechanical problems such as cardiac arrhythmias. Autopsy statistics indicate that the overall incidence of persistent left superior vena cava is 0.3%. The incidence rises to 3–4% in patients with congenital cardiac anomalies. Approximately 80% of affected individuals also have a patent right superior vena cava.

Contrary to policy, the initial chest radiograph, which had a critical bearing on subsequent events, was not read by an experienced radiologist immediately after it was developed. The image remained in the ICU; it was not actively retrieved for reading within a time frame in which the pericardial tamponade could have been prevented. This violates the national quality assurance guidelines of the members of the European Union, which are subsidiary to the guidelines of Council of the European Union and require that radiographic examinations be interpreted promptly and that the findings be documented in a written report that is archived in a suitable form (see interdisciplinary excursion, "Guidelines of the Council of the European Union on Radiation Protection," p. 217).

References and Further Reading

Booth SA, Norton B, Mulvey DA. Central venous catheterization and fatal cardiac tamponade. Br J Anaesth 2001; 87: 298–302

Collier PE, Ryan JJ, Diamond DL. Cardiac tamponade from central venous catheters report of a case and review of the English literature. Angiology 1984; 35: 595–600

Council of the European Union. Council Directive 96/29/EURA-TOM of 13 May 1996 laying down basic safety standards for the protection of the health of workers and the general public against the danger arising from ionizing radiation. http://ec.europa.eu/energy/nuclear/radioprotection/doc/legislation/9629_en.pdf (accessed January 10, 2011)

Council of the European Union. Council Directive 97/43/EURA-TOM of 30 June 1997 on health protection in individuals against the dangers of ionizing radiation in relation to medical exposure, and repealing Directive 84/466/Euratom. http://ec.europa.eu/energy/nuclear/radioprotection/doc/legislation/9743_en.pdf (accessed January 10, 2011)

Kamola PA, Seidner DL. Peripherally inserted central catheter malposition in an persistent left superior vena cava. J Infus Nurs 2004; 27: 181–184

Kao CL, Chang JP. Malposition of a catheter in the persistent left superior vena cava. A rare complication of totally implantable venous devices. J Cardiovasc Surg 2003; 44: 145–147

Leibowitz AB, Haplpern NA, Lee M-H, Iberti TJ. Left-sided superior vena cava: a not-so-unusual vascular anomaly discovered during central venous and pulmonary artery catheterization. Crit Care Med 1992; 20: 1119–1122

Lonnqvist P-A, Olsson GL. Persistent left superior vena cava–an unusual location of central venous catheters in children. Intensive Care Med 1991; 17: 497–500

Sarodia BD, Stoller JK. Persistent left superior vena cava: case report and literature review. Persp Care 2000; 45: 411–416

Sheep RE, Guiney WB. Fatal cardiac tamponade. JAMA 1982; 248: 1632–1635

Ying Z-Q, Ma J, Xu G, et al. Double superior vena cava with a persistent left superior vena cava. Intern Med 2008; 47: 679–680

Normal Postoperative Findings/Mediastinal Mass

History and Clinical Findings

Chest radiographs were taken in a 31-year-old woman who presented with a 4-week history of cough, lethargy, and fatigue. As a child she had undergone surgery to correct a tetralogy of Fallot, and since then she had experienced no cardiac problems. A mass in the upper left mediastinum was diagnosed from the chest radiograph (**Fig. 2.12**).

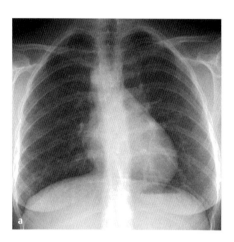 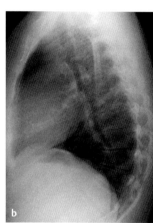

Fig. 2.12 a, b   Chest radiographs. The radiography report described a mass in the upper left mediastinum. As a child the patient had undergone surgical correction of tetralogy of Fallot via a sternotomy. The film shows kyphosis of the lower thoracic spine and thoracolumbar junction.

Further Case Summary

MRI was performed to exclude a mediastinal tumor. The images showed a right descending aorta as a normal congenital variant with otherwise normal postoperative findings (**Fig. 2.13**).

Error Analysis and Strategy for Error Prevention

The pathoanatomy caused by the cardiac anomaly and right descending aorta was not recognized when the frontal chest radiograph was interpreted (**Figs. 2.14, 2.15; Table 2.1**). The right descending aorta and pulmonary stenosis resulted in an unusual superimposed view of the pulmonary artery (**Fig. 2.16**), which was misinterpreted as a mediastinal mass. This error could have been avoided by comparison with the lateral radiograph (**Fig. 2.12 b**), which did not show a mediastinal mass, and by analyzing the postoperative pathoanatomy in the image.

References and Further Reading

Fogel MA. Principles and Practice of Cardiac Magnetic Resonance in Congenital Heart Disease: Form, Function and Flow. Hoboken, NJ: Wiley Blackwell; 2010

Myerson SG, Francis J, Neubauer S. Cardiovascular Magnetic Resonance. Oxford Specialist Handbooks in Cardiology. Oxford: Oxford University Press; 2010

Schoepf JU. CT of the Heart. Principles and Applications. Totowa, NJ: Humana Press; 2005

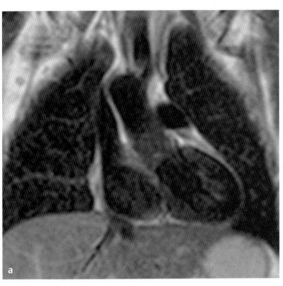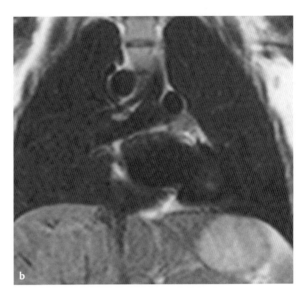

Fig. 2.13 a, b MRI. Coronal T2-weighted TSE images without contrast medium show normal postoperative findings.

a Anterior mediastinum.
b Middle mediastinum.

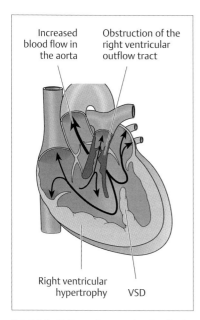

Fig. 2.14 Pathoanatomy and pathophysiology of the tetralogy of Fallot. VSD, ventricular septal defect.

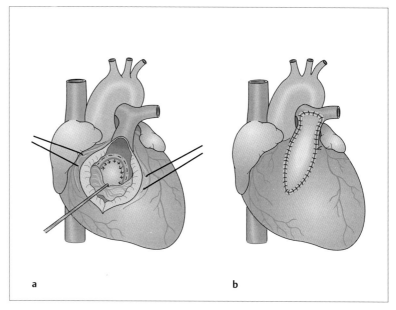

Fig. 2.15 a, b Surgical correction of the tetralogy of Fallot.
a The VSD is repaired with a Dacron or PTFE patch.
b The pulmonary arteriotomy is enlarged and closed with a transannular patch after removal of the hypertrophic trabeculae.

Table 2.1 Characteristic features of the tetralogy of Fallot on chest radiographs

Pathoanatomy and pathophysiology	Findings on frontal chest radiograph
Normal cardiac size and configuration or enlargement of the right ventricle (pressure overload and resistance hypertrophy due to infundibular pulmonary stenosis)	■ Normal cardiac size and configuration ■ *Or* widening of the heart at the ventricular level toward the left side ■ Elevation and rounding of the cardiac apex (coer en sabot)
Enlargement of the atria (volume overload)	
Pulmonary artery hypoplasia	■ Indentation of the lateral border of the descending aorta and left atrium caused by the hypoplastic pulmonary artery segment
Decreased pulmonary blood flow	■ Small caliber of pulmonary vessels ■ Decreased vascular markings in the periphery of the lung
Right descending aorta (approximately 20% of cases)	■ Aorta descends to the right of the thoracic spine

Tetralogy of Fallot

Tetralogy of Fallot is a common congenital cardiac anomaly, accounting for approximately 10–15% of cases of congenital cardiac anomaly. It has four main pathoanatomic features: a ventricular septal defect (VSD); infundibular or valvular pulmonary stenosis; right ventricular hypertrophy; and dextroposition of the anterior cruciate ligament origin. Its hemodynamic features depend mainly on the degree of obstruction of the right ventricular outflow tract. The sole embryonic defect consists of an anterior displacement of the right ventricular infundibular septum. The infundibular septum, which is normally directed backward, downward, and to the right, assumes a forward, upward, and leftward orientation when tetralogy of Fallot is present. As a result, the infundibular septum, which is fused with the ventricular infundibular fold and forms the crista terminalis, does not attach between the anterior and posterior limbs of the septal band but is placed in front of the anterior limb. This leaves a vacant area between the anterior and posterior septal bands, resulting in a VSD and narrowing of the infundibulum and/or the pulmonary valve.

Approximately one-third of patients have associated cardiovascular anomalies: peripheral pulmonary stenosis (20–28%), hypoplasia (20%) or aplasia (2%) of the (left) pulmonary artery, an atrial septal defect or patent foramen ovale (50%, "pentalogy of Fallot"), a second VSD (5%), a right aortic arch (20–30%), and coronary anomalies (4–5%).

The VSD is usually large, resulting functionally in a common chamber. The distribution of blood flow to the pulmonary and systemic circulations depends on the degree of obstruction of the right ventricular outflow tract and on systemic arterial resistance. Postnatal pulmonary blood flow remains adequate as long as the ductus arteriosus is patent. After closure of the ductus, arterial saturation declines in proportion to the degree of right ventricular outflow obstruction. Body growth may cause further narrowing of the right ventricular outflow tract. Decreased pulmonary blood flow leads to hypotrophy of the left atrium and left ventricle. Since cardiac output to the systemic circulation is low, the blood in the periphery of the body becomes so oxygen-depleted that it cannot be fully saturated during its next pass through the lung. The oxygen tension in the systemic circulation assumes a lower level than normal, resulting in peripheral cyanosis. The persistent hypoxic state causes bone marrow stimulation and, given the limited iron storage capacity of the blood, leads to microcytic hypochromic anemia and eventual polycythemia once adaptation has occurred.

Infants and small children already manifest respiratory distress during exertion. Children often assume a typical squatting posture, which improves pulmonary blood flow by increasing the resistance in the systemic circulation.

In principle, surgery is indicated for every child with tetralogy of Fallot because the VSD will not close spontaneously and the infundibular stenosis tends to progress. The only interventional options are palliative measures or adjuncts to operative treatment such as stent implantation in the ductus arteriosus or angioplasty for peripheral pulmonary stenosis. Symptomatic children are operated between the third and fourth months of life, asymptomatic children during the first year of life. Without surgery, 70% of affected children would die before 10 years of age.

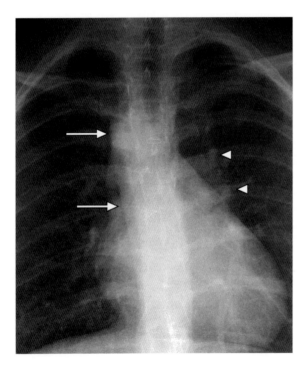

Fig. 2.16 Frontal chest radiograph. The superimposed pulmonary trunk and left pulmonary artery (arrowheads) were misinterpreted as a mediastinal tumor. Note the right aortic arch and right descending aorta (arrows). Magnified view of **Fig. 2.12 a**.

Pneumonia/ Pulmonary Venous Congestion/ Pulmonary Emphysema

History and Clinical Findings

An 86-year-old man was referred for chest radiography. The clinical question was "Change in infiltrates?".

The radiology report described bilateral basal pleural adhesions, dilatation of the left ventricle, an indurated focus in the left upper lobe, and a metallic foreign body in the chest wall (**Fig. 2.17**).

Pulmonary venous congestion and infiltrates were excluded.

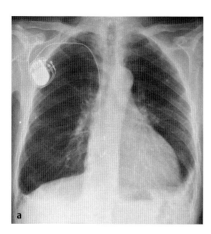 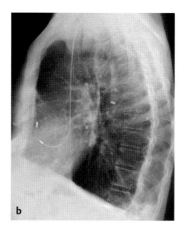

Fig. 2.17 a, b Chest radiographs were interpreted as showing bilateral basal pleural adhesions, dilatation of the left ventricle without pulmonary venous congestion, an indurated focus in the left upper lobe, and a metallic foreign body in the right chest wall.

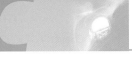

Further Case Summary

Because of the discrepancy between clinical findings (declining inflammatory markers, diminishing productive cough, normal pacemaker function) and radiographic findings, the attending cardiologist reviewed 6-week-old chest radiographs in which the same radiologist had described extensive infiltrates in the left lower lobe and lingula, milder infiltrates in the right lower lobe, and concomitant pleural effusions consistent with pleuropneumonia (**Fig. 2.18**).

Error Analysis and Strategy for Error Prevention

The following errors were made in interpreting the chest radiographs:

- Attention was not given to the patient's history on the referral form.
- The findings of prior examinations were disregarded.
- The following misinterpretations were made during image analysis:
  - Flattening of the diaphragm was not recognized in the lateral view as the cardinal sign of pulmonary emphysema (**Fig. 2.19**).
  - Pleural effusion vs. pleural adhesion was not considered in the differential diagnosis of the well-defined opacities in the costophrenic angles.
  - The linear opacities in the left lower lobe were missed.

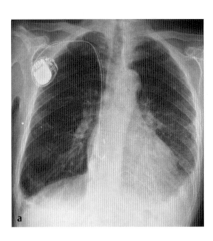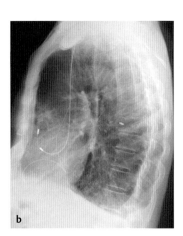

Fig. 2.18 a, b Prior radiographs 6 weeks old were interpreted as bilateral congestive pneumonia with pleural effusions.

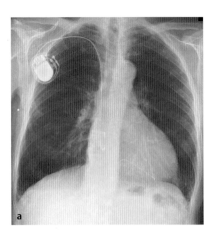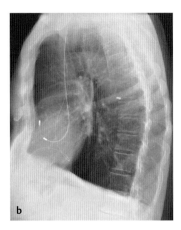

Fig. 2.19 a, b Chest radiograph 3 months later documents regression of pulmonary congestion, pleural effusions and infiltrates. Findings are consistent with pulmonary emphysema.

Pneumonia/Tumor/Cavity

History and Clinical Findings

An 88-year-old woman with dementia was transferred from a nursing home to a hospital due to high fever. The chest radiograph taken during the night shift was initially interpreted as normal (**Fig. 2.20**). Since the patient had no clinical or laboratory signs of inflammation, she was returned to the nursing home the following morning.

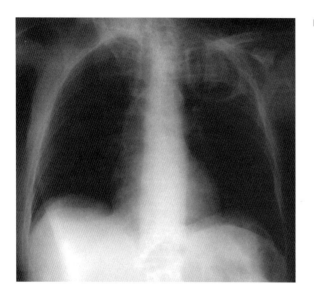

Fig. 2.20   Chest radiograph on hospital admission.

Further Case Summary

The next morning the chest film was interpreted by a radiologist, who noted a thick-walled cavity in the upper lobe of the left lung (**Fig. 2.21 b**). This finding was new relative to a prior examination 3 months earlier (**Fig. 2.21 a**). The differential diagnosis included open tuberculosis and a fungal infection. The necrotic degeneration of a bronchial carcinoma was considered unlikely because of the brief course. The patient was rehospitalized and isolated due to the infection risk. CT confirmed the finding on the chest radiograph, showing infiltration and cavitation in the left upper lobe (**Fig. 2.22 a**). Since no acid-fast rods or fungi were detected in sputum or bronchial washings, a CT-guided biopsy was taken from the posterior wall of the cavity and this confirmed tuberculosis (**Fig. 2.22 b**).

Error Analysis and Strategy for Error Prevention

Missing the cavity in the left upper lobe is an error of interpretation. Since no abnormalities were found, the patient was returned to the nursing home without waiting for the radiology report the next morning and without a request for an immediate reading by teleradiology. This would have allowed for more rapid quarantining of the patient.

In the case shown in **Fig. 2.23**, the changes caused by acute pulmonary tuberculosis were initially missed as well. The patient had been referred for CT-guided percutaneous biopsy of a pulmonary nodule (**Fig. 2.23 c**). During planning of the biopsy, fresh nodular opacities were noted in the apex of the right lung. Since the morphologic lung findings were consistent with tuberculosis, the biopsy was postponed and more specific testing was initiated. Microbiology confirmed the diagnosis of pulmonary tuberculosis.

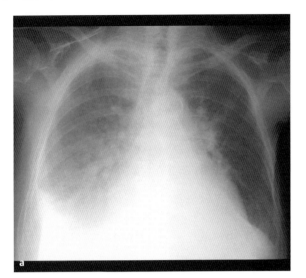

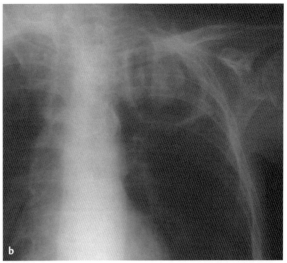

Fig. 2.21 a, b Radiographic follow-up.

a Prior chest radiograph 3 months earlier showed left ventricular decompensation with pulmonary venous congestion and bilateral pleural effusions, more pronounced on the right side than on the left.

b Current examination (magnified view of the lesion in **Fig. 2.20**) shows cardiac recompensation with a cavity and new infiltrates in the left upper lobe.

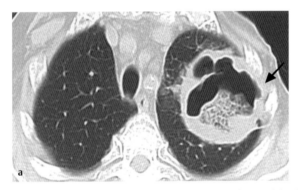

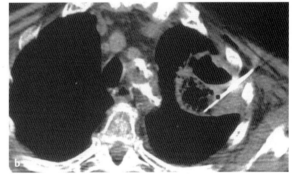

Fig. 2.22 a, b Axial CT demonstrates a cavity in the left upper lobe that is in broad contact with the chest wall (arrow in **a**). **b** CT-guided biopsy.

References and Further Reading

Hopewell PC. Tuberculosis and other mycobacterial diseases. In: Mason RJ, Broaddus VC, Murray JF, Nadel JA, eds. Murray and Nadel's Textbook of Respiratory Medicine. 4th ed. Philadelphia: Elsevier Saunders; 2005: 979–1043

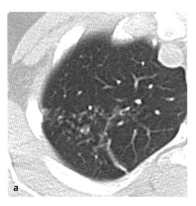
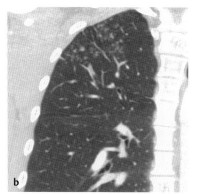
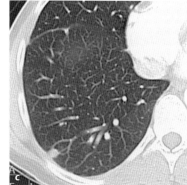

Fig. 2.23 a–c The patient was referred for CT-guided biopsy of the right lower lobe for a suspected lung malignancy (**c**).

a Axial scan through the right upper lobe.
b Coronal reformatted image of the upper right lung.
c Axial scan through the right lower lobe.

Tuberculosis (TB)

The current incidence of pulmonary tuberculosis worldwide is 140/100 000 population/year, with a reported mortality rate of 19/100 000 population/year. The respective figures für Europe are 47/100 000 and 7/100 000 inhabitants/year and for the Americas 29/100 000 and 2/100 000 inhabitants/year. TB is usually acquired by the inhalation of ubiquitous acid-fast mycobacteria that are pathogenic to humans. The lung is most commonly affected (approximately 86 % of cases), followed by the lymph nodes (7 %) and urogenital tract (4 %).

Detection of the causative organism. The causative mycobacteria of tuberculosis are detected by light and fluorescent microscopic examination of sputum, bronchial secretions, urine, or biopsy material and by polymerase chain reaction (PCR) testing. If microscopy fails to detect mycobacteria in clinically suspicious cases, the samples should be cultured on specific media. Culture tests require 3–5 weeks. Open TB is present when causative organisms can be identified in sputum, urine, feces, or fistula discharge.

Postprimary TB. This form develops in immunocompromised patients who have had a primary infection that resolved years or decades earlier. Mycobacteria still present in the primary complex gain access to the bloodstream and spread by the hematogenous route, seeding primarily to the lungs. The ratio of the virulence of the mycobacteria to the host resistance determines the pattern of lung involvement. In patients who still have fairly good host defenses, pneumonic foci most commonly develop in the apicoposterior segment of the upper lobe and the apical segment of the lower lobe. These "Simon foci" may coalesce and undergo cavitation (Assmann foci) or may become encapsulated and calcify. The apical segments are sites of predilection because of their slightly lower local oxygen tension, relatively low perfusion, and reduced lymphatic drainage. Assmann foci that undergo cavitation are a frequent cause of open TB. Immunocompromised patients may develop miliary TB consisting of numerous productive pneumonic foci distributed throughout both lungs, predominantly in the upper lobes. Severely immunocompromised patients may develop Landouzy septicemia (sepsis tuberculosa acutissima), which is characterized by extensive tissue necrosis and usually has a fatal outcome.

Productive lesions. Productive lesions consist of infiltrating epithelioid and giant cells rimmed by lymphocytes. The lesions usually range from 1 to 2 mm in diameter. Separate productive lesions may coalesce. Lesions that undergo central caseation and liquefaction and communicate with a draining bronchus form tuberculous cavities, from which necrotic material is coughed up, aspirated, or swallowed. Relatively fresh cavities are surrounded by pneumonic infiltrates.

Abscesses and cavities. Abscesses that do not communicate with the bronchial system—like nonspecific, undrained abscesses—rarely present radiographically as a rounded opacity within an infiltrate. The abscess wall appears on postcontrast CT as an enhancing ring that surrounds nonenhancing contents. The cavities have the same attenuation as air on CT scans. Tuberculous bronchitis is characterized by a wall-thickened draining bronchus that is already visible on plain chest films. The cavity wall shows irregular thickening during the acute inflammatory phase. Tuberculous cavities and neoplastic cavities are indistinguishable by their imaging appearance, as both entities have irregular, thickened walls, air–fluid levels, and perifocal infiltrates. Equivocal cases should be investigated by biopsy, therefore.

References and Further Reading

World Health Organization (WHO). Tuberculosis. Fact Sheet No. 104, November 2010. http://who.int/mediacentre/fact-sheets/fs104/en/ (accessed December 28, 2010)

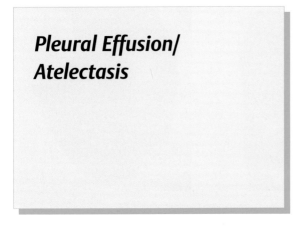

Pleural Effusion/Atelectasis

History and Clinical Findings

A 58-year-old woman with advanced multiple sclerosis was admitted to the ICU with clinical suspicion of pneumonia. Her supine chest radiograph was described as showing a basal pleural effusion tracking toward the apex of the left lung (**Fig. 2.24**). Ultrasound-guided needle aspiration was recommended to investigate the cause of the effusion.

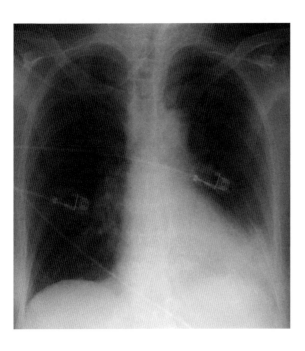

Fig. 2.24 Supine chest radiograph, interpreted as showing a left pleural effusion. The film also shows a left jugular vein catheter, nasogastric tube, ECG leads, and an extracorporeal catheter superimposed over the upper right lung.

Further Case Summary

A chest radiograph taken the following day (**Fig. 2.25**) showed atelectasis of the left lung, which was attributed to mucous plugging of the left main bronchus. Subsequent bronchoscopy confirmed occlusion of the left main bronchus by mucus, which was removed by suction. A chest radiograph taken the next day documented the regression of findings (**Fig. 2.26**).

Error Analysis and Strategy for Error Prevention

The differential diagnosis of the initial chest radiograph was between atelectasis and pneumonic infiltration of the lingula (**Table 2.2**). The signs of diminished left lung volume supported a diagnosis of atelectasis. Misinterpretations of this kind can be avoided by a systematic image analysis with routine evaluation of all anatomical and clinical details.

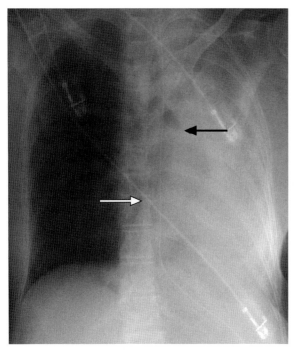

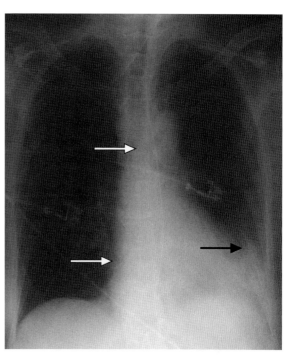

Fig. 2.25 Chest radiograph 1 day later shows atelectasis of the left lung with displacement of the heart and mediastinum toward the left side (white arrow) and cutoff of the left main bronchus (black arrow). Monitoring and support devices are still visible.

Fig. 2.26 Chest radiograph 2 days later. Atelectasis of the lingula appears as a patchy opacity projected over the lower left lung (black arrow). The heart and trachea are again centered in the chest (white arrows).

Table 2.2 Morphologic criteria for differentiating among atelectasis, infiltrate, and pleural effusion on chest radiographs

Criterion	Atelectasis	Pneumonic infiltrate	Pleural effusion
Shape of opacity	Patchy	Focal or patchy	Patchy
Parenchymal margins	Indistinct	Indistinct	Sharp
Displacement of mediastinum and diaphragm	Absent or ipsilateral	Absent or contralateral	Absent or contralateral

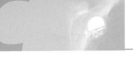
Pneumonic Infiltrates/ Pulmonary Metastases

History and Clinical Findings

A 26-year-old woman with no serious prior illnesses was admitted with a 4-week history of fever and hemoptysis. The patient claimed that a chest radiograph taken by her family doctor 2 weeks earlier had shown infiltrates in both lungs. Current radiographic examination confirmed focal opacities in both lungs, which were interpreted as pneumonia (**Fig. 2.27**). Laboratory tests revealed leukocytosis and an elevated ESR. The patient's symptoms did not improve in response to antibiotic therapy. A chest radiograph 4 days later showed progression of the infiltrates (**Fig. 2.28**), at which time the patient was placed on a different antibiotic.

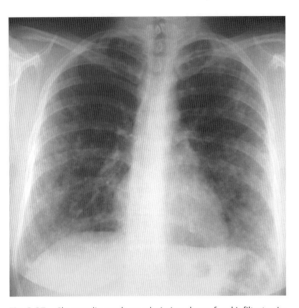

Fig. 2.27 Chest radiograph on admission shows focal infiltrates in both lungs, which were interpreted as pneumonia.

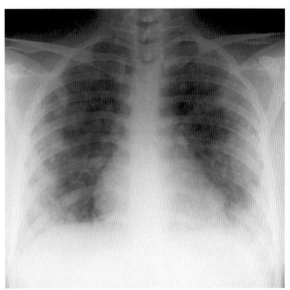

Fig. 2.28 Chest radiograph 4 days later.

Further Case Summary

When her condition did not improve, another chest radiograph and thoracic CT scans were obtained after an additional 5 days (**Fig. 2.29**). CT showed a hypodense mass in the right atrium with extension to the right ventricle, focal infiltrates in the periphery of both lungs, and hypodense nodules in the liver. Vasculitis, cardiac thrombi, a cardiac tumor, and metastases were considered as possible etiologies. An open lung biopsy revealed pulmonary metastases from rhabdomyosarcoma. Experimental chemotherapy was unsuccessful, and the patient died a few days later. Autopsy revealed pulmonary, hepatic, and ovarian metastases from a rhabdomyosarcoma arising in the right atrium.

Error Analysis and Strategy for Error Prevention

Focal (nodular) opacities are a nonspecific finding. Primary alveolar diseases as well as primary interstitial processes and their combinations may lead to focal opacities, resulting in a broad differential diagnosis (**Table 2.3**).

Resistance to antibiotic therapy did not support a diagnosis of uncomplicated pneumonia. At least in retrospect the increasing prominence of the right atrium on the chest radiographs was an indication ot the right atrial tumor (**Fig. 2.30**). The final chest radiograph was an unnecessary adjunct to thoracic CT scans.

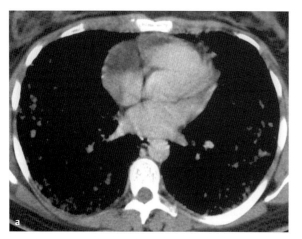 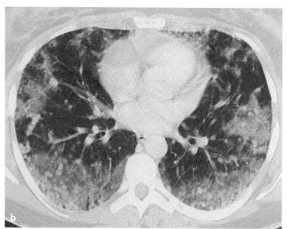

Fig. 2.29 a, b Thoracic CT scans show a rhabdomyosarcoma in the right atrium and ventricle with disseminated pulmonary metastases.

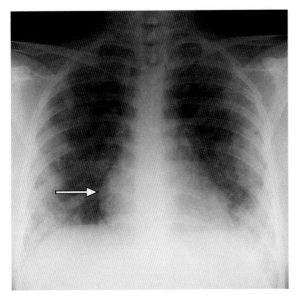

Fig. 2.30 Chest radiograph 4 days after hospitalization shows focal subpleural infiltrates in both lungs and prominence of the right atrium (arrow) caused by tumor growth.

Table 2.3 Differential diagnosis of focal pulmonary opacities

Infectious etiology
■ Bacterial pneumonia
■ Tuberculosis
■ Viral pneumonia
■ Fungal pneumonia
■ Parasitic diseases
■ Exogenous allergic alveolitis
■ Sarcoidosis
■ Connective-tissue disease

Neoplastic etiology
■ Metastases
■ Malignant lymphoma
■ Bronchoalveolar carcinoma
■ Carcinomatous lymphangitis

Miscellaneous
■ Idiopathic pulmonary fibrosis
■ Langerhans cell histiocytosis
■ Pneumoconioses
■ Alveolitis due to toxic inhalation
■ Amyloidosis
■ Hemosiderosis
■ Aspiration
■ Intrapulmonary hemorrhage

References and Further Reading

Fraser RS, Muller NL, Coleman N. Fraser and Pare's Diagnosis of Diseases of the Chest. Philadelphia: WB Saunders; 1999

Prokop M, van der Molen A. Heart. In: Prokop M, Galanski M, eds. Computed Tomography of the Body. Stuttgart: Thieme; 2003

Intrapleural Fat/ Pleural Effusion/ Pulmonary Infiltrate

History and Clinical Findings

A 56-year-old man was referred for thoracic CT because he had recovered from clinically diagnosed pneumonia 4 weeks earlier and now his laboratory inflammatory markers were elevated again. He also had a low-grade fever. The most significant CT findings were a pericardial effusion with a maximum thickness of 1 cm and an encapsulated effusion in the oblique fissure of the left lung (**Fig. 2.31**). Pulmonary infiltrates were not described.

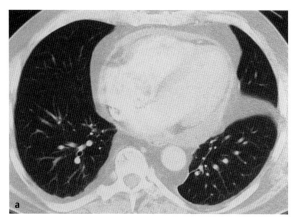 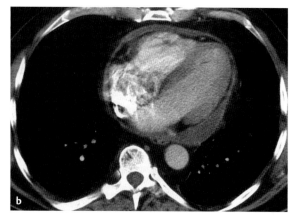

Fig. 2.31 a, b   Thoracic CT scans prompted a diagnosis of pericardial effusion and an "encapsulated effusion" in the oblique fissure of the left lung.

Further Case Summary

The presumed interlobar effusion consisted of fatty deposits in the basal interlobar fissure. This is a normal variant. Mediastinal lipomatosis was also present. The diagnosis of pericardial effusion was correct.

Error Analysis and Strategy for Error Prevention

The following rules were disregarded during image analysis:

- Use of multiple window settings. Unlike the pericardial effusion, the presumed interlobar pleural effusion was not visible with a mediastinal window because it had the same attenuation as mediastinal, epicardial, and subcutaneous fat (approximately −100 HU). When viewed with a mediastinal window (window width 400 HU, window level 40 HU), the pleural deposits had the same uniform black appearance as lung tissue.

- Analysis of topographic anatomy and pathoanatomy. Thickening of the oblique fissure was in continuity with the thickened fibrofatty tissue of the mediastinum.
- Attenuation values within the interlobar fissure were not determined. CT is the only imaging modality that yields objective data on density. MRI and ultrasound interpretation are based purely on a visual assessment of relative gray-scale information. Thus, CT is better than MRI and ultrasound for evaluating the quality of tissues and fluids present within the scanned volume.

Hounsfield Scale and Window Settings

In CT data acquisition, relative attenuation values are measured after the x-rays have passed through the object of interest. A computer relates these attenuation values to the x-ray absorption of water, yielding quantitative image data. In the Hounsfield scale, named for its inventor, the x-ray absorption of water provides the basic reference point and is defined as zero. Structures of higher density (greater x-ray absorption) are assigned positive attenuation values, while structures of lower density (less x-ray absorption) are assigned negative values. The scale usually spans a range of 4000 Hounsfield units (HU). The HU values determined for each pixel in the image matrix are converted to a gray scale. The various shades of gray are then used to produce an image showing the density distribution of the scanned structures.

Because the human eye can distinguish fewer than 100 shades of gray, encoding the full range of gray-scale values would yield a low-contrast image that would be unsuitable for diagnostic analysis. Acceptable contrast resolution is achieved by selecting a portion of the density scale, called the "window," and distributing it over the full range of gray-scale values. This range of displayed HU values is called the window width, and the center of that range is called the window level. The window width and level are set to the density range of greatest diagnostic interest. Density values below the window setting appear black in the image, while values above the window appear white. Given the complex anatomy of all body regions, the image data should be documented using various combinations of settings in order to fully utilize all the diagnostic information contained in the digital image data set.

References and Further Reading

Prokop M. Principles of CT, spiral CT, and multislice CT. In: Prokop M, Galanski M, eds. Computed Tomography of the Body. Stuttgart: Thieme; 2003

Aortic Dissection/ Aortic Wall Hematoma/ Mediastinal Hematoma

History and Clinical Findings

A 66-year-old woman with no prior history of aortic disease was referred for coronary angiography. Considerable resistance was met when the catheter was advanced into the aorta. After the procedure the patient complained of pressure and pain in the jugular fossa and behind the upper sternum. She stated that her complaints were aggravated by swallowing. Due to clinical suspicion of an aortic dissection, CT angiography of the thoracoabdominal aorta was performed during the night shift on an emergent basis (**Fig. 2.32**). The following conditions were diagnosed:

- Aortic dissection extending from the aortic arch to the aortic bifurcation
- Up to 50% narrowing of the true lumen of the descending thoracic aorta
- Celiac trunk, superior mesenteric artery, and both renal arteries arising from the true lumen

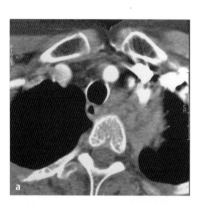
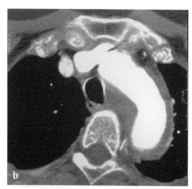
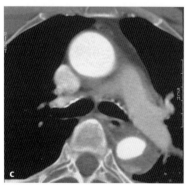
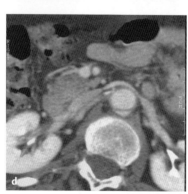

Fig. 2.32 a–d CT angiography shows an aortic dissection from arch to bifurcation. The right renal artery arises from the true lumen.

Further Case Summary

Because the patient was clinically stable, it was decided that an endovascular intervention or surgery was not indicated. Her complaints improved during the next few days. Daily chest radiographs showed slight widening of the upper mediastinum (**Fig. 2.33**).

CT angiography at 3-week intervals showed that the false lumen in the descending thoracic aorta was no longer perfused and had become reapproximated to the aortic wall (**Fig. 2.34**). The widening and diffusely increased density of the fibrofatty tissue in the upper mediastinum and about the aortic arch, initially missed at CT angiography, were also regressing along with the earlier shift of the upper trachea and esophagus toward the right side.

Error Analysis and Strategy for Error Prevention

The patient's complaints (pressure and pain aggravated by swallowing), the widening and diffusely increased density of the upper mediastinum (**Fig. 2.32 a, b**), lateralization of the upper esophagus (**Fig. 2.32 a, b**), and shift of the upper trachea toward the right side (**Fig. 2.32 a**) had been disregarded in the emergency situation. All of these findings were suggestive of bleeding into the upper mediastinum.

The extravasation was apparently caused by injury to the aortic wall at the level of the aortic arch caused by ad-

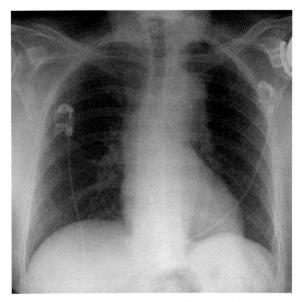

Fig. 2.33 Chest radiograph 3 days after CT shows slight widening of the upper mediastinum.

vancement of the cardiac catheter along the false channel. Active arterial bleeding was not detected. The symptoms resolved completely over the next few days as the hematoma was reabsorbed.

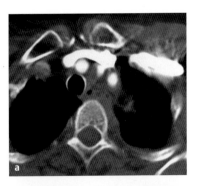
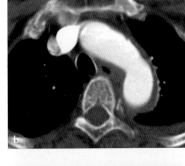
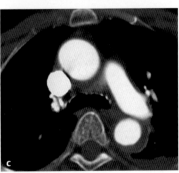
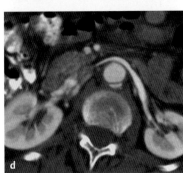

Fig. 2.34 a–d CT angiography 3 weeks after cardiac catheterization. The upper part of the false lumen is no longer visualized compared with initial CT angiography (**c**). The mediastinal hemorrhage has undergone significant resorption and regression (**a, b**). Aortic dissection persists at the infrarenal level (**d**).

Perforated Aortic Dissection/ Venous Mediastinal Hemorrhage

History and Clinical Findings

A 75-year-old man was transferred to the ICU from a different hospital at approximately 03:00 with a suspected perforated aortic aneurysm. When admitted to the other hospital, the patient had complained of acute pain radiating between the scapulae. He also manifested pallor and cold sweats. His blood pressure was 90/75 mm Hg. ECG, laboratory tests, and abdominal ultrasound were negative. A chest radiograph had raised suspicion of a dissecting thoracic aortic aneurysm. A ruptured aneurysm of the aortic arch was diagnosed elsewhere by thoracic CT (**Fig. 2.35**). The images from the CT examination were interpreted as follows by the radiologist on duty and discussed with the cardiac surgeon:

- Ectasia of the aortic arch to < 4.5 cm in diameter
- Mural thrombus in the descending aorta
- Kinking of the descending thoracic aorta
- Bleeding into the mediastinal fat (widening and increased density of the mediastinal fibrofatty tissue cranial to the aortic arch and caudal to the left main bronchus)
- No perforation or dissection of the aorta

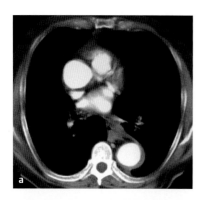
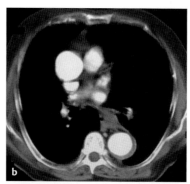
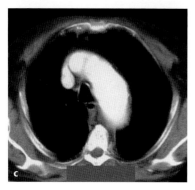
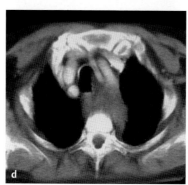

Fig. 2.35 a–d Thoracic CT. Initial report described ectasia of the aortic arch (**c**), a mural thrombus in the descending aorta (**a, b**), bleeding into the mediastinal fat (**d**), and an absence of aortic dissection or perforation. On further analysis, the density about the posterolateral circumference of the descending thoracic aorta is dystelectatic lung resulting from pulsation-induced damage to the lung parenchyma bordering on the aorta (**a, b**).

Further Case Summary

Because the patient was hemodynamically unstable, transesophageal echocardiography (TEE) was not performed. Instead, surgery was performed the same night because of the patient's clinical presentation and the prior suspicion of a ruptured aortic aneurysm. In the course of the operation, the entire ascending aorta, aortic arch, and origins of the supra-aortic arteries were dissected free. The ascending aorta was found to be dilated, but there was no evidence of a perforation or dissection. Afterward it was assumed that the patient had a venous mediastinal hemorrhage.

Error Analysis and Strategy for Error Prevention

The radiologist on duty had interpreted the CT scans correctly. Except for the diffuse increase in mediastinal density, none of the radiologic signs of a perforated aortic aneurysm listed in **Table 2.4** was present.

References and Further Reading

Batra P, Bigoni B, Manning J, et al. Pitfalls in the diagnosis of thoracic dissection at CT angiography. Radiographics 2000; 20: 309–320

Shiga T, Wajima Z, Apfel CC, Inoue T, Ohe Y. Diagnostic accuracy of TEE, helical CT and MRI for suspected thoracic aortic dissection. Systematic review and meta-analysis. Arch Intern Med 2006; 166: 1350–1356

Table 2.4   Signs of a perforated thoracic aortic aneurysm

Direct signs	Indirect signs

■ Diffuse increased density of mediastinal fibrofatty tissue with:
  — A long area of contact with the aneurysm or dissection
  — Signs of mass effect
  — Mediastinal widening
■ Contrast extravasation from the aorta after IV contrast administration
	■ Aortic aneurysm (thoracic diameter > 5 cm, intraluminal thrombosis)
	■ Aortic dissection
	■ Pleural effusion (usually on the left side)
	■ Pericardial effusion

Table 2.5   Meta-analysis of the diagnostic accuracy of TEE, spiral CT, and MRI for suspected aortic dissection. The data indicate mean values and range of values. (Source: Shiga et al. 2006.)

	Sensitivity (%)	Specificity (%)	Positive likelihood ratio	Negative likelihood ratio
TEE	98 95–99	95 92–97	14 6–33	0.04 0.02–0.08
CT	100 96–100	98 87–99	14 4–46	0.02 0.01–0.11
MRI	98 95–99	98 95–100	25 11–57	0.05 0.03–0.10

Accuracy of TEE, Spiral CT, and MRI in the Diagnosis of Aortic Dissection

In 2006, Shiga et al. published a meta-analysis on the diagnostic accuracy of TEE, spiral CT, and MRI in patients with suspected aortic dissection. The analysis covered published English-language reports that met the following criteria: prospective data acquisition, consecutive patient recruitment, use of at least one of the three imaging techniques, results stated in absolute values, clear identification of the diagnostic reference standard, quality grades, and blinded interpretation.

The authors reviewed 10 studies on TEE published between 1991 and 2001 involving a total of 631 patients, three studies on CT in 117 patients from 1995 to 2003, and seven studies on MRI in 392 patients from 1989 to 2000. They found that even with the older generations of equipment used in the studies, all three imaging modalities yielded equally reliable results for confirming or excluding aortic dissection (**Table 2.5**). No further publications are available on the relative accuracies of modern CT and MRI technologies.

Normal Mediastinum/ Pseudotumor/ Malignant Lymphoma/ Lymph Node Metastases

History and Clinical Findings

A 46-year-old man presented at a dermatology clinic with a flare-up of eczematous skin lesions. He had had a prior history of acneiform dermatosis and eczema for 6 years, during which time a diagnosis of pyoderma gangrenosum had been considered. This is an ulcerating skin disease that has a prevalence of 0.3% in the general population and may be associated with malignancies and immune dysfunction. The patient had also been diagnosed with thrombophilia marked by recurrent thrombosis in the deep veins of the upper and lower extremities. A chest radiograph, taken to exclude a neoplasm, was considered to show no abnormalities except for a left-sided pleural effusion (**Fig. 2.36**).

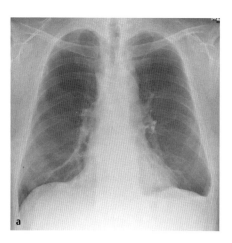
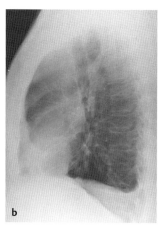

Fig. 2.36 a, b The chest radiograph was interpreted as normal except for a left-sided pleural effusion.

Further Case Summary

On further inquiry from dermatology, it was discovered that widening of the upper mediastinum had been missed. The differential diagnosis was expanded to include a primary or secondary malignant mediastinal tumor. Further investigation by CT revealed a venous anomaly (**Fig. 2.37**). The superior vena cava was not present in this patient. Contrast medium flowed through the subclavian vein into a large-caliber vessel that descended along the left side of the mediastinum. This vein ran to the diaphragm at the left cardiac border and crossed between the ventricle and diaphragm to the right side, where it drained into the inferior vena cava. Venous collaterals were additionally present in the upper mediastinum. Subsequent comparison with a prior examination done 2 years earlier showed that these features were already present at that time, though to a less prominent degree (**Fig. 2.38**).

Error Analysis and Strategy for Error Prevention

Initial interpretation of the chest radiograph had missed the widening and double outlines of the left upper mediastinum and the increased density of the aortopulmonary window (**Fig. 2.39 a**). Increased density of the anterior upper mediastinum had also been missed in the lateral radiograph (**Fig. 2.39 b**).

Mediastinal tumors are often discovered incidentally, as in the present case. Given the relatively large volume of the mediastinum, some time is needed before the mass begins to compress adjacent structures. Common symptoms are retrosternal tenderness, persistent cough, dyspnea, palpitations or other cardiac sensations, hoarseness, and/or dysphagia. The differential diagnosis is broad because all three germ layers contribute to the mediastinum during embryonic development and because major anatomic landmarks (the aorta, vena cava, esophagus, trachea, thoracic duct, nerves) traverse the mediastinum. The differential diagnosis may be narrowed by the history, mediastinal tumor site, tumor attachment, and associated imaging findings in other organs. In the present case, the radiographic detection of a mass in the anterior and

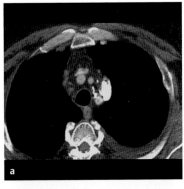
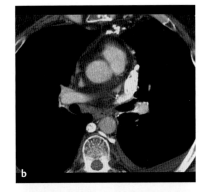
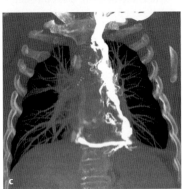
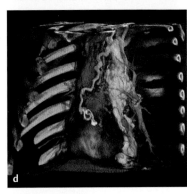

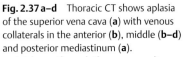

Fig. 2.37 a–d Thoracic CT shows aplasia of the superior vena cava (**a**) with venous collaterals in the anterior (**b**), middle (**b–d**) and posterior mediastinum (**a**).

a Axial scan through the upper mediastinum.

b Axial scan through the middle mediastinum.

c Coronal reformatted maximum-intensity projection (MIP) of the middle mediastinum.

d Volume-rendered image.

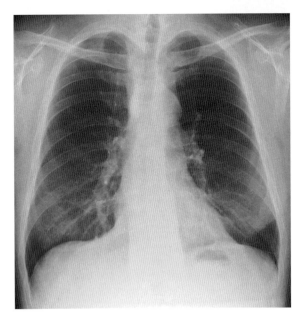

Fig. 2.38 Prior chest radiograph 2 years earlier showed mediastinal widening (vascular pseudotumor).

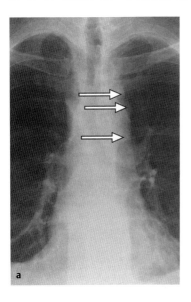
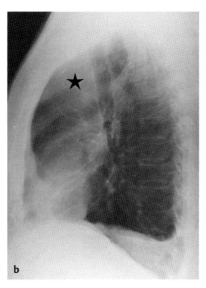

Fig. 2.39 a, b Current chest radiographs (**Fig. 2.36**). The widening and double outlines of the left upper mediastinum (upper arrows) and increased density of the aortopulmonary window (lower arrow) indicate the mediastinal mass in panel **a**. The vascular pseudotumor has caused increased density of the anterior upper mediastinum in panel **b** (★).

Radiographic Signs of Mediastinal Masses

Anterior mediastinum. When tumors of the anterior mediastinum have reached sufficient size, they cause mediastinal widening that blends with the cardiac border on frontal chest radiographs. The lateral view shows a retrosternal opacity that may coalesce with the anterior cardiac border and ascending aorta if the mass is abutting those structures.

Middle mediastinum. Middle mediastinal masses of sufficient size correlate with widening and increased density of the corresponding mediastinal compartment. A distance of more than 4 mm between the trachea and esophagus in the lateral radiograph establishes the presence of a mass. Thickening of the retrotracheal line (lateral view) to more than 4 mm, displacement of the azygoesophageal line (frontal view), and obliteration of the aortopulmonary window also signify a mediastinal mass.

Posterior mediastinum. Tumors of the posterior mediastinum appear as paravertebral opacities separate from the cardiac border on frontal radiographs due to their different object–film distance. Masses in contact with the posterior aortic arch and descending aorta appear to blend with the aortic border in both the frontal and lateral projections.

mid-upper mediastinum prompted the CT diagnosis of a venous collateral circulation, which explained the large vessel passing through the left middle mediastinum on the chest radiograph.

Aplasia of the vena cava, possibly accompanied by recurrent venous thrombosis secondary to antiphospholipid antibody syndrome, was assumed to be the cause of the venous collaterals. Vascular occlusive disease in antiphospholipid syndrome almost always has a thrombotic cause and is not due to vascular inflammation. The following sets of findings are suggestive of an antiphospholipid syndrome:

- Venous thrombosis at an unusual site (axillary, renal, portal, caval, retinal)
- Recurrent episodes of venous thrombosis in the absence of predisposing factors, especially in young patients
- Stroke, myocardial infarction, peripheral gangrene, or ischemia of visceral organs in patients who have no risk factors for atherosclerosis
- Habitual abortion

References and Further Reading

Levasseur P, Kaswin R, Rojas-Miranda A, et al. Profile of surgical tumors of the mediastinum. Apropos of a series of 742 operated patients. Nouv Presse Med 1976; 5: 2857–2859

Marchevsky AM, Kaneko M. Surgical Pathology of the Mediastinum. 2nd ed. New York: Raven; 1992

Shimosato Y, Mukai K. Tumors of the mediastinum. In: Atlas of Tumor Pathology, Series 3, Fascicle 21. Washington DC: Armed Forces Institute of Pathology; 1997

Follow-up of Thymoma

density in the anterior upper mediastinum. The lesion had infiltrated the upper lobes of both lungs. A review of available images showed that the mass had been missed 2 years earlier on chest films and on MR images that included the superior thoracic aperture. MRI had been performed as part of a scientific study and was not done at that time to investigate the patient's symptoms.

The patient underwent a thymectomy that included a partial resection of both upper lobes and patch grafting of the innominate vein. Histology revealed a B2 thymoma showing some progression to well-differentiated thymic carcinoma (**Table 2.6**). Disease extent was classified as Masaoka stage III (**Table 2.7**). No lymphogenous or hematogenous metastasis was present at the time of surgery.

Since the operation, the patient has had follow-up thoracic CT scans scheduled at intervals of 6 months to 1 year. Illustrative images are shown in **Fig. 2.40**. Each of the scans was interpreted as showing normal postoperative findings with areas of scar induration.

History and Clinical Findings

The patient, a 56-year-old male at the time of diagnosis, presented for CT scans to investigate the cause of retrosternal pressure. Thoracic CT showed a mass of soft-tissue

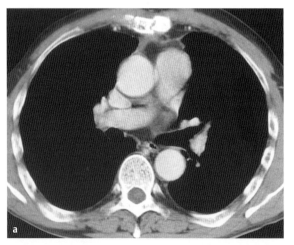

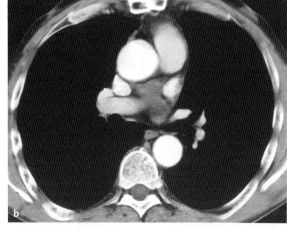

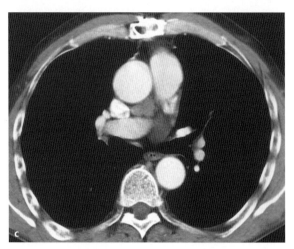

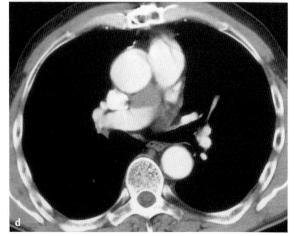

Fig. 2.40 a–d CT follow-ups. The density in the transverse pericardial sinus was interpreted as postoperative induration. Status post sternotomy.

a Six months after thymectomy.
b One year and 6 months after thymectomy.
c Two years and 6 months after thymectomy.
d Four years after thymectomy.

Thymoma

Epidemiology. Thymomas are malignant tumors. They comprise approximately 0.2–1.5% of all malignancies. A mass lesion in the anterior mediastinum is most commonly a thymoma (approximately 50% of patients), malignant lymphoma, or embryonal tumor (approximately 25%). Thymomas are most prevalent in the fourth to sixth decades but may occur at any age. Males and females are affected equally.

Clinical manifestations. There are no typical early symptoms. Approximately 30% of patients are asymptomatic at initial diagnosis. Symptoms in approximately 40% of patients result from the mass effects of the tumor (chest pain, cough, dyspnea). Symptoms in approximately 30% of patients are systemic (fatigue, weight loss), while symptoms in another 30% result from a paraneoplastic syndrome (myasthenia gravis). Approximately one-half of thymic neuroendocrine tumors (<5% of all tumors of the anterior mediastinum) have endocrine activity.

Classification and prognosis. Thymomas arise from the epithelial cells of the thymus. The WHO classification of 1999 is based on the histomorphology of the neoplastic epithelial cells and the nonneoplastic lymphocytic component (**Table 2.6**). The principal types are classified as A, AB, B, and C. Type C thymomas are also termed thymic carcinoma. The well-differentiated thymic carcinomas cited in older classifications are unrelated to true thymic carcinoma and are described as type B3 thymomas in the newer classification. Approximately 10% of thymomas are classified as type A, 20% as type AB, 60% as type B,

and 10% as type C. The 20-year survival rates are 80–100% for types A, AB, and B1; 35–60 % for type B2; and 0% for type C.

The most widely used staging classification for thymomas was introduced by Masaoka in 1981 (**Table 2.7**). Approximately 40% of patients have stage I disease at initial surgery, 25% are at stage II, 25% are at stage III, and 10% are at stage IV. Approximately 90% of the less aggressive types A, AB, and B1 thymomas are at Masaoka stage I or II. The 5-year survival rates are 89–100% at stage I, 70–100% at stage II, 50–85 % at stage III, and 42% at stage IV.

Treatment. The treatment of choice is surgery. Resections with clear margins yield significantly better survival times than subtotal resections (debulking). When dealing with higher tumor stages, debulking offers a survival advantage over conservative options (biopsy, chemotherapy, radiotherapy). Radical lymph node dissection is mandatory in patients with thymic carcinoma.

Recurrence. Most recurrences of thymoma are local. The average incidence of tumor recurrence is 23% (minimum 4%, maximum 46%). The average interval between initial diagnosis and local recurrence is 5.5 years (range from 2 to 16 years). Up to two-thirds of all recurrences are resectable, and clear margins are achieved in approximately 60% of cases. The reported 10-year survival rates after recurrent tumor surgery are 63% for R0 resections (histologically clear margins) and 6% (0–11%) for R1 resections (histologically positive margins with no metastases) or R2 resections (grossly positive margins and/or metastases).

Table 2.6 WHO classification of thymic tumors (adapted from Rosai and Sobin 1999)

WHO type	Histology
A	A tumor composed of a population of neoplastic thymic epithelial cells having spindle/oval shape, lacking nuclear atypia, and accompanied by few or no non-neoplastic lymphocytes
AB	A tumor in which foci having the features of type A thymoma are admixed with foci rich in lymphocytes.
B1	A tumor which resembles the normal functional thymus in that it combines large expanses having an appearance practically indistinguishable from normal thymic cortex with areas resembling thymic medulla
B2	A tumor in which the neoplastic epithelial component appears as scattered plump cells with vesicular nuclei and distinct nucleoli among a heavy population of lymphocytes. Perivascular spaces are common and sometimes very prominent. A perivascular arrangement of tumor cells resulting in a palisading effect may be seen.
B3	A tumor predominantly composed of epithelial cells having a round or polygonal shape and exhibiting no or mild atypia. They are admixed with a minor component of lymphocytes, resulting in a sheetlike growth of the neoplastic epithelial cells.
C	Thymic carcinoma

Table 2.7 Masaoka staging of thymic tumors (adapted from Masaoka 1981)

Stage	Histology
I	Microscopically encapsulated and microscopically no capsular invasion
II	1) Macroscopic invasion into surrounding fatty tissue of mediastinal pleura, or 2) microscopic invasion into capsule
III	Macroscopic invasion into neighboring organ
IV	IV a Pleural or pericardial dissemination IV b Lymphogenous or hematogenous metastasis

Further Case Summary I

Scans obtained 4½ years after the thymectomy detected a recurrence of thymic carcinoma located between the posterior wall of the aorta and the root of the pulmonary artery (**Figs. 2.41, 2.42**). In retrospect, this tumor was already detectable on CT follow-up at 1½ years (**Fig. 2.40 b**) and had gradually enlarged since that time. It was visible not only in an axial scan but also in three adjacent scans since the 3-year follow-up.

The median sternotomy was reopened for resection of the recurrent tumor. It was found at operation that pericardial invasion had occurred at the pericardial reflection. The affected portion of the pericardium was removed and the sac was closed with a Gore-Tex patch. The resection margins were histologically clear (R0 resection).

The second surgery was followed by an uneventful postoperative course. In the seventh and ninth years after the primary operation for thymic carcinoma, two malignant melanomas were removed from the left side of the neck, and additional CT follow-ups were performed at 6-month intervals (**Fig. 2.43**). The major findings were postoperative sequelae consisting of indurated scar tissue at the operative site, indurated areas in the right lower lobe, and a pericardial effusion in both apical upper lobes. Two and a half years after removal of the recurrent tumor (**Fig. 2.43 e, f**), a pleural-based soft-tissue tumor was found abutting the right mediobasal lower lobe. Because this finding was unchanged relative to the prior examination at 1½ years, it was classified as benign.

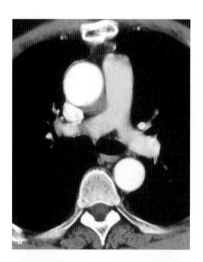
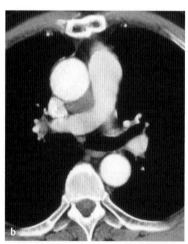
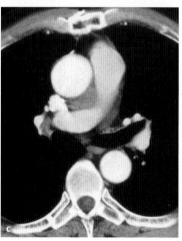
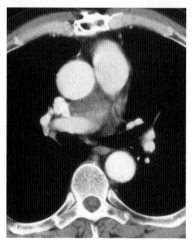

Fig. 2.41 a–d CT follow-up 4½ years after thymectomy. The scans indicate a local recurrence in the transverse pericardial sinus.

Further Case Summary II

Gradual size progression was noted thereafter, and two masses of soft-tissue density arising from the right mediastinal pleura were diagnosed 5½ years after the second operation (**Fig. 2.44**). Retrospective analysis of the CT series over an extended period revealed that circumscribed areas of pleural thickening were visible at the location of the two primary tumors just 6 months after the second operation (**Fig. 2.43 a, b**). Initially these areas had been classified as surgery-related changes. Since pleural metastasis was suspected, the chest was reopened through a right posterolateral approach, and the mediastinal and parietal pleura were partially removed along with the metastases. Histology confirmed pleural metastases from the previously diagnosed B2 thymoma with features of well-differentiated thymic carcinoma. An ulcerating malignant melanoma of the knee was resected 2½ years after removal of the recurrence. The follow-up care was without evidence for a tumor recurrence for the last 1½ years.

Error Analysis and Strategy for Error Prevention

The mediastinal tumor was missed on MRI of the shoulder and chest radiographs 2 years before the thymectomy, as the patient had no symptoms of a mediastinal process and attention was not directed toward the mediastinum.

Detection of the metastases at CT follow-ups was delayed because each current examination was compared with the CT examination directly preceding it. Because tumor growth occurred at a very slow rate, no significant morphologic image changes were perceived at the 6- to 12-month intervals. Tumor growth dynamics could be appreciated only by comparing the images with earlier prior examinations. This particularly applies to detection of the two pleural metastases.

CT-guided biopsy of the pleural masses was withheld due to an expressed concern that the procedure might lead to disseminated pleural metastasis.

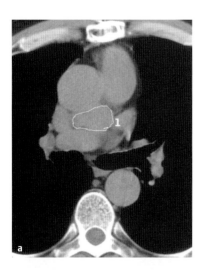
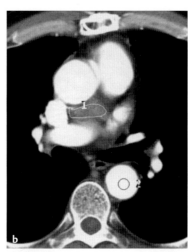
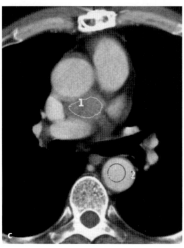
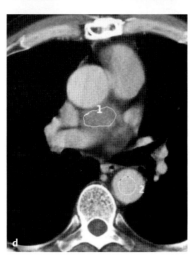

Fig. 2.42 a–d Qualitative perfusion study of the recurrent tumor 4½ years after thymectomy. Scans acquired at intervals before and after contrast injection demonstrate early, intense enhancement due to tumor neoangiogenesis.

a Unenhanced scan acquired before IV administration of a contrast bolus. Mean tumor density is 37 HU ± 12 HU.

b Early arterial phase following an IV contrast bolus. Mean tumor density is 71 HU ± 11 HU.

c Scan acquired 22 seconds after **b**. Mean tumor density is 76 HU ± 11 HU.

d Scan acquired 62 seconds after **c**. Mean tumor density is 64 HU ± 11 HU.

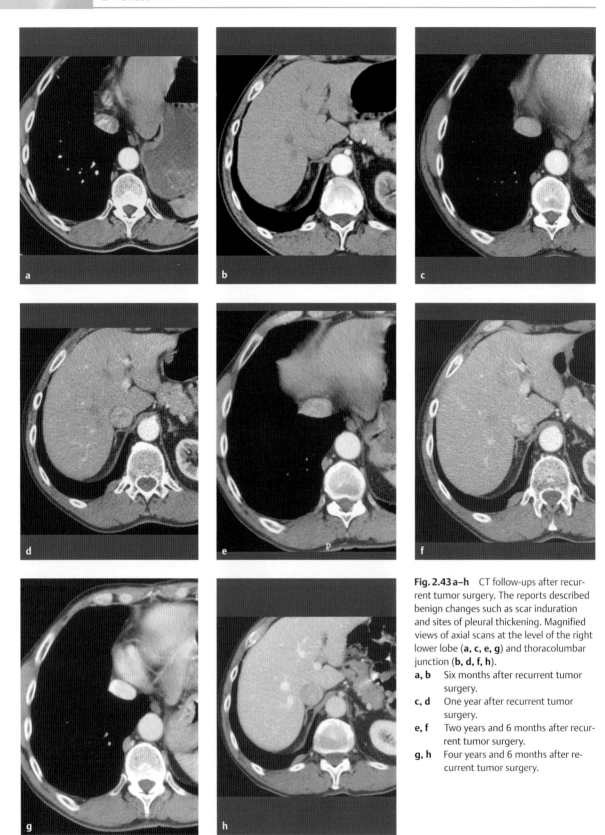

Fig. 2.43 a–h CT follow-ups after recurrent tumor surgery. The reports described benign changes such as scar induration and sites of pleural thickening. Magnified views of axial scans at the level of the right lower lobe (**a, c, e, g**) and thoracolumbar junction (**b, d, f, h**).

a, b Six months after recurrent tumor surgery.
c, d One year after recurrent tumor surgery.
e, f Two years and 6 months after recurrent tumor surgery.
g, h Four years and 6 months after recurrent tumor surgery.

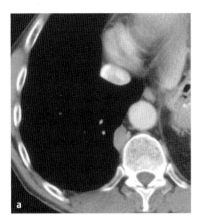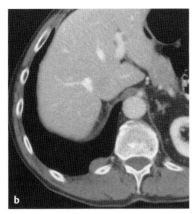

Fig. 2.44 a, b Detection of pleural metastasis 5½ years after recurrent tumor surgery.

References and Further Reading

Kondo K. Optimal therapy for thymoma. J Med Invest 2008; 55: 17–28

Masaoka A, Monden Y, Nakahana K, Tanioka T. Follow-up study of thymomas with special reference to their clinical stages. Cancer 1981; 48: 2485–2492

Matsumoto K, Ashizawa K, Tagawa T, Nagayasu T. Chest wall implantation of thymic cancer after computed tomography-guided core needle biopsy. Eur J Cardiothoracic Surg 2007; 32: 171–173

Okumura M, Shinichiro M, Fujii Y, et al. Clinical and functional significance of WHO classification on human thymic epithelial neoplasm. Am J Surg Pathol 2001; 25: 103–110

Rosai J, Sobin LH. Histological Typing of Tumors of the Thymus. 2nd ed. Berlin: Springer; 1999

Srirajaskanthan R, Toubanakis C, Dusmet M, Caplin ME. A review of thymic tumors. Lung Cancer 2008; 60: 4–13. doi:10.1016/j.lungcan.2008.01.014

Wright CD. Management of thymomas. Crit Rev Oncol Hematol 2008; 65: 109–120

Sarcoidosis/ Bronchial Carcinoma/ Malignant Lymphoma

History and Clinical Findings

A 48-year-old man in subjective good health had undergone chest radiography elsewhere as part of a routine examination. The x-ray report expressed suspicion of a central bronchial carcinoma. The patient was referred to an outpatient oncology unit for further evaluation and treatment. Physical examination and a complete blood count showed no abnormalities. The principal finding on thoracic CT was a right perihilar mass of soft-tissue density with a maximum diameter of approximately 3 cm (**Fig. 2.45**). Multiple lymph nodes with maximum diameters of 2–4 cm were found in the right hilar region and in the middle and upper mediastinum, predominantly on the right side. The diagnostic impression was a central bronchial carcinoma with ipsilateral hilar and mediastinal lymph node involvement. CT scans of the neck revealed normal-sized bilateral lymph nodes that were presumed to show reactive changes. Positron emission tomography with [18F]fluorodeoxyglucose (FDG/PET) showed increased uptake in all CT-positive areas.

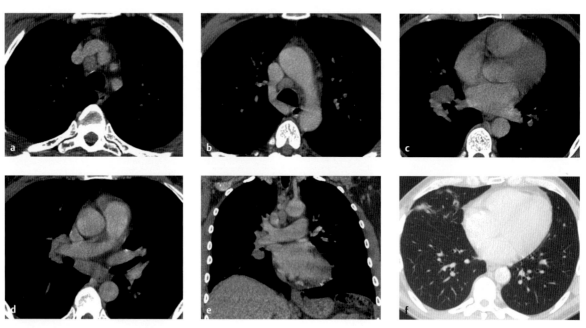

Fig. 2.45 a–f Thoracic CT scans. The report described a perihilar mass of soft-tissue density in the apical segment of the right lower lobe (**c, d**), enlarged right hilar (**d**) and mediastinal lymph nodes (**a, b, d, e**) and linear densities in the middle lobe, consistent with areas of dystelectasis or poststenotic pneumonia (**f**).

Further Case Summary

Bronchoalveolar brush cytology revealed inflammatory granulomas consistent with sarcoidosis. There was no evidence of carcinoma. Serum values for interleukin-2 receptors and ACE (angiotensin-converting enzyme) were elevated at 1350 kU/L (normal range is 223–710 kU/L) and 72 U/L (normal range is 8–52 U/L), respectively (**Fig. 2.46**). A comprehensive review of cytologic and laboratory chemical results yielded a diagnosis of acute stage I sar-

coidosis (**Table 2.8**). The densities in the middle lobe were interpreted as areas of dystelectasis. Because the patient had normal lung function and because acute stage I pulmonary sarcoidosis has a reported spontaneous remission rate of 55–90%, depending on the study cited, treatment was withheld. The patient was placed under the care of internists elsewhere, who reported that the pulmonary and lymph node findings normalized in subsequent months, confirming the diagnosis.

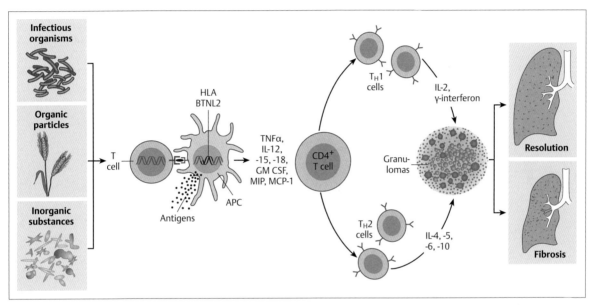

Fig. 2.46   Current concept on the mechanism of granuloma formation in sarcoidosis (after Iannuzzi et al. 2007). APC: antigen-presenting cells, TNF-α: tumor necrosis factor α, MIP-1: macrophage inflammatory protein 1, MCP-1: monocyte chemotactic protein 1, GM CSF: granulocyte-macrophage colony-stimulating factor.

Table 2.8   Radiographic staging of pulmonary sarcoidosis

Stage	Features
0	No abnormalities on chest radiographs
I	Bilaterally symmetrical hilar and/or mediastinal lymph node enlargement. Pulmonary involvement is usually detectable by histology and cytology but is not yet visible on radiographs
IIA	Diffuse pulmonary involvement accompanied by hilar and/or mediastinal lymphadenopathy
IIB	Diffuse pulmonary involvement without lymph node enlargement. Radiographs typically show bilateral reticulonodular opacities smaller than 5 mm distributed symmetrically in the middle lung zones. Frequent ground-glass opacities signify a florid alveolitis or incipient fibrosis
III	Pulmonary fibrosis

Error Analysis and Strategy for Error Prevention

The typical imaging appearance of stage I sarcoidosis consists of bilaterally symmetrical bihilar and mediastinal lymph node enlargement, whereas the lymphogenous spread of central bronchial carcinoma appears as a perihilar mass of soft-tissue density with predominantly ipsilateral mediastinal lymph node enlargement. In the case described here, then, the asymmetrical lymph node involvement suggested a central bronchial carcinoma or possibly a malignant lymphoma. The eccentric location of the lobar, segmental, and subsegmental lymph nodes (12R, 13R, 14R) in the fibrofatty hilar tissue and the broad differential diagnosis of solitary pulmonary nodules could have suggested other diseases as well, however (**Fig. 2.47 a, b, Table 2.9**).

FDG/PET was performed to investigate the presumed lung cancer. This imaging modality detects changes in glucose metabolism, regardless of whether the increased activity has a malignant, inflammatory, or other cause. In the present case, the PET study supplied no additional information. Even in the case of non–small-cell lung cancer, FDG/PET would not have been indicated due to the definitive hilar and mediastinal findings revealed by CT (see interdisciplinary excursions "Metabolic imaging: positron emission tomograph", p. 289 and "Image fusion with hybrid systems," p. 295).

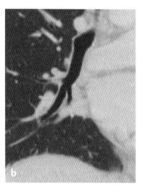

Fig. 2.47 a, b

a   Regional lymph node classification based on the American Thoracic Society mapping scheme (modified by Mountain et al. 1997). Not included in this map are lymph node stations 1R and 1L (highest level of the right and left mediastinal lymph nodes), 3 (prevascular and retroesophageal lymph nodes), 5 (subaortic lymph nodes in the aortopulmonary window), and 6 (para-aortic lymph nodes, ascending aorta, phrenic).

Ao	aorta
PA	pulmonary artery
7	Subcarinal lymph nodes
8	Paraesophageal lymph nodes
9R, 9L	Lymph nodes along the right and left pulmonary ligament
10R, 10L	Right and left hilar lymph nodes
11R, 11L	Right and left interlobar lymph nodes
12R, 12L	Right and left lobular lymph nodes
13R, 13L	Right and left segmental lymph nodes
14R, 14L	Right and left subsegmental lymph nodes

b   Reformatted image of the right lower lobe bronchus and enlarged subsegmental lymph nodes 12R, 13R, and 14R.

Sarcoidosis

Definition and epidemiology. Sarcoidosis is a chronic inflammatory multisystem disease of unknown etiology (genetic disposition, toxic exposure) that is characterized histologically by noncaseating epithelioid-cell granulomas composed of histiocytes, giant cells, and lymphocytes. The most frequent sites of involvement are the mediastinal and hilar lymph nodes (>95% of patients), lung (75%), liver (55%), spleen (25%), eyes (20%), and skin (15%). The incidence in Central Europe is 10–20 cases per 100 000 population with a peak age incidence between the second and fourth decades.

Clinical manifestations. Approximately one-half of patients are asymptomatic in the early stages of the disease. Typical symptoms are fever, weakness, dry cough, dyspnea (often only on exertion), and retrosternal pain. Many acute cases are self-limiting and respond well to corticosteroids. Classified as radiographic stage 0/I to IIA (Löffgren syndrome), these cases present with fever, elevated ESR, CRP and ACE, erythema nodosum, polyarthralgia, and arthritis. Additionally, there are primary chronic recurring and progressive forms (radiographic stages IIB to III) that are more refractory to treatment and culminate in approximately 20% of cases in pulmonary fibrosis that is fatal or necessitates a lung transplant.

Diagnosis. Sarcoidosis is often an incidental finding on chest radiographs. Generally, there is no need for CT because the clinical and radiographic features of stage I and IIA cases are definitive. If necessary, the presumptive diagnosis can be confirmed cytologically and/or histologically. Biopsy may be omitted in cases where a confident clinical and radiographic diagnosis can be made, histopathology would not significantly alter treatment or prognosis, or tissue sampling is contraindicated.

Table 2.9 Causes of mediastinal and hilar lymph node enlargement

Frequent	Rare
■ Tuberculosis	■ Infectious mononucleosis
■ Pneumonia	■ Wegener granulomas
■ Sarcoidosis	■ Erythema nodosum
■ Pneumoconiosis	■ Nonspecific lymphadenitis
■ Histoplasmosis	■ Fungal diseases
■ Metastases	■ Idiopathic
■ Malignant lymphoma	

References and Further Reading

Iannuzzi MC, Rybicki BA, Teirsteinn AS. Sarcoidosis. N Engl J Med 2007; 357: 2153–2165

Mountain CF. Revisions in the international system for staging lung cancer. Chest 1997; 111: 1710–1717

Wasfi Y, Newman LS. Sarcoidosis. In: Mason RJ, Broaddus VC, Murray JF, Nadel JA, eds. Murray and Nadel's Textbook of Respiratory Medicine. 4th ed. Philadelphia: Elsevier Saunders; 2005: 1634–1655

Thrombosis due to Thrombophilia/ Hodgkin Disease, Non-Hodgkin Lymphoma/ Thymoma/ Thymic Carcinoma

History and Clinical Findings

A 22-year-old woman was referred by a cardiothoracic surgery unit for abdominal CT scans to investigate an "indeterminate" mediastinal mass detected by CT. She presented clinically with bilateral enlargement of cervical lymph nodes and distended neck veins, raising suspicion of non-Hodgkin lymphoma (NHL). Abdominal CT revealed bilateral pleural effusions. Additional findings were focal nodular hyperplasia in segment IV of the liver and zonal fatty infiltration adjacent to the falciform ligament. There was no evidence of venous collaterals or enlarged lymph nodes.

Due to the limited quality of the thoracic scans, a CT examination of the neck, chest, and abdomen was performed 5 days later for the purpose of planning a lymph node biopsy or thoracotomy (**Fig. 2.48**). The principal findings were as follows:

- Thrombus in the right internal jugular vein and superior vena cava.
- Lymphedema in the thoracic and cervical soft tissues.
- Bilateral enlargement of numerous submental, cervical, and nuchal lymph nodes due to an unknown cause.
- Soft-tissue mass in the upper mediastinum—most likely a remnant of the thymus. A definite etiologic classification could not be made.

An iliac crest biopsy showed no abnormalities. An excisional biopsy taken from a parajugular lymph node posterior to the right sternocleidomastoid muscle indicated histologically and immunohistochemically benign changes (plasmacytosis, reticulohistiocytosis, fibroblast activation). The pathologist questioned whether the sample was representative. Corticosteroid therapy was instituted based on a clinical diagnosis of benign lymphadenopathy. Despite the lymphadenopathy, the thrombus in the superior vena cava, which extended into the right jugular vein, was attributed to laboratory-confirmed thrombophilic risk factors (elevated serum lipoprotein A).

Three months later the patient returned to the cardiothoracic surgery unit because MRI performed elsewhere showed a mass in the anterior upper mediastinum that had progressed since the previous CT examination (**Fig. 2.49**). A preoperative chest radiograph confirmed the finding (**Fig. 2.50**).

Exploratory thoracotomy through a median sternotomy revealed a firm tumor that had infiltrated the superior vena cava, the innominate vein, both subclavian veins, the aortic arch, the pericardium, and the upper lobes of both lungs. The residual thymus itself was poorly demarcated. Intraoperative frozen-section histology raised suspicion of thymic carcinoma (differential diagnosis: malignant non-Hodgkin lymphoma of the B-cell type, B-NHL). Because the lesion was technically inoperable, only a large biopsy was obtained.

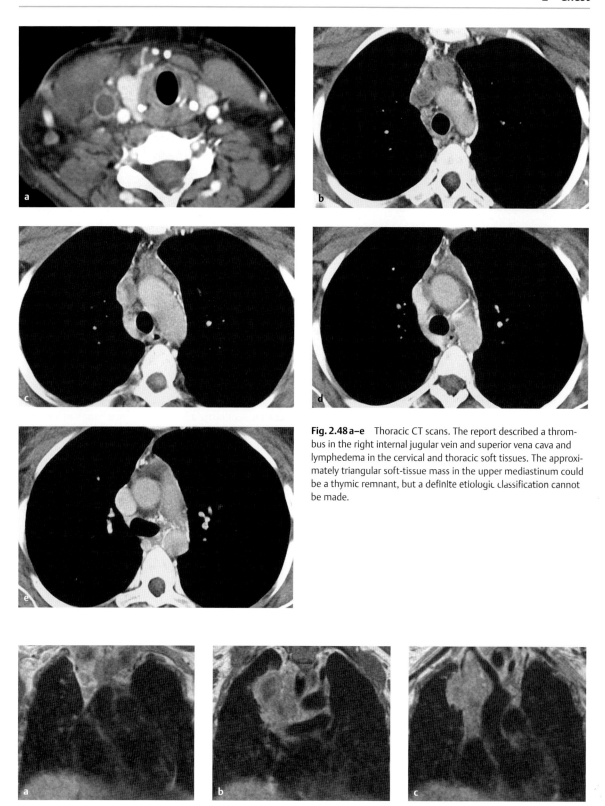

Fig. 2.48 a–e Thoracic CT scans. The report described a thrombus in the right internal jugular vein and superior vena cava and lymphedema in the cervical and thoracic soft tissues. The approximately triangular soft-tissue mass in the upper mediastinum could be a thymic remnant, but a definite etiologic classification cannot be made.

Fig. 2.49 a–c MRI shows a centrally necrotic tumor in the anterior upper mediastinum with associated obstruction of the superior vena cava.

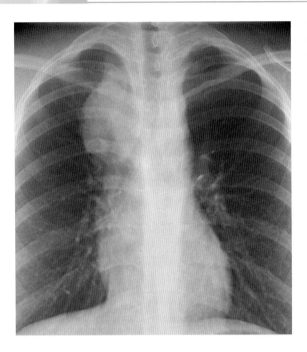

Further Case Summary

Histologic evaluation of the biopsy material was difficult due to extensive necrosis. Finally the pathologist and reference pathologist agreed on a diagnosis of high-grade mediastinal (thymic) large-cell non-Hodgkin lymphoma of the B-cell type, that is, primary NHL originating from the thymus (**Table 2.10**).

Tumor remission was achieved with several months of chemotherapy. The tumor was still in remission when the patient was seen 2 years later.

Error Analysis and Strategy for Error Prevention

The thrombosis was caused by a high-grade B-NHL originating from the thymus. On initial interpretation of the clinical and CT findings, it was assumed that a single disease entity was responsible for all the enlarged lymph nodes. The different findings in different organ regions did not support this interpretation, however. The cervical and nuchal lymph nodes were solid and showed intense contrast enhancement (**Fig. 2.48a**). The axillary lymph nodes showed central fatty infiltration. The mediastinal lesions were predominantly necrotic and showed peripheral ring enhancement (**Figs. 2.48b–e, 2.49**).

While no imaging modality can positively distinguish between neoplastic and inflammatory lymphadenopathy (**Table 2.11**, see p. 114), it seemed highly unlikely that the same underlying disease could account for such a variety of morphologic lymph node changes. Also, the mediastinal masses made it implausible that the superior vena cava thrombosis was due entirely to thrombophilia. Restriction of blood flow due to extrinsic compression of the vessel lumen was a far more likely explanation.

Table 2.10 WHO classification of malignant lymphomas (adapted from Jaffe et al. 2001)

B-cell neoplasms	T-cell and NK-cell neoplasms
Precursor B-cell neoplasms ■ Precursor B-lymphoblastic leukemia/lymphoma	**Precursor T-cell neoplasms** ■ Precursor T-lymphoblastic leukemia/lymphoma ■ Blastic NK-cell lymphoma
Mature B-cell neoplasms ■ Chronic lymphatic leukemia/small lymphocytic lymphoma ■ B-cell prolymphocytic lymphoma ■ Lymphoplasmacytic lymphoma ■ Splenic marginal zone lymphoma ■ Hairy cell leukemia ■ Plasma cell myeloma ■ Solitary plasmacytoma of bone ■ Extranodal marginal zone B-cell lymphoma of mucosa-associated lymphoid tissue (MALT lymphoma) ■ Nodal marginal zone B-cell lymphoma ■ Follicular lymphoma ■ Mantle-cell lymphoma ■ Burkitt lymphoma/leukemia ■ Diffuse large B-cell lymphoma 　*Morphologic variants* 　– Centroblastic large-cell B-cell lymphoma 　– Immunoblastic B-cell lymphoma 　– T-cell or histiocyte-rich B-cell lymphoma 　– Plasmablastic B-cell lymphoma 　*Clinical subtypes* 　– Mediastinal (thymic) large B-cell lymphoma 　– Primary effusion lymphoma 　– Intravascular large B-cell lymphoma	**Mature T-cell neoplasms** ■ T-cell prolymphocytic leukemia ■ T-cell large granular lymphocytic leukemia ■ Aggressive NK-cell leukemia ■ Adult T-cell leukemia/lymphoma ■ Extranodal NK/T-cell lymphoma, nasal type ■ Enteropathy-type T-cell lymphoma ■ Hepatosplenic T-cell lymphoma ■ Subcutaneous panniculitis-like T-cell lymphoma ■ Mycosis fungoides ■ Sezary syndrome ■ Primary cutaneous anaplastic large-cell lymphoma ■ Peripheral T-cell lymphoma, unspecified ■ Angioimmunoblastic T-cell lymphoma ■ Anaplastic large-cell lymphoma **T-cell proliferations of uncertain malignant potential** ■ Lymphomatoid papulosis
B-cell proliferations of uncertain malignant potential ■ Lymphomatoid granulomatosis ■ Post-transplant lymphoproliferative disorder (PTLD), polymorphic	**Hodgkin lymphoma** ■ Nodular lymphocyte-predominant Hodgkin lymphoma ■ Classical Hodgkin lymphoma

Table 2.11 Criteria for the benign/malignant differentiation of mediastinal lymphadenopathy

Criterion	Benign	Malignant
Related topographically to the lymphatic drainage of lung malignancies	No	Yes
Minimum short-axis diameter	<8–15 mm	>8–15 mm
Ratio of long-axis to short-axis diameter	>2	<2
Fat in the hilar notch	Yes	No
Parenchyma	Homogeneous	Inhomogeneous
Calcifications	Possible	Possible
Necrosis	Possible	Possible
Capsule outline	Regular	Irregular
Contrast enhancement	Yes	Yes
Increased metabolic activity (FDG/PET)	Yes	Yes

Mediastinal Tumors

Clinical manifestations. Mediastinal masses are usually asymptomatic and are discovered incidentally. Pain, cough, dyspnea, fever, recurrent laryngeal nerve palsy, Horner syndrome, or distended neck veins due to rapid onset of superior vena cava compression are the cardinal symptoms of mediastinal malignancies. More gradual obstruction of the superior vena cava is often clinically silent owing to the development of collaterals.

Thymomas. Masses in the anterior mediastinum are often thymomas, teratogenic tumors, and malignant lymphomas. After 20 years of age, the parenchyma of the thymus is normally replaced by fatty tissue (involution). Epithelial thymic tumors (thymomas) are the most common tumor of the anterior mediastinum in middle-aged patients. Noninvasive and invasive thymomas (thymic carcinoma) are distinguished by their growth characteristics. Thymomas may metastasize within the chest. Approximately 50% of patients have myasthenia gravis, and 10% develop a paraneoplastic syndrome.

Malignant lymphomas. Secondary mediastinal tumors include metastases and involvement by a malignant lymphatic systemic disease. Malignant lymphomas account for approximately 20% of mediastinal masses in adults. Mediastinal involvement usually occurs in the setting of disseminated disease. It is present in two-thirds of patients with an initial diagnosis of Hodgkin disease and in one-half of patients with an initial diagnosis of non-Hodgkin lymphoma (NHL). Hodgkin disease is the most common malignant lymphoma affecting the mediastinum. It is characterized by contiguous spread arising from the supraclavicular and cervical lymph nodes. NHLs spread by the hematogenous route, with typical sparing of the mediastinum. Although multiple lymph node regions are involved in approximately 80% of cases at initial diagnosis, only 10–15% of NHL patients develop a mediastinal tumor. NHLs with mediastinal bulk (> 5 cm in diameter) consist mainly of the more malignant histologic subtypes. High-grade B-cell lymphomas are predominant in adults.

In the WHO classification, mediastinal (thymic) large-cell B-cell lymphoma, which originates in the anterior mediastinum, is classified as a clinical subtype of diffuse large-cell B-cell lymphoma (**Table 2.10**). The latter entity is a mature B-cell neoplasm that comprises the largest group of NHLs (approximately 30%). With suitable tumor size and location, a percutaneous biopsy can often confirm the diagnosis since CT guidance allows for accurate placement of the biopsy needle (**Fig. 2.51**). Repeated biopsies can be taken through the guide sheath to supply adequate material for the pathoanatomic differentiation of lymphomas.

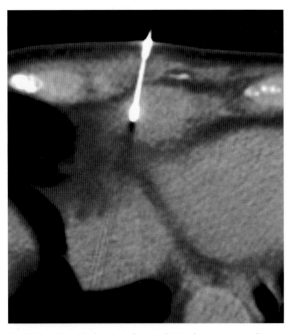

Fig. 2.51   CT-guided paracardiac mediastinal percutaneous biopsy.

References and Further Reading

Hesselmann V, Zähringer M, Krug B, et al. Computed-tomography guided percutaneous core needle biopsies of suspected malignant lymphomas: impact of biopsy, lesion and patient parameters on diagnostic yield. Acta Radiol 2004; 45: 641–645

Jaffe ES, Harris NL, Stein H, Variman JW, eds. World Health Organization Classification of Tumours. Pathology and Genetics of Tumours of Haematopoietic and Lymphoid Tissues. Lyon: IARC Press; 2001

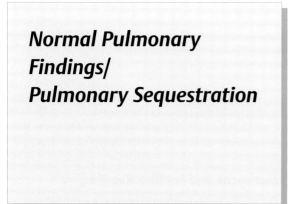

Normal Pulmonary Findings/ Pulmonary Sequestration

History and Clinical Findings

A 21-year-old Moroccan man had a 1-week history of a flulike infection with a productive cough. He had no known significant prior illnesses. Serologic tests showed an elevated WBC at 13 000/mm³ and elevated CRP at 100 mg/L. Since pneumonia was suspected, a PA chest radiograph was obtained and was interpreted as normal (**Fig. 2.52**). Contrary to guidelines, a lateral radiograph was omitted due to concerns about radiation exposure.

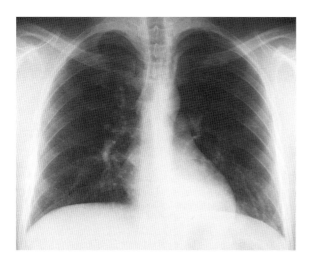

Fig. 2.52   The PA chest radiograph was interpreted as normal.

Further Case Summary

Given the impressive clinical and laboratory findings, the patient was evaluated by thoracic CT, which showed a pulmonary sequestration in the left lower lobe associated with secondary pneumonia (**Fig. 2.53**).

Error Analysis and Strategy for Error Prevention

The patient's clinical symptoms were most likely the result of a "simple" infection rather than the pulmonary sequestration. The indistinct medial outline of the left hemidiaphragm and the "double contour" density projected over the cardiac silhouette were caused by pneumonic infiltrate in the posterobasal segment (segment 10) of the left lower lobe (**Figs. 2.54, 2.55**). This infiltrate was obscured in the frontal radiograph by the superimposed lower mediastinum and upper abdomen. Given the impressive clinical and laboratory findings, it was correct to omit a lateral chest radiograph, which would have shown the lower lobe infiltrate, and proceed directly to thoracic CT, which identified the pneumonia as secondary by additionally demonstrating the aberrant bronchial artery.

References and Further Reading

Fraser RS, Muller NL, Coleman N. Fraser and Pare's Diagnosis of Diseases of the Chest. Philadelphia: WB Saunders; 1999

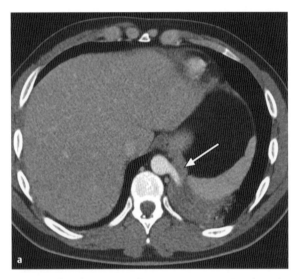 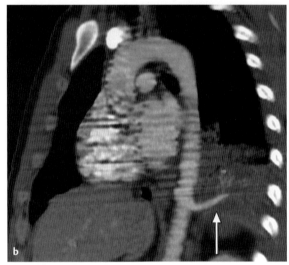

Fig. 2.53 a, b Thoracic CT. Pulmonary sequestration is indicated by a pathognomonic aberrant bronchial artery arising from the aorta and supplying the left lower lobe (arrow) accompanied by secondary lower lobe pneumonia.

a Axial scan at the level of the thoracolumbar junction.
b Reformatted sagittal image.

Pneumonia and Pulmonary Sequestration

Primary vs. Secondary Pneumonia

Pneumonia may be described as primary, occurring in a previously healthy individual, or as secondary, occurring in a patient with preexisting pulmonary or systemic disease that predisposes to pulmonary inflammation.

Pulmonary Sequestration

The term "pulmonary sequestration" denotes a congenital anomaly in which the affected lung segment does not communicate with the bronchial system or pulmonary artery.

A pathognomonic feature of this condition is that the sequestered lung segment receives its arterial supply from an aberrant bronchial artery arising from the infra- or supradiaphragmatic aorta. Venous drainage is variable and may be to the pulmonary veins, portal vein, or vena cava. The posterior segment of the left lower lobe is most commonly affected. Pulmonary sequestration may also be bilateral, however. Pulmonary sequestra may be supplied by a separate branch of the descending thoracic aorta or abdominal aorta. Communication with the bronchial tree is absent or ineffectual. The infection of a healthy pulmonary sequestration displays the histologic features of constrictive bronchiolitis and is uncommon. Since most pulmonary sequestra appear radiographically as homogeneous wedge-shaped or elliptical densities, they require differentiation from solid pulmonary masses. Other sequestra may present as cystic changes in the lower lobe. The diagnosis is considered to be established when conventional or CT angiography shows an aberrant bronchial artery supplying the sequestered segment.

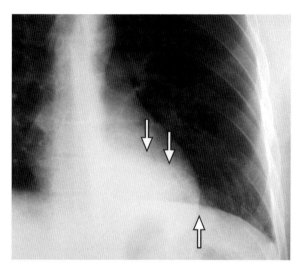

Fig. 2.54 Magnified view of the cardiac shadow in **Fig. 2.52** shows a retrocardiac density (double contour, upper arrows) associated with an indistinct medial outline of the left hemidiaphragm (lower arrow) caused by infiltrate in segment 10 of the left lower lobe.

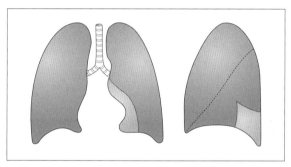

Fig. 2.55 Pneumonia in segment 10 of the left lower lobe.

Pulmonary Involvement by Lymphoma/ Pneumonia/ Abscess

History and Clinical Findings

A 70-year-old woman was hospitalized with pleuropneumonia in the lower lobe of the left lung. When the pneumonia did not resolve with antibiotics, CT scans of the chest and upper abdomen were obtained. The principal CT findings were a left-sided pleural effusion, splenomegaly, and a focal hypodense splenic lesion. An elective splenectomy was performed without complications (**Fig. 2.56**). Histology yielded a diagnosis of high-grade non-Hodgkin lymphoma of the B-cell type (subclassification: diffuse large-cell B-cell lymphoma, see **Table 2.10**). In subsequent weeks the patient underwent two chemotherapy cycles while antibiotic therapy was continued. The pneumonia did not regress. When a chest radiograph was taken 10 weeks postoperatively, air collections with air–fluid levels projected over the lower left lung were found within the density that had been attributed to pleuropneumonia (**Fig. 2.57**). This finding was attributed to a perioperative defect in the diaphragm that allowed the stomach to herniate into the chest. Multiple CT examinations during the next 3 weeks showed similar changes (**Fig. 2.58**).

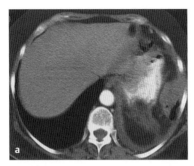
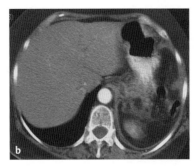
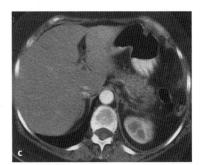

Fig. 2.56a–c CT scans of the upper abdomen approximately 1 week after splenectomy were considered to show a left pleural effusion with otherwise normal postoperative findings.

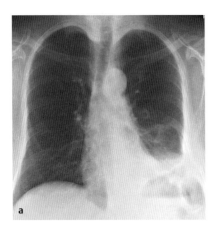
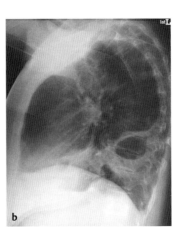

Fig. 2.57a, b Chest radiographs 10 weeks after splenectomy. The opacity in the left lower lobe was interpreted as a gastrothorax.

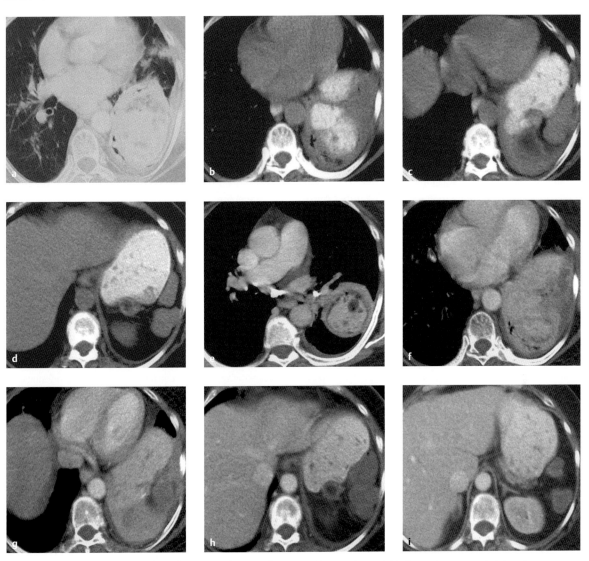

Fig. 2.58 a–i CT scans 13 weeks after splenectomy show a well-circumscribed cavity in the lower left thorax filled with fluid and air. Interpretation: herniation of the stomach into the chest.

a–d Unenhanced CT after oral contrast administration.
e–i CT after IV contrast administration.

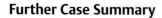

Further Case Summary

When clinical symptoms persisted, an oral contrast examination of the stomach (**Fig. 2.59**) was performed 12 days after the last CT scans (**Fig. 2.58**). This study showed extravasation of the water-soluble contrast agent through a leak in the gastric fundus. The agent passed through the diaphragm, pleural space, and parenchyma of the left lower lobe into the lower lobe bronchus and trachea. This finding was interpreted as opacification of the herniated stomach with the formation of a gastrobronchial fistula.

Subsequent surgery revealed a necrotic cavity in the lower lobe of the left lung extending to the upper retroperitoneum and eroding the lower lobe bronchi, diaphragm, and gastric fundus. The left lower lobe, portions of the stomach, and portions of the pancreas were resected. Histology of the surgical specimens showed diffuse infiltration by non-Hodgkin lymphoma with areas of focal necrosis. Acute granulocytic pneumonia was also present. In summary, the gross and microscopic findings were consistent with a transdiaphragmatic fistula between the left pleural cavity and left upper abdomen caused by the high-grade non-Hodgkin lymphoma.

The patient died 5 months later. The autopsy report described extensive lymphomas in both lungs, in the heart and mediastinum, and in the retroperitoneum. Recurrent pulmonary emboli were also noted. A lymphoma-associated reduction of gas-exchange surface area in the lung was cited as the cause of death.

Error Analysis and Strategy for Error Prevention

The following errors of interpretation were made:
- The differential diagnosis of pulmonary infiltrates unresponsive to antibiotics for 10 weeks should include carnifying pneumonia, a lung abscess that does not communicate with the bronchial tree, and a lung malignancy (bronchial carcinoma, bronchioalveolar carcinoma, malignant lymphoma, metastasis). The course is not consistent with an "uncomplicated" bacterial, viral, or fungal pneumonia. The differential diagnosis should have been narrowed further by the clinical symptoms and findings (inflammatory markers, detection of the causative organism in sputum or blood culture, associated findings). Splenic involvement by high-grade non-Hodgkin lymphoma would have explained the lung findings as pulmonary invasion by non-Hodgkin lymphoma.
- The diagnosis of gastric herniation through a perioperative defect in the diaphragm, based on the detection of new intrapulmonary air collections with air-fluid levels, was also implausible. Injury to the diaphragm is very unlikely to occur during an elective, uncomplicated splenectomy. CT one week after the splenectomy showed a normal postoperative appearance of the upper abdomen (**Fig. 2.56**). A pulmonary abscess or tumor eroding the central airways would have been a better differential diagnosis.
- CT misinterpretation of the intrathoracic cavity also ignored the fact that the stomach, including the fundus, was situated below the diaphragm as it was in the initial postoperative CT scans (**Figs. 2.56, 2.58**).

A similar error was made in a 59-year-old woman with metastatic colon cancer (**Fig. 2.60**). This patient had undergone a right-sided colectomy with adjuvant chemotherapy 2 years earlier for a perforated adenocarcinoma of the ascending colon with peritoneal carcinomatosis. The tumor was staged as pT4 N2 (12 of 26 extirpated lymph nodes were positive) M0 G3. The postoperative course was initially uneventful. Four weeks before the illustrated images were obtained, the patient developed dyspnea and a mild fever. She received a clinical and radiographic diagnosis of bilateral pneumonia (most likely differential diagnosis: aspergillus pneumonia). Enlarged mediastinal lymph nodes detected by CT were interpreted as an inflammatory response, and the enlarged retroperitoneal lymph nodes were considered to have an unknown cause (**Fig. 2.60 b, c**). Despite intensive care, the patient died 2 weeks later from respiratory failure. Autopsy revealed metastatic colon cancer in both lungs and in the lymph nodes. Two-thirds of the lung parenchyma had been destroyed. The radiologic diagnosis was incorrect because the liver—ordinarily the first filter for the hematogenous spread of colon carcinoma drained by the superior mesenteric vein—had been spared.

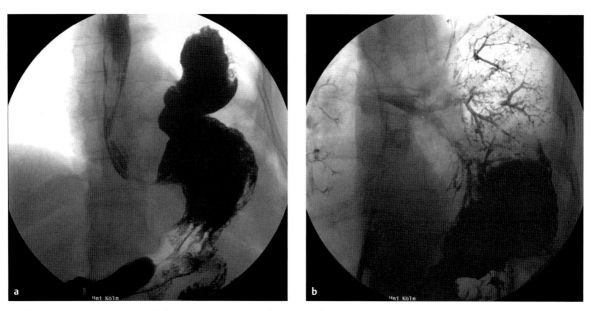

Fig. 2.59 a, b Fluoroscopically guided contrast examination of the stomach. Contrast medium opacifies an intrathoracic cavity via a defect in the gastric fundus (**a**) and passes from the cavity into the central bronchial tree (**b**).

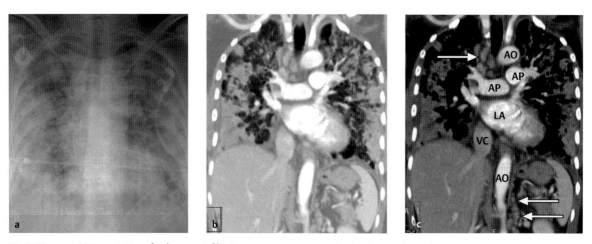

Fig. 2.60 a–c Misinterpretation of pulmonary infiltrates as pneumonia in a different, 59-year-old patient.

a Supine chest radiograph.

b, c Coronal reformatted CT image 5 days later. AO: aorta, AP: pulmonary artery, LA: left atrium, VC: inferior vena cava, arrows: enlarged lymph nodes.

Bronchial Carcinoma/ Inflammatory Pseudotumor

History and Clinical Findings

An 81-year-old woman with a persistent cough was referred for outpatient chest radiography by her family doctor. She gave a childhood history of tuberculosis and claimed that she had had several chest radiographs in recent years, which had shown no abnormalities. The current chest radiograph showed a mass in the medial portion of the middle lobe, which was considered suspicious for a neoplasm (**Fig. 2.61**). Subsequent CT confirmed a rounded density in the medial segment of the middle lobe with spicules radiating into the surrounding lung parenchyma (**Fig. 2.62**). Peripheral bronchial carcinoma was considered to be the most likely diagnosis. The differential diagnosis also included an inflammatory pseudotumor, which was considered less likely given the history, the regular calibers of the bronchi traversing the mass, and the scarring and induration that was present in both lower lobes. No abnormalities were found at subsequent bronchoscopy.

The family doctor referred the patient, whose clinical condition was unchanged, for additional chest radiographs 1 month and 6 months later. These films showed no further changes, leading to the presumptive diagnosis of an inflammatory pseudotumor (**Fig. 2.63**).

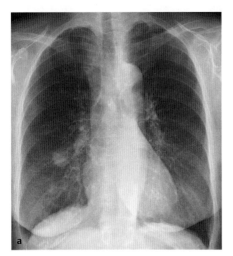

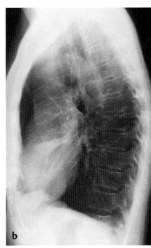

Fig. 2.61 a, b Chest radiograph shows a well-circumscribed opacity approximately 3 cm in diameter in the medial segment of the middle lobe.

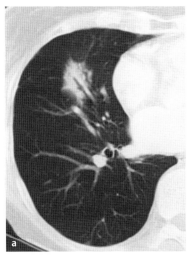 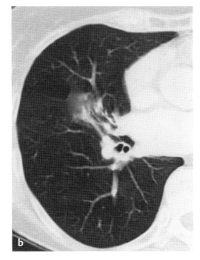 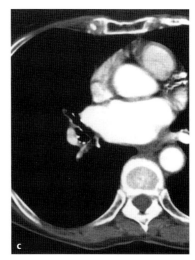

Fig. 2.62 a–c   Thoracic CT scans on the same day show a spiculated density in the medial segment of the middle lobe. The hilum at the periphery of the mass appears normal (**a**).

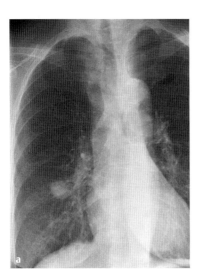 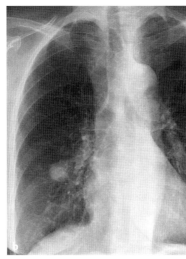

Fig. 2.63 a, b   The opacity appears unchanged in follow-ups.
a   One month later.
b   Six months later.

Further Case Summary

Dyspnea recurred 2 years later, prompting a new referral for chest radiographs and thoracic CT (**Fig. 2.64**). Both examinations showed enlargement of the mass in the middle lobe, additional nodules in the middle lobe and both lower lobes, and a new right-sided pleural effusion. Bronchoscopy revealed a small-cell bronchial carcinoma. The patient died from disseminated disease 2½ years after the initial chest radiographs.

Error Analysis and Strategy for Error Prevention

Peripheral lung cancers appear radiographically as rounded opacities with ill-defined margins. Absence of change in the size or configuration of a nodular lesion over a 1- to 2-year period does not exclude lung cancer, especially in elderly patients in whom tumor growth often proceeds more slowly than in younger patients due to lower rates of cell division. Whenever possible, then, previous images should be consulted for comparison with more recent films.

The following criteria support the suspicion of *bronchial carcinoma:*

- Risk profile
- Diameter >3 cm
- Ill-defined margins

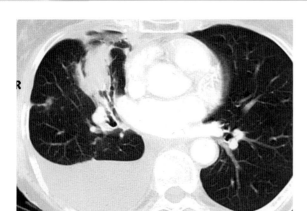
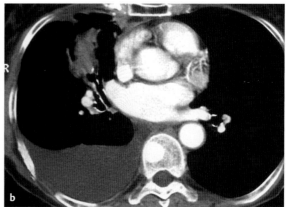

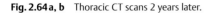

Fig. 2.64 a, b Thoracic CT scans 2 years later.

- Notched margin (vascular pole of the tumor)
- Radiating spicules due to carcinomatous lymphangitis
- Linear extensions to the pleura
- An eccentric intratumoral cavity with irregular outlines

The diagnosis of a *benign lung tumor* is likely only if:
- the volume and configuration of the tumor have remained unchanged for at least 2 years relative to prior images;
- coarse calcifications are present (hamartoma); or
- negative, fat-equivalent attenuation values are found (lipoma).

Otherwise there is no radiologic study (showing morphology and perfusion) or nuclear medicine study (showing metabolic activity) that can supply a specific, noninvasive diagnosis. It is desirable, therefore, to obtain histologic confirmation by performing an endoscopic transbronchial biopsy or CT-guided percutaneous biopsy (for lesions near the chest wall).

A patent bronchial system does not exclude lung cancer. The false-negative finding at bronchoscopy was due either to the absence of an endoluminal tumor component or a predominantly submucous pattern of tumor growth that was concealed by the intact mucosa. In either case the high index of radiologic suspicion should have prompted a CT-guided biopsy after bronchoscopy to establish the diagnosis.

References and Further Reading

American College of Radiology. American College of Radiology Appropriateness Criteria. Thoracic Imaging. Solitary Pulmonary Nodule. http://www.acr.org/SecondaryMainMenu-Categories/quality_safety/app_criteria/pdf/ExpertPanelonThoracicImaging.aspx (accessed November 10, 2010)

Prakash UBS. Bronchoscopy. In: Mason RJ, Broaddus VC, Murray JF, Nadel JA, eds. Murray and Nadel's Textbook of Respiratory Medicine. 4th ed. Philadelphia: Elsevier Saunders; 2005: 617–650

Pue C, Pacht E. Complications of fiberoptic bronchoscopy at a university hospital. Chest 1995; 107: 430–432

CT-Guided Lung Biopsy

The sensitivity and specificity of CT-guided percutaneous lung biopsy are greater than 90%. Potential complications are pneumothorax (≤ 30% of biopsies), which usually does not require treatment, and hemoptysis (≤ 10%).

Bronchoscopy

According to a meta-analysis, transbronchial biopsy has a sensitivity of 74% in the diagnosis of central bronchial carcinoma. Brush cytology has a sensitivity of 59% and bronchial washings has sensitivity of 48%, resulting in a collective sensitivity of 88% when all three methods are used. The sensitivities reported for central lung cancer are as follows: transbronchial biopsy 46%, brush cytology 52%, bronchial washings 43%, and a collective sensitivity of 69%. Transbronchial biopsy has a sensitivity of 33% for detecting tumors smaller than 2 cm and 62% for detecting tumors larger than 2 cm.

A retrospective study found that bronchoscopy had a 0.5% morbidity rate and 0.8% mortality rate when flexible bronchoscopes were used. In a series of 173 consecutive transbronchial biopsies, 4% of the patients developed pneumothorax, while 3% had significant bleeding (> 50 mL).

Normal Radiographic Findings/ Bronchopneumonia/Scar/ Bronchial Carcinoma

History and Clinical Findings

A 56-year-old woman, who was a heavy smoker, regularly received chest radiographs elsewhere to screen for lung cancer. Two films taken 3 years apart were interpreted as normal (**Fig. 2.65**).

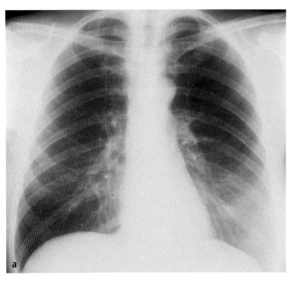

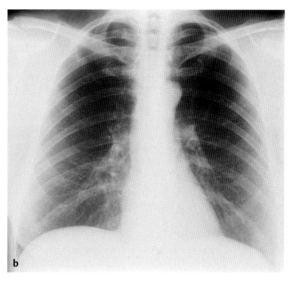

Fig. 2.65 a, b These chest radiographs were interpreted as normal. **b** Follow-up at 3 years.
a Initial examination.

Further Case Summary

Four years later she had another screening examination, which showed a focal opacity in the right upper lobe (**Fig. 2.66**). In retrospect, the opacity was already visible in the two earlier radiographs, although it was less conspicuous at that time. Axial CT confirmed the finding and validated suspicion of peripheral bronchial carcinoma (**Fig. 2.67**). The patient underwent an upper lobectomy and adjuvant radiotherapy. Histologic analysis of the surgical specimen indicated a pT2 M0 R0 G2–3 adenocarcinoma. One year later, hematogenous metastases appeared in the left lung. The further course is unknown.

Error Analysis and Strategy for Error Prevention

The opacity projected over the apical segment of the right upper lobe was missed in the first two radiographic examinations. The finding was still subtle at that time (**Figs. 2.68, 2.69**). It was missed because there was little contrast between the tumor and its surroundings due to the smaller lesion diameter and because the lesion was obscured by the superimposed anterior segment of the second rib and posterior segment of the fourth rib.

Surveillance programs in asymptomatic smokers for the early detection of lung cancer have been discussed since the 1970s, since only early tumor stages are amenable to a curative resection that can improve survival. Large-scale studies during the 1980s and 1990s showed that chest radiographs and sputum cytology—alone or in combination—do not provide acceptable accuracy in the detection of small, asymptomatic lung cancers.

The medical and economic benefits of *lung cancer screening* using low-dose CT technology are currently being evaluated. CT using lower-than-normal exposure levels (low-dose CT) has proven to be more accurate than chest radiographs in the detection of small lung tumors. The CT screening of high-risk patients is not currently recommended, however, because there is no conclusive evidence that the early detection of lung cancer can lower mortality rates. On the other hand, low-dose CT may be an appropriate screening tool in older, asymptomatic patients with carcinophobia and a corresponding risk profile.

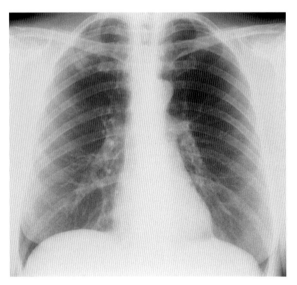

Fig. 2.66 Chest radiograph 7 years after the initial examination shows a 2-cm opacity with indistinct margins in the right upper lobe. In retrospect, the lesion was already visible on the two previous radiographs.

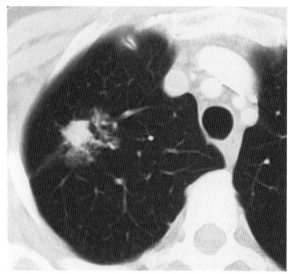

Fig. 2.67 Thoracic CT shows a density with indistinct margins in the apical segment of the right upper lobe with extensions to the pleura. Lesion histology confirmed bronchial carcinoma.

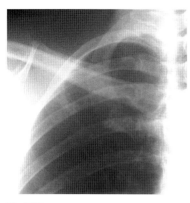

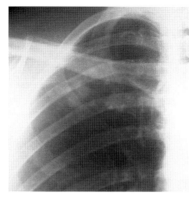

Fig. 2.68 Magnified view of the second chest radiograph (**Fig. 2.65 a**).

Fig. 2.69 Magnified view of the third chest radiograph (**Fig. 2.65b**).

Fig. 2.68

Fig. 2.69

Definition of Terms

- **Screening:** The examination of asymptomatic individuals in a normal population for the detection of premalignant lesions and curable cancer stages
- **Surveillance:** The examination of persons in a subgroup at high risk for a particular disease
- **Early detection:** The examination of individuals for the purpose of secondary disease prevention

- **Primary prevention:** Adopting a certain lifestyle with the goal of preventing disease
- **Secondary prevention:** The treatment of premalignant lesions with the goal of preventing the development of a malignant tumor
- **Tertiary prevention:** Follow-up

Peripheral Lung Cancer I

Epidemiology and prognosis. Lung cancer (bronchial carcinoma, bronchogenic carcinoma) is the third most common cause of death in high-income countries after coronary heart disease and stroke. The prognosis is poor, with an estimated 5-year survival rate of 5–15% averaged over all tumor stages. The early detection and resection of lung cancers offers the only prospect for a cure or a significant increase in survival. More than 80% of lung cancer patients are smokers. The latent period between initial smoke inhalation and clinical manifestations of lung cancer is measured in decades. Clinical symptoms often do not appear until the tumor has reached an advanced stage.

Histology. Fifteen percent to 30% of lung cancers are peripheral carcinomas that develop in the mucosa of the small bronchi. Initially they grow by local expansion, growing at a slower rate than central lung cancers. The majority of these tumors are adenocarcinomas. Squamous-cell and small-cell carcinomas are less common. From a clinical therapeutic and prognostic standpoint, squamous cell carcinoma, adenocarcinoma, and non–small-cell lung cancer (NSCLC) are considered separately from small-cell lung cancer (SCLC). Adenocarcinoma, the third most common histologic subtype, usually develops in the submucous glands of the peripheral lung.

Imaging. Peripheral lung cancers appear radiographically as round to oval opacities with indistinct margins. Segmental and subsegmental atelectasis results from endobronchial tumor spread or from a ventilation defect that occurs when the tumor narrows the corresponding bronchial segments. Early tumor stages present on initial examination are difficult to classify. Unfortunately, the results of lung cancer screenings indicate a false-negative rate as high as 90% for early-stage lesions (see p. 99). The absence of change in lesion size and configuration over a 1-year period does not exclude lung cancer. Lesions must be larger than 5 mm in diameter to be detectable on chest radiographs. But even larger tumors are often missed due to superimposed pulmonary, mediastinal, and chest-wall structures.

References and Further Reading

Austin JHM, Romney BM, Goldsmith LS. Missed bronchogenic carcinoma: radiographic findings in 27 patients with a potentially resectable lesion evident in retrospect. Radiology 1992; 182: 115

Forrest JV, Friedman PJ. Radiologic errors in patients with lung cancer. West J Med 1981; 134: 485

Heelan RT, Flehinger BJ, Melamed MR, et al. Non–small-cell lung cancer: results of the New York Screening Program. Radiology 1984; 151: 289

Muhm JR, Miller WE, Fontana RS, Sanderson DR, Uhlenhopp MA. Lung cancer detected during a screening program using four-month chest radiographs. Radiology 1983; 148: 609

Peterson KA, DiSario JA. Secondary prevention: screening and surveillance of persons at average and high risk for colorectal cancer. Hematol Oncol Clin North Am 2002; 16: 841–865

Stitik FP, Tockman MS. Radiographic screening in the early detection of lung cancer. Radiol Clin North Am 1978; 16: 347

World Health Organization (WHO) Cancer. Work sheet No. 297 February 2009. http://www.who.int/mediacentre/factsheets/fs310/en/ (accessed December 28, 2010)

Bronchial Carcinoma/ Pulmonary Metastasis/ Indurated Pleural Focus/ Rib Metastasis/ Encapsulated Pleural Effusion

History and Clinical Findings

A 72-year-old woman presented with Fontaine stage IIb peripheral arterial occlusive disease. A heavy smoker, the patient had no complaints other than a chronic cough due to COPD. Chest radiographs taken on hospital admission showed the following (**Fig. 2.70**):

- Pulmonary emphysema
- Anterobasal pleural fibrosis
- Linear opacity projected over the anterior part of the right fourth rib, most likely an area of focal pleural induration; may require follow-up, depending on clinical findings

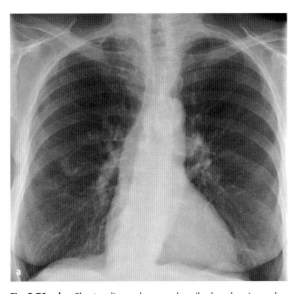
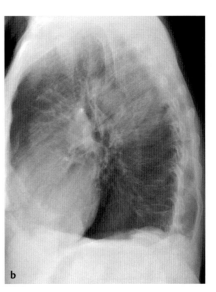

Fig. 2.70a, b Chest radiographs were described as showing pulmonary emphysema, anterobasal pleural fibrosis, and a linear opacity projected over the anterior part of the right fourth rib, mostly like an area of pleural induration. Follow-up was recommended, depending on clinical findings.

Further Case Summary

Stenosis of the left popliteal artery was treated by PTA (percutaneous transluminal angioplasty), resulting in improvement of intermittent claudication, and the patient was discharged. She presented again 18 months later, again complaining of limited walking distance. Chest radiographs taken at that time showed enlargement of the mass in the apical segment of the right lower lobe, raising the possibility of a peripheral bronchial carcinoma (**Fig. 2.72**). The films also showed a new patchy opacity arising from the pleura and located in the lateral portion of the lower left lung, identified as an encapsulated pleural effusion. CT confirmed a tumor in the apical segment of the right lower lobe and destruction of the left seventh rib with a significant soft-tissue component (**Fig. 2.71**). Histology confirmed a peripheral small-cell lung cancer with rib involvement. The patient was referred for palliative chemotherapy.

Error Analysis and Strategy for Error Prevention

The following errors were made:

- The "linear" opacity described in the initial chest radiograph was intrapulmonary rather than pleural, as indicated by the accompanying lateral view (**Fig. 2.73**).
- A new pulmonary or pleural mass is always suspicious for a tumor and thus requires further investigation. This should be stated explicitly in the written report.
- The patchy pleural opacity seen on the second chest radiograph could not have been an encapsulated pleural effusion because the lateral portion the left seventh rib showed destructive changes and the pleura at the ipsilateral costophrenic angle appeared normal.

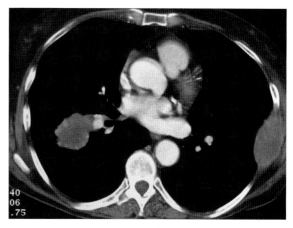

Fig. 2.71 CT confirmed a mass in the apical segment of the right lower lobe. A chest wall tumor is visible on the left side.

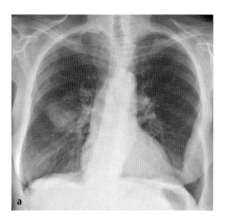

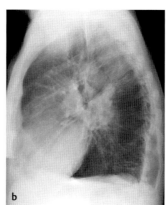

Fig. 2.72 a, b Chest radiographs 1½ years later document enlargement of the mass in the apical segment of the right lower lobe and a new, patchy pleural opacity in the left laterobasal region.

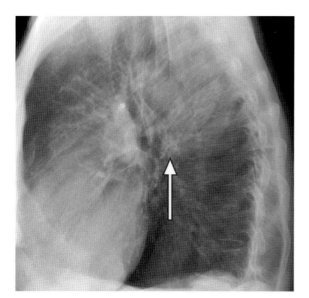

Fig. 2.73 Initial lateral chest radiograph. The arrow indicates a tumor in the apical segment of the lower lobe.

References and Further Reading

Fraser RS, Muller NL, Coleman N. Fraser and Pare's diagnosis of diseases of the chest. Philadelphia: WB Saunders; 1999

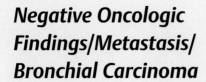

Negative Oncologic Findings/Metastasis/ Bronchial Carcinoma

History and Clinical Findings

A 61-year-old woman had been diagnosed 6 years earlier with a Clark level II superficial spreading melanoma (SSM), tumor thickness 1.3 mm, which was excised. The chest radiographs shown in **Fig. 2.74** and **Fig. 2.75** were obtained during follow-up and were interpreted as normal.

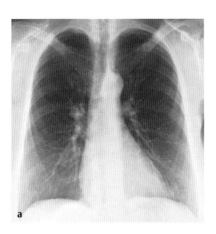
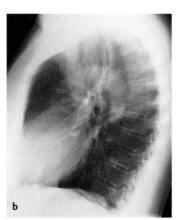

Fig. 2.74 a, b Initial chest radiographs were interpreted as normal.

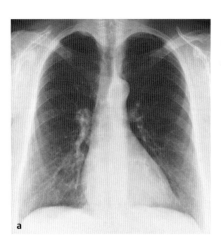
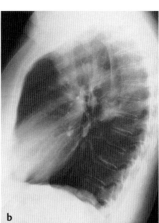

Fig. 2.75 a, b Radiographs taken 1 year later were also interpreted as normal.

Further Case Summary

Seven months after the last chest radiographs, additional films were taken to investigate a persistent cough. They showed a 3-cm mass located in the central portion of the right lung. The tumor was surgically removed by a bilobectomy. Histology identified the lesion as a stage pT2 N0 G2 R0 bronchioalveolar carcinoma. Seven years after the lung surgery, the patient was diagnosed with breast cancer. It was accompanied by diffuse osteolytic metastasis in the axial skeleton, which was identified by CT-guided biopsy as being metastatic to the breast cancer.

Error Analysis and Strategy for Error Prevention

Asymmetry of the upper pole of the right hilum in the frontal view (**Fig. 2.76a**) and the opacity projected over the apical lower lobe segment in the lateral view (**Fig. 2.76b**) had been missed on the initial radiographs. The findings were slowly progressive during the observation interval.

Missed Pulmonary Nodules

Epidemiologic Data

Since the 34th Congress of the American Radiological Society (now RSNA) in 1949, the percentage of lung cancers missed on chest radiographs at respected radiology centers has been estimated at 26–90%, despite all technological advances.

As part of the Memorial Sloan-Kettering Lung Cancer Screening Program in New York, a total of 10040 smokers underwent an annual chest radiographic examination from 1978 to 1982 (Heelan et al. 1984). One-year-old radiographs were available in 78 of the 102 patients in whom screening had detected lung cancer, and radiographs 2 years old were available in 47 of the patients. The correct finding had been missed in 65% of the patients with 1-year prior radiographs (51 of 78) and in 45% of the patients with 2-year prior radiographs (21 of 47).

As part of the Cooperative Early Lung Cancer Detection Program of the National Cancer Institute, the Mayo Clinic conducted a prospective randomized study on lung cancer screening in smokers from 1971 to 1982. The 4618 participants received chest radiographs and sputum analysis at 4-month intervals (Muhm et al. 1983). Lung cancer was detected radiographically in 92 patients. On retrospective analysis, it was found that 75 of the 92 cancers (82%) were detectable on prior radiographs.

Causes

Numerous factors can contribute to pulmonary nodules being missed on chest radiographs. They include the sensory physiology of the eye, viewing time, room lighting, the distance from the eye to the x-ray image, the internal decision-making system of the radiologist, the type of equipment used, the image documentation system, examination technique, available data on history and clinical presentation, and the lesion and its location (size, margins, texture, density, contrast with surrounding structures, complexity of surrounding structures). Individual case analysis reveals multifactorial causes.

Sensory physiology of the eye. When reading a chest radiograph, the viewer performs a complex series of unconscious eye movements. The direction of gaze, which is centered on the fovea, jumps from point to point in quick movements called saccades. "Fixation" refers to the resting points between saccades. The gaze must be fixed for an average duration of 350 milliseconds in order for the viewer to perceive an object at the fovea and detect it via sensory pathways. Perception is limited during the last 40 milliseconds before a new saccade. Pulmonary nodules are optimally detected at a fixation time of 300 milliseconds. The optimum fixation time for detecting normal surrounding structures is 480 milliseconds.

But this is true only if the object of interest is centered on the fovea. This field encompasses a cone-shaped area whose boundaries deviate 2.0° to 2.8° from the direction of the central ray. The detection rate is reduced by half if the location of the object differs by 5° from the fovea-centered direction of gaze. Approximately 300 fixations are required for a complete visual evaluation of both lungs without gaps. Normally, however, a viewer will perform only 80–120 fixations while reading an x-ray image, although experienced readers generally require fewer fixations than beginners in order to detect an abnormality. This means that large portions of the lungs are not scanned by the fovea during a typical viewing. It is reasonable to assume that this deficit is partially offset by the fact that the peripheral portions of the retina cover an approximately 240° field of view during one fixation, with poorer spatial resolution than the fovea, and that the direction of the next saccade is unconsciously shifted toward possible abnormalities. The accuracy of visual detection by the peripheral retina increases with the angular proximity of the object to the central foveal direction of gaze. The processes described above are not under the conscious control of the individual viewer.

Viewing time. Kundel and Nodine (1975) showed that radiologists who viewed chest radiographs with only a 200-millisecond "flash" were able to achieve surprisingly high diagnostic accuracy with a true-positive detection rate of 70% for pulmonary nodules 1 cm in size. The true-positive rate rose to 97% when the reader was allowed unlimited viewing time. Oestmann et al. (1988) showed their participants 40 normal chest films (category A), 40 chest films with lung cancers that were difficult to detect (category B), and 40 chest films with conspicuous lung cancers (category C). The participants were four independent readers who respectively viewed the films for a period of 0.25 seconds, 1 second, 4 seconds, and ad libitum. The authors found that the rate of true-positive findings was 74% in category B and 98% in category C, even with unlimited viewing time, with a false-positive rate of 20%. In this study scenario, then, 2% of the "conspicuous" lung lesions were not detected.

Fatigue. By contrast, viewer fatigue appears to have considerably less impact on reading accuracy. Christensen et al. (1977) had 14 radiologists read 25 radiographs of a chest phantom with 73 pulmonary nodules in a rested condition and after 15 hours of work. The interval between the two sessions was 1 month. The authors found no statistically significant difference in detection rates between the two sessions.

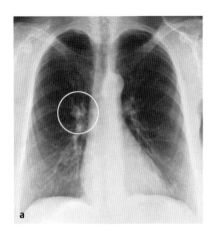 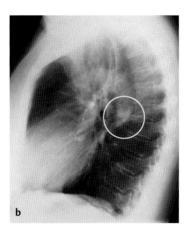

Fig. 2.76 a, b Analysis of the radiographic examination (**Fig. 2.74**). The tumor is outlined with a circle.

References and Further Reading

Austin JHM, Romney BM, Goldsmith LS. Missed bronchogenic carcinoma: radiographic findings in 27 patients with a potentially resectable lesion evident in retrospect. Radiology 1992; 182: 115

Berlin L. Does the "missed" radiographic diagnosis constitute malpractice? Radiology 1977; 123: 523

Berlin L. Malpractice and radiologists, update 1986: an 11.5-year perspective. AJR 1986; 147: 1291

Berlin L. Reporting the "missed" radiologic diagnosis: medico-legal and ethical considerations. Radiology 1994; 192: 183

Berlin L, Berlin JW. Malpractice and radiologists in Cook County, IL: trends in 20 years of litigation. AJR 1995; 165: 781

Berlin L, Hendrix RW. Malpractice issues in radiology. Perceptual errors and negligence. AJR 1998; 170: 863

Brogdon BG, Kelsey CA, Moseley RD. Effect of fatigue and alcohol on observer performance. AJR 1978; 130: 971

Christiansen EE, Dietz GW, Murry RC, Moore JG. The effect of fatigue on resident performance. Radiology 1977; 125: 103

Forrest JV, Friedman PJ. Radiologic errors in patients with lung cancer. West J Med 1981; 134: 485

Heelan RT, Flehinger BJ, Melamed MR, et al. Non–small-cell lung cancer: results of the New York screening program. Radiology 1984; 151: 289

Hessel SJ, Herman PG, Swensson RG. Improving performance by multiple interpretations of chest radiographs: effectiveness and costs. Radiology 1978; 127: 589

Kundel HL, Nodine CF. Interpreting chest radiographs without visual search. Radiology 1975; 116: 527

Kundel HL, Revesz G. Lesion conspicuity, structured noise, and film reader error. AR 1976; 126: 1233

Kundel HR, Nodine CF, Carmody D. Visual scanning, pattern recognition and decision-making in pulmonary nodule detection. Invest Radiol 1978; 13, 175

Muhm JR, Miller WE, Fontana RS, Sanderson DR, Uhlenhopp MA. Lung cancer detected during a screening program using four-month chest radiographs. Radiology 1983; 148: 609

Oestmann JW, Greene R, Kusher DC, Bourgouin PM, Linetsky L, Llewelly HJ. Lung lesions: correlation between viewing time and detection. Radiology 1988; 166: 451

Stitik FP, Tockman MS. Radiographic screening in the early detection of lung cancer. Radiol Clin N Am 1978; 16: 347

Swensson RG, Hessel SJ, Herman PG. Omissions in radiology: faulty search or stringent reporting criteria. Radiology 1977; 123: 563

Thomas EL. Search behavior. Radiol Clin N Am 1969; 7: 403

Woodring JH. Pitfalls in the radiologic diagnosis of lung cancer. AJR 1990; 154: 1165

Yerushalmy J. The statistical assessment of the variability in observer perfection and description of radiographic pulmonary shadows. Radiol Clin N Am 1969; 7: 381

Solitary Pulmonary Metastasis from an Unknown Primary/ Benign Pseudotumor/ Peripheral Bronchial Carcinoma

History and Clinical Findings

A 59-year-old man had been receiving outpatient treatment for chronic obstructive lung disease for some years. A chest radiograph obtained in this setting showed a new elliptical opacity projected over the lateral midzone of the right lung (**Fig. 2.77**). CT confirmed a mass of soft-tissue density in the lateral segment of the middle lobe, which did not transgress the pleura of the horizontal fissure (**Fig. 2.78**). The differential diagnosis was considered to include a benign pseudotumor, a solitary metastasis from an unknown primary tumor, and a peripheral bronchial carcinoma. Because the lesion respected the visceral and parietal pleura of the horizontal fissure, it was classified as a benign pseudotumor.

Two years later a follow-up chest radiograph was obtained in an outpatient setting (**Fig. 2.79**). The opacity was unchanged in its size and shape, appearing to confirm the earlier diagnosis of a benign pseudotumor.

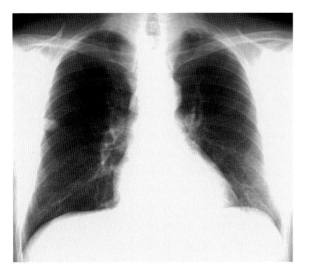

Fig. 2.77 Chest radiograph shows an elliptical opacity projected over the lateral segment of the middle lobe.

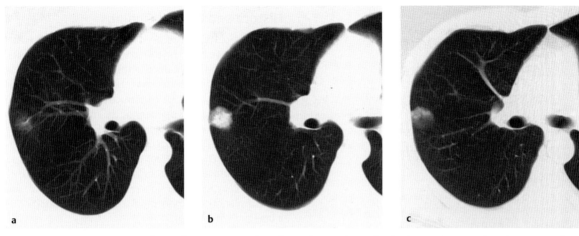

Fig. 2.78 a–c   Thoracic CT scans taken at the same time as the radiograph in **Fig. 2.77**. The density was interpreted as a benign pseudo-tumor due to its connection with the pleura.

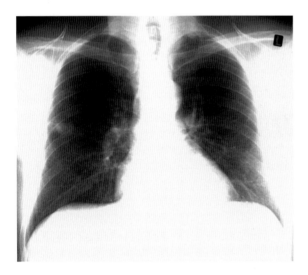

Fig. 2.79   Findings at 2-year follow-up are unchanged, apparently confirming the diagnosis of a benign tumor.

Further Case Summary

One year later the patient presented with night sweats, lethargy, and a weight loss of 8 kg. A new chest radiograph showed increased volume of the tumor in the middle lobe, which was now infiltrating the anterior basal segment of the upper lobe. Enlargement of the right hilum was also noted (**Fig. 2.80**). CT additionally showed mediastinal and bilateral hilar lymph nodes up to 2 cm in diameter, enlargement of the left adrenal gland, and three enhancing masses in the cerebral parenchyma with perifocal edema. The pulmonary mass was investigated by CT-guided biopsy. Histopathology revealed a moderately differentiated nonkeratinizing squamous cell carcinoma, which was staged as a T2 N2 M1 lesion (adrenal and cerebral metastases). The tumor was considered inoperable due to hematogenous and lymphogenous metastasis, and chemotherapy with carboplatin and paclitaxel was instituted.

Error Analysis and Strategy for Error Prevention

Barring contraindications to tumor excision (previous or associated cardiopulmonary or oncologic diseases, etc.), newly detected pulmonary nodules more than 1.5 cm in diameter require histologic evaluation in all patients because the resection of a peripheral bronchial carcinoma at an early stage is the only treatment that can potentially cure the disease or significantly prolong survival (see p. 90, p. 93, and p. 96). Additionally, there have been at least isolated reports of significant increases in survival time following the surgical removal of pulmonary metastases from certain cancers in other organs (malignant melanoma, renal cell carcinoma, colon cancer, etc.).

Because the lesion in this case was approximately 2 cm in diameter and was close to the chest wall, CT-guided percutaneous lung biopsy should have been offered. Sensitivity and specificity rates greater than 95% have been

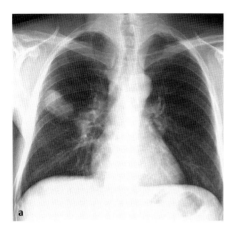
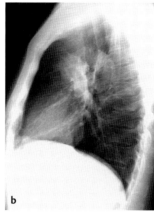

Fig. 2.80 a, b Follow-up films 3 years later show progression of tumor size and widening of the right hilum. CT additionally showed bilateral hilar and mediastinal lymph node metastases. Histopathology identified the tumor as a moderately differentiated nonkeratinizing squamous cell carcinoma.

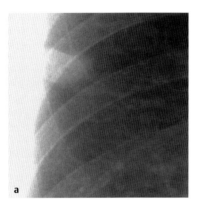
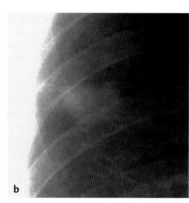

Fig. 2.81 a, b Magnified views of the first two chest radiographs. In each case the differential diagnosis did not include lung cancer. Since the volume of a tumor increases exponentially with its diameter, tumor enlargement is easily missed in early stages.
a First chest radiograph.
b Follow-up radiograph 2 years later.

reported for this procedure (see p. 92). Pneumothorax and hemoptysis that do not require treatment are the most frequent complications and occur in ≤ 30% and ≤ 10% of cases, respectively. For this reason, the American College of Radiology states that solitary pulmonary nodules larger than 10 mm in diameter should be investigated by CT-guided biopsy. For solitary nodules smaller than 5 mm, annual CT follow-ups are recommended on the basis of study experience with lung cancer screening by CT.

The following errors were made in image interpretation and diagnostic analysis of the first two chest radiographs (**Fig. 2.81**):
- Even the first examination showed radiating spicules and linear extensions from the tumor to the pleura as evidence of carcinomatous lymphangitis.
- Although the tumor initially respected the pleural boundary, this does not prove that it is benign. It means only that the surrounding lung parenchyma was easier to infiltrate than the relatively tough pleura.
- Lack of change in the size and configuration of a pulmonary nodule over a 2-year period does not exclude lung cancer (see p. 90). Assuming a constant doubling time, the volume of the tumor increases exponentially. Thus, a change in the volume of a small tumor can be difficult to appreciate in a two-dimensional image. An increase in the volume of a larger tumor is more obvious because the volume of the lesion increases with the cube of its radius. Moreover, a number of hormonal, immunologic, genetic, and environmental factors can influence tumor growth, causing the growth rate to slow or accelerate during the individual course of the disease. Modern CT software includes algorithms for the automatic volumetry of pulmonary masses, providing greater accuracy in the quantification of volume changes.
- Bronchial carcinoma and pulmonary metastases are common differential diagnoses of an uncalcified pulmonary nodule more than 1.5 cm in diameter (see **Table 2.12**).

Clinical manifestations. Lung cancer is the leading cause of cancer deaths throughout the world. As a rule, clinical symptoms do not appear until the tumor has reached an advanced stage. Nonspecific symptoms include anorexia, weight loss, and fatigue, while more specific manifestations are productive cough, hemoptysis, dyspnea, and pain. A refractory post-stenotic pneumonia may develop as an initial sign. Paraneoplastic syndromes are rare. Brachialgia, arm paralysis, and Horner syndrome (miosis, ptosis, enophthalmos) are suggestive of a Pancoast tumor. Hoarseness suggests infiltration of the recurrent laryngeal nerve, while dysphagia reflects invasion of the esophagus.

Histology. Squamous cell carcinoma is the most common histologic subtype of lung cancer, accounting for 30–40% of cases. These tumors develop mainly from the epithelium of the segmental and subsegmental bronchi and occur predominantly in the peripheral airways. In advanced stages, an imbalance between tumor growth and blood supply leads to tumor necrosis with ulceration and cavitation. From a clinical therapeutic and prognostic standpoint, squamous cell carcinoma and non–

small-cell lung cancer (NSCLC) are considered separately from small-cell lung cancer (SCLC).

Except for rapidly proliferating small-cell tumors, lung cancers are extremely variable in their proliferative behavior, regardless of histologic subtype. Doubling rates from 2 months to 1.5 years have been described for NSCLC in cell cultures.

Treatment and prognosis. According to a meta-analysis of 9387 patients with stage IIIB or IV NSCLC in which cisplatin-based chemotherapy was compared with palliative supportive care, the mean survival time for the chemotherapy arm was 7 months compared with 5 months for the supportive-care arm. The 1-year survival rate was 24% for the chemotherapy arm and 15% for the supportive-care arm.

At the time of initial diagnosis, 30% of the NSCLC patients had stage IIIB disease (inoperable due to metastatic involvement of contralateral mediastinal lymph nodes) and 40% already had stage IV disease (distant metastases). The remaining 30% of cases were distributed approximately equally between stages IA and IIIA.

References and Further Reading

Alberg AJ, Yung RC, Samet JM. Epidemiology of lung cancer. In: Mason RJ, Broaddus VC, Murray JF, Nadel JA, eds. Murray and Nadel's Textbook of Respiratory Medicine. 4th ed. Philadelphia: Elsevier Saunders; 2005: 1328–1356

American College of Radiology. American College of Radiology Appropriateness Criteria. Thoracic Imaging. Solitary Pulmonary Nodule. http://www.acr.org/SecondaryMainMenu-Categories/quality_safety/app_criteria/pdf/ExpertPanelonThoracicImaging/SolitaryPulmonary-NoduleDoc10.aspx (accessed December 27, 2010)

Non–small-cell Lung Cancer Collaborative Group. Chemotherapy in non–small-cell lung cancer: a meta-analysis using updated data on individual patients from 52 randomized clinical trials. Br Med J 1995; 311: 899–909

Takahashi T, Sidransky D. Biology of lung cancer. In: Mason RJ, Broaddus VC, Murray JF, Nadel JA, eds. Murray and Nadel's Textbook of Respiratory Medicine. 4th ed. Philadelphia: Elsevier Saunders; 2005: 1311–1327

Table 2.12 Differential diagnosis of solitary pulmonary nodules

Etiology	Common	Rare
Infectious	▪ Granuloma ▪ Tuberculoma	▪ Chronic pneumonia ▪ Aspergilloma ▪ Abscess ▪ Echinococciosis
Neoplastic	▪ Adenoma ▪ Hamartoma ▪ Peripheral bronchial carcinoma ▪ Hematogenous metastasis	▪ Fibroma ▪ Neurinoma ▪ Lipoma ▪ Kaposi sarcoma ▪ Malignant lymphoma ▪ Malignant fibrous histiocytoma
Miscellaneous		▪ Interlobar effusion ▪ Arteriovenous malformation ▪ Bronchogenic cyst ▪ Pulmonary sequestration ▪ Pseudonodules (projection radiography)

Lung Cancer/Scar Tissue

History and Clinical Findings

A 67-year-old hospital administrator had a 5-year history of peripheral neuropathy with pronator weakness of the foot and peripheral paresthesias. His symptoms remained constant over time. He was known to have an inflammatory bowel disease in the setting of histologically confirmed vasculitis. Because the differential diagnosis included a paraneoplastic syndrome, chest radiographs were obtained at a different hospital. Until 11 years ago, the patient had smoked two packs of cigarettes a day. Otherwise his history and clinical examination were normal. The principal finding in his chest radiograph was a focal opacity projected over the left midzone (**Fig. 2.82**).

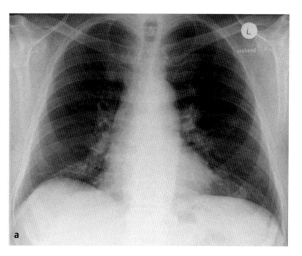
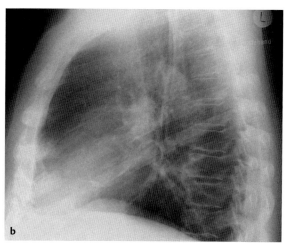

Fig. 2.82 a, b Frontal chest radiograph (**a**) shows a focal opacity projected over the fourth rib on the left side. The lateral radiograph (**b**) does not provide a nonsuperimposed view of the lesion.

Thoracic and abdominal CT was performed 26 days later to investigate the radiographic density. The scans confirmed a nodular density 1.2 cm in diameter in the left upper lobe with spicules radiating into the surrounding parenchyma (**Fig. 2.83 a**). The differential diagnosis included peripheral bronchial carcinoma and scar tissue.

Normal-sized lymph nodes, some showing central fatty infiltration, were found in the upper and middle mediastinum and were interpreted as benign (**Fig. 2.83 b, c**). The patient was presented with the option of CT-guided biopsy to establish a diagnosis.

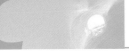

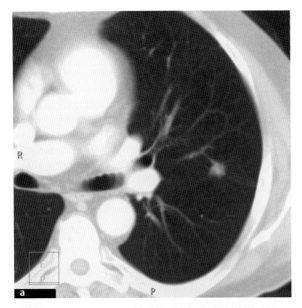

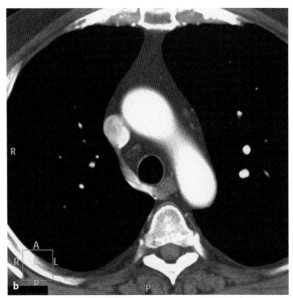

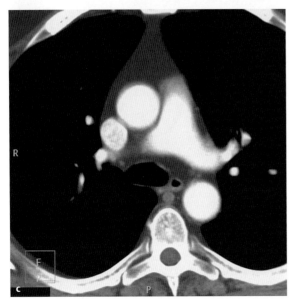

Fig. 2.83 a–c Thoracic CT scans 26 days after the chest radiographs (**Fig. 2.82**) confirm a rounded, spiculated mass in the left upper lobe (**a**). Lymph nodes in the upper and middle mediastinum are of normal size, with some showing central fatty infiltration (**b, c**).
a Left upper lobe, pulmonary window.
b Upper mediastinum, mediastinal window
c Middle mediastinum, mediastinal window.

One week later a PET/CT examination was performed elsewhere to investigate the etiology of the pulmonary mass and exclude metastasis. The test involved the sequential IV administration of FDG (PET contrast agent for characterizing local glucose metabolism) and an iodinated CT contrast agent (to define tumor perfusion). Scan coverage extended from the skull base to the thighs. The CT part of the examination confirmed the lesion detected by CT scans taken 1 week earlier. The PET portion of the hybrid study showed an area of increased uptake projected over the mass in the left upper pulmonary lobe (**Fig. 2.84**). The intensity of tracer uptake was measured

and was found to have a standard uptake value (SUV) of 2.2. Increased uptake was also found throughout the colon, showing an SUV of 11.4 increasing to 16.9 on delayed scans. In summary, the PET/CT examination showed no evidence of malignancy. Given the low intensity of tracer uptake in the left upper lobe, the finding was attributed to postinflammatory changes. Follow-up at 4 months was recommended as a precaution. The increased uptake in the colon was attributed to colitis.

CT follow-up was performed 10 weeks later at a different institution. The written report described an identical appearance of the mass in the left upper lobe. For this rea-

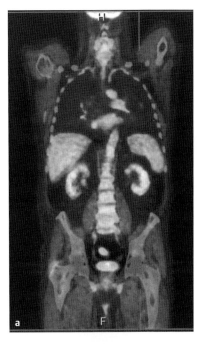

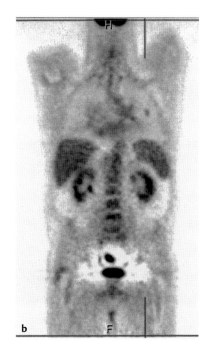

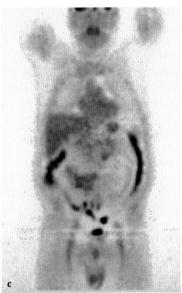

Fig. 2.84 a–c PET shows focal increased uptake at the location of the CT-detected mass in the left upper lobe, with an SUV of 2.2 (**a, b**). Increased uptake is also present in the ascending colon and descending colon, with respective SUVs of 11.4 and 16.9 (**c**).
a PET/CT fusion image.
b PET sectional image.
c PET sectional image.

son, the lesion was again interpreted as nonsuspicious for malignancy. A 3-month follow-up was recommended.

Six months later, the patient underwent CT angiography of the coronary arteries to exclude coronary heart disease and check the status of the mass in the left upper lobe. Coronary calcifications and stenoses were excluded. The mass in the left upper lobe and the mediastinal lymph nodes showed no change in size or configuration relative to previous studies. Because of its rounded shape, the

spicules radiating from the mass into the subpleural space, and the absence of other lung changes suggestive of scarring, the lesion was considered strongly suspicious for peripheral bronchial carcinoma, and CT-guided biopsy was advised. The status of the mediastinal lymph nodes was interpreted as inconclusive.

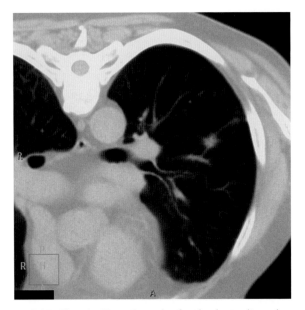

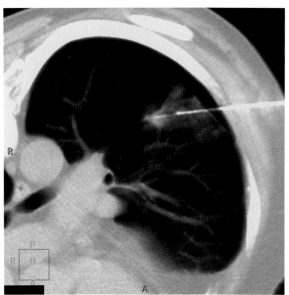

Fig. 2.85 Thoracic CT scan 9 months after the chest radiographs (**Fig. 2.82**). The rounded, spiculated mass in the left upper lobe appears unchanged relative to prior images.

Fig. 2.86 CT-guided biopsy of the mass in the left upper lobe, with the needle trough positioned for tissue sampling. The small pleural air collection subsequently resolved without treatment.

Further Case Summary

CT-guided biopsy was performed another 4 weeks after the last CT study (**Figs. 2.85, 2.86**). Preinterventional CT scans for planning the procedure showed no change relative to previous studies (**Fig. 2.85**). A postinterventional air collection in the pleural space was several millimeters wide and resolved spontaneously without treatment (see "CT-guided lung biopsy/bronchoscopy," p. 92). Histologic evaluation of the specimen revealed bronchoalveolar carcinoma. The tumor was removed by an atypical segmental resection. The hilar and mediastinal lymph nodes were found to be negative at operation. Six months of postoperative CT follow-ups to date have shown no further evidence of disease.

Error Analysis and Strategy for Error Prevention

Pulmonary nodules can be definitely classified as benign only if they show no enlargement over at least a 2-year period and contain coarse calcifications. Otherwise, any pulmonary mass in an adult should be considered suspicious for lung cancer until proven otherwise (see p. 90, and p. 101). The accuracy of the history, clinical findings, and imaging parameters in the characterization of pulmonary nodules has been rigorously investigated. Aspects in favor of malignancy are: age > 70 years, diameter > 3 cm, SUV > 2.5, enhancement > 15 UH, irregular margins, and a history of malignancy (Winer-Muram 2006).

In the case presented here, several factors were suggestive of malignancy: age ≥ 50 years, history of smoking, peripheral neuropathy, lesion location in the upper lobe, and the presence of spiculations. For this reason the initial CT examination should have been followed by CT-guided biopsy to establish a histologic diagnosis.

The fact that the SUV measured at FDG/PET was 2.5 or less does not exclude lung cancer for several reasons:

- Bronchoalveolar carcinomas, low-grade adenocarcinomas, and carcinoid tumors of the lung usually differ from the far more common histologic subtypes of bronchial carcinoma in their low to moderate metabolic activity, leading to relatively little focal uptake of fluorodeoxyglucose (FDG). The lack of progression of CT findings over a 9-month period also reflects the relatively slow growth rate of bronchoalveolar cancers (see p. 98).

- The radiotracer FDG is a nonspecific indicator of local glucose metabolism. A focal increase of glucose metabolism may be found in association with benign conditions (inflammations, injuries) as well as malignant diseases (carcinomas, sarcomas, metastases) (see "Metabolic imaging by positron emission tomography," p. 289).

- The diameter of the tumor, at 1.2 cm, was at the geometrical threshold of detection by PET imaging, which is limited by the pixel edge length of the detector (3.6 mm in clinical PET scanners) and is defined as ≥ 1.0 cm.

Accordingly, the reported sensitivity and specificity of FDG/PET in the diagnosis of bronchial carcinoma are only in the range of 83–97% and 69–100%, respectively.

Besides confidence level, the strategic considerations that are involved in the diagnostic investigation of an indeterminate pulmonary nodule should also include the level of radiation exposure. In the case presented here, repeating the abdominal CT scans during the whole-body PET/CT examination (not a low-dose protocol) one week after the initial CT scans was associated with an exposure dose of 5–6 mSv. This repetition was not medically indicated because it supplied redundant information and thus conflicted with atomic energy regulations (see "justified indication," p. 217). The exposure of 9–15 mSv caused by follow-up thoracic CT could also have been avoided.

References and Further Reading

American College of Radiology (ACR). American College of Radiology ACR Appropriateness Criteria ®. Solitary Pulmonary Nodule. http://www.acr.org/SecondaryMainMenuCategories/quality_safety/app_criteria/pdf/ExpertPanelonThoracicImaging/SolitaryPulmonaryNoduleDoc10.aspx (accessed December 27, 2010)

Christensen JA, Nathan MA, Mullan BP, Hartmann TE, Swensen SJ, Lowe VJ. Characterization of the solitary pulmonary nodule: 18F-FDG/PET versus nodule-enhancement CT. AJR 2006; 187: 1361–1367

Erasmus JJ, Mc Adams HP, Patz EF Jr, Colemann RE, Ahuja V, Goodman PC. Evaluation of primary pulmonary carcinoid tumors using FDG/PET. AJR 1998; 170: 1369

Higashi K, Ueda Y, Deki H, et al. Fluorine-18-FDG/PET imaging is negative in bronchioalveoar lung carcinoma. J Nucl Med 1998; 39: 1016–1020

Winer-Muram HT. The solitary pulmonary nodule. Radiology 2006; 239: 34–47

Inflammatory Pseudotumor/ Bronchial Carcinoma

History and Clinical Findings

A 42-year-old woman was hospitalized for treatment of a spontaneous pneumothorax. She had a prior history of several such events, each of which resolved with conservative treatment. Thoracic CT scans were obtained to search for subpleural emphysematous bullae, which predispose to pneumothorax (risk of rupture) and can be resected (**Fig. 2.87**). The principal CT findings were a left-sided peripheral pneumothorax with a maximum thickness of 2 cm and a subpleural bulla 5 mm in diameter located in the apical segment of the left upper lobe. Additionally, the apical segment of the left lower lobe contained a rounded density with a maximum diameter of 1.5 cm and linear extensions radiating into the surrounding lung tissue. It was considered suspicious for carcinoma. Staging concluded with cranial and abdominal CT scans, which showed no evidence of metastasis. The peripheral pneumothorax was managed by suction drainage. The planned resection of the apical segment of the upper lobe to remove the bulla was extended to include a lower lobectomy.

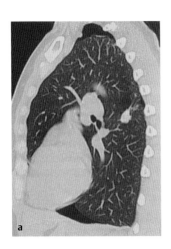 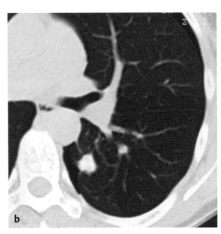

a

b

Fig. 2.87 a, b   Thoracic CT shows a round, 1.5-cm soft-tissue mass with irregular margins in the apical segment of the left lower lobe. The lesion was interpreted as bronchial carcinoma. Pneumothorax is also present.
a Sagittal reformatted image of the left lung.
b Magnified axial view of the apical segment of the left lower lobe.

Further Case Summary

On further consultation, it was decided to investigate the mass in the left lower lobe by CT-guided biopsy in order to detect or exclude a benign lesion (**Fig. 2.88**). Histologic analysis of the biopsy material indicated a healing stage of pneumonia with no evidence of malignancy. Six weeks later the inflammatory pseudotumor appeared unchanged in its size and configuration. In week 7 the apical segment of the left upper lobe was surgically resected without complications. New onset of chest pain in week 9 was investigated by CT, which showed a decrease in the size of the mass in the apical segment of the left lower lobe (**Fig. 2.89**). A pneumothorax was excluded. Imaging findings could not establish a cause for the new complaints.

Error Analysis and Strategy for Error Prevention

During etiologic classification of the mass in the left lung, it was not considered that solitary pulmonary nodules are frequently benign in patients without an underlying malignant disease. This is particularly true in younger patients and nonsmokers. Ill-defined margins may be seen with inflammatory pseudotumors as well as carcinomas and metastases. Linear extensions radiating from the lesion margins may be caused by granulation or scar tissue forming along lymphatics and interstitial septae and do not always indicate centrifugal tumor spread (carcinomatous lymphangitis). An etiologic diagnosis cannot be established for solitary lung tumors without several years' follow-up or biopsy. For this reason, solitary masses

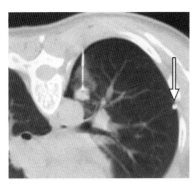 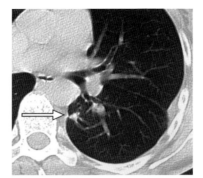

Fig. 2.88 CT-guided biopsy in the supine position. The scan shows minimal medial expansion of the pleural space resulting from the biopsy. Pleural drain (arrow).

Fig. 2.89 CT follow-up 9 weeks later shows decreased size of the inflammatory pseudotumor and the formation of a pleural adhesion (arrow).

Fig. 2.88 **Fig. 2.89**

should be investigated by biopsy in cases that cannot be followed and reviewed for more than 2 years and if the results are likely to have therapeutic implications. An excellent minimally invasive option is CT-guided percutaneous biopsy (see p. 90 and p. 96). Biopsies have an inherent uncertainty factor in excluding malignancy, however, and it must be certain that representative material is obtained. This can be confirmed only by the imaging documentation of correct needle placement. False-negative results of transbronchial and transcutaneous biopsies are discussed on page 92. When technically feasible and compatible with individual risk, multiple biopsies should be taken from one lesion to increase statistical accuracy, as in the case of breast biopsies.

References and Further Reading

Fraser RS, Muller NL, Coleman N. Fraser and Pare's Diagnosis of Diseases of the Chest. Philadelphia: WB Saunders; 1999

Normal Mediastinal and Hilar Findings/Scars/ Recurrence of Bronchial Carcinoma/Lymph Node Metastases/Appropriate Diagnosis/Overdiagnosis

History and Clinical Findings

A 56-year-old man who had undergone chemotherapy for non–small-cell lung cancer (NSCLC) was referred for radiographic follow-up (**Fig. 2.90**). He complained of new pain in the left anterior hemithorax, making it necessary to exclude pleural effusion and osteolytic changes. Chest radiographs showed the following:

- Plaque or effusion in the left costophrenic angle
- Widening of the right upper mediastinum, considered mostly likely due to patient rotation
- "Fullness" of the right hilum
- No pulmonary masses

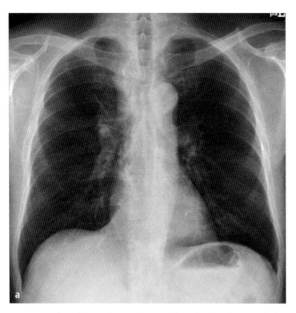 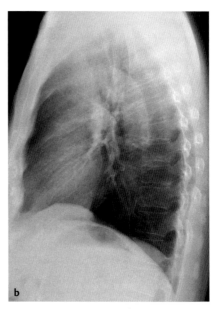

Fig. 2.90 a, b   Chest radiographs were described as showing slight widening of the right upper mediastinum caused by slight patient rotation to the left, along with "fullness" of the right hilum.

Further Case Summary

The clinicians did not consider the radiographic findings to be suspicious for cancer. Since there was clinical suspicion of tumor progression, the patient was scheduled for additional chest films 7 weeks later (**Fig. 2.91**) as well as CT scans of the neck, chest, and abdomen (**Fig. 2.92**).

CT showed an approximately 2-cm mass that was infiltrating the right hilum from the posterior side and was interpreted as a recurrence of central bronchial carcinoma. Lymph nodes up to 3 cm in diameter with central necrosis were also noted in the right mid- and upper mediastinum. The findings were confirmed by the further clinical and CT course.

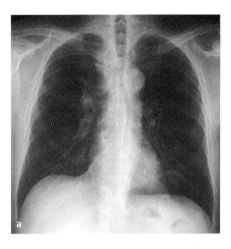
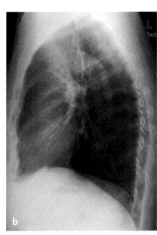

Fig. 2.91 a, b Chest radiographs 7 weeks after **Fig. 2.90** show progressive widening of the right upper mediastinum. The mass projected over the upper pole of the right hilum appears unchanged. Diagnosis: recurrence of central bronchial carcinoma in the right lung with hilar and mediastinal lymph node metastases.

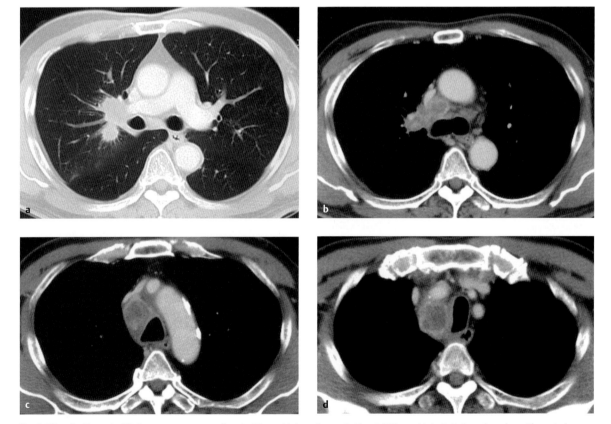

Fig. 2.92 a–d Thoracic CT shows a recurrence of central bronchial carcinoma in the right lung. Metastatic lymph nodes with central necrosis are visible in the right mid- and upper mediastinum.

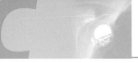
Error Analysis and Strategy for Error Prevention

Concomitant chest radiographs and CT scans were not indicated, as the chest films were unlikely to add any information to the thoracic CT study.

The following errors were made in interpreting the chest radiographs:

- **No systematic analysis of image morphology.** The accuracy of radiographic interpretation can be improved by evaluating the structures in a standard sequence: costophrenic angle, diaphragm, heart, mediastinum, large vessels, trachea and central tracheobronchial tree, hila, lungs, pleura, skeleton, chest wall, neck, and abdomen. This sequence should be followed in both the frontal and lateral views.
- **Mixing description and interpretation.** Because image analysis did not proceed systematically, key morphologic findings were not placed in a coherent differential diagnostic context.
- **No significant body rotation in the frontal view.** Patient rotation in the sagittal plane causes asymmetric distances from the medial ends of the clavicles to the spinous process of the T3 vertebra. But the discrepancy in **Fig. 2.90a** is too small to cause projection-related pseudowidening of the upper mediastinum.

- **Failure to recognize a mass at the upper pole of the right hilum.** Elevation of the right hilum is abnormal and signifies a hilar or perihilar mass or a change in lung volume (dystelectasis or atelectasis of the right upper lobe).

Images from another patient in **Fig. 2.93** also illustrate the difficulties of detecting a central bronchial carcinoma on chest films. The right paramediastinal mass was missed in the first two radiographic examinations (**Fig. 2.93a–d**). The presumptive diagnosis was made from radiographs taken 11 months after the first examination (**Fig. 2.93e, f**) and was confirmed by CT (**Fig. 2.93g**).

The following example also shows that the limited diagnostic information furnished by projection radiographs and the late utilization of CT can delay the diagnosis of diseases with prognostic implications. The patient in **Fig. 2.94** had been diagnosed with stage IIIB nodular sclerosing Hodgkin disease.

A complete remission was achieved for several years with mantle field radiation and combination chemotherapy. Follow-up in this patient included annual chest radiographs. The new widening of the left upper mediastinum shown in **Fig. 2.94b** was missed during interpretation. Three months later the patient complained of back pain, and CT scans showed a tumor with associated bone de-

---

Mediastinal Lymph Node Metastases

Lymph node metastases are the most frequent cause of mediastinal masses. Intrathoracic tumors (lung cancer, esophageal cancer) undergo antegrade metastasis via lymphatic pathways to the dependent mediastinal lymph nodes. Further metastasis occurs via anastomotic connections to contralateral hilar and mediastinal lymph nodes and via the thoracic duct to the left brachiocephalic vein.

Clinical manifestations. Tumors of the mediastinal lymph nodes remain clinically silent for some time. Compression or invasion of key structures leads to dyspnea, dysphagia, hoarseness (recurrent laryngeal nerve palsy), neuralgia, and diaphragmatic dysfunction (phrenic nerve palsy). Frequent complications are superior vena cava obstruction, necrotizing bacterial pneumonia, fungal pneumonia, and atypical viral pneumonia.

Imaging. All imaging modalities are limited by a lack of tissue specificity (see **Tab. 2.11**, p. 81). No imaging study can detect micrometastases in normal-sized lymph nodes. The differential diagnosis of enlarged lymph nodes is based on indirect criteria such as relationship to lymphatic drainage, pulmonary or pleural disease, and the size and texture of lymph nodes. The history, clinical manifestations, and associated imaging findings such as extrathoracic lymph node enlargement and diseases of the lung, pleura, or skeleton can narrow the differential diagnosis.

Enlarged pericardial, retrosternal, and retrocrural lymph nodes are suspicious for malignancy because they do not drain the regions affected by inflammatory lung or pleural diseases. Enlarged lymph nodes that drain the region occupied by a malignant tumor are more likely to be metastatic than enlarged

nodes located outside that region. Bilateral enlargement of mediastinal and hilar lymph nodes is most likely due to malignant lymphoma or sarcoidosis.

Lymph node size is an uncertain benign/malignant criterion because the parenchyma of normal-sized lymph nodes draining a malignancy contains micrometastases in <15% of cases, while moderate enlargement has an inflammatory cause in <30% of cases. The likelihood of metastasis or malignant lymphoma increases with nodal size. Empirically, mediastinal lymph nodes ≥10 mm in diameter are suspicious for malignancy. This does not apply to lymph nodes located near the carina or azygos vein, which are still considered normal if their maximum transverse diameter is less than 15 mm.

Because neoplasms generally infiltrate the fatty tissue in the hilum of lymph nodes, the presence of *fibrofatty tissue in the hilar notch* suggests that the lymph node is benign. Calcifications may signify osteogenic metastasis (osteosarcoma, ovarian carcinoma, bronchioalveolar carcinoma), but other frequent causes are chemoradiation, tuberculosis, histoplasmosis, sarcoidosis, silicosis, or amyloidosis. Coarse flecks of calcifications suggest an inflammatory or granulomatous cause but are also seen after chemoradiation.

Reactive inflammatory lymph nodes and malignant lymphomas often show homogeneous enhancement up to 20 HU on postcontrast CT. More intense enhancement would be consistent with hypervascular metastases from renal cell carcinoma, thyroid cancer, or small-cell lung cancer. Central necrosis in metastatic or tuberculous lymph nodes creates a peripheral or ring pattern of enhancement.

struction in the left posterior mediastinum (**Fig. 2.95**). Histology after CT-guided biopsy revealed a fibrous synovial sarcoma. The mesenchymal malignancy may have developed as a late sequel to radiotherapy. CT follow-ups for the early detection of secondary neoplasms due to Hodgkin disease (common: breast and bronchial carcinoma, sarcoma) are not currently mandated by national and international guidelines.

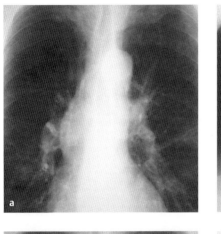

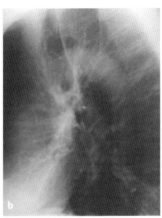

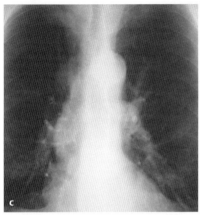

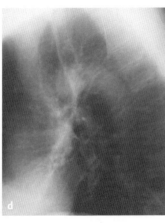

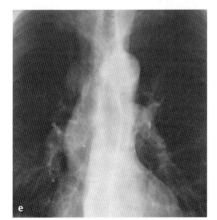

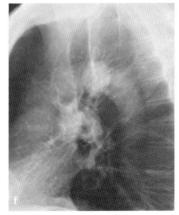

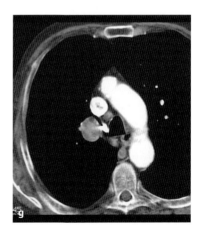

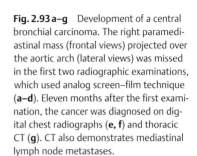

Fig. 2.93 a–g Development of a central bronchial carcinoma. The right paramediastinal mass (frontal views) projected over the aortic arch (lateral views) was missed in the first two radiographic examinations, which used analog screen–film technique (**a–d**). Eleven months after the first examination, the cancer was diagnosed on digital chest radiographs (**e, f**) and thoracic CT (**g**). CT also demonstrates mediastinal lymph node metastases.

a, b Initial chest radiographs.

c, d Chest radiographs 10 months after the initial examination.

e, f Digital chest radiographs 11 months after the initial examination.

g Axial CT scan 11 months after the initial examination.

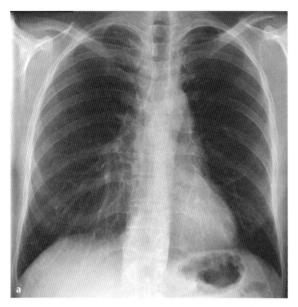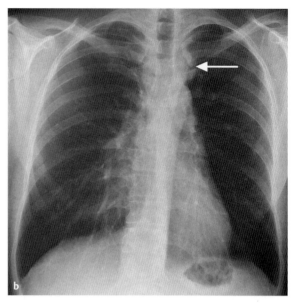

Fig. 2.94 a, b The patient is a 43-year-old man diagnosed with stage IIIB nodular sclerosing Hodgkin disease in 1986. Remission was achieved with mantle field radiation and chemotherapy, and follow-ups were scheduled.

a Chest radiograph taken in 2006 shows no mediastinal abnormalities.
b Chest radiograph 13 months later visualizes widening of the left upper mediastinum (arrow).

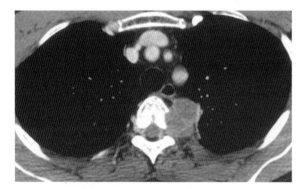

Fig. 2.95 CT shows a correlative mass of soft-tissue density in the left posterior mediastinum that has destroyed adjacent vertebral bodies and invaded the intervertebral foramen.

References and Further Reading

American College of Radiology. ACR Appropriateness Criteria. Follow-up of Hodgkin's Disease. http://www.acr.org/SecondaryMainMenuCategories/quality_safety/ app_criteria/ pdf/ (accessed November 10, 2010)

Dystelectasis/Ischemia/ Pneumonia/ Carcinomatous lymphangitis/ARDS

History and Clinical Findings

A 61-year-old woman was admitted for operative treatment of a tumor in the upper lobe of the right lung. Chest radiography showed a rounded opacity with indistinct margins in the anterior segment of the right upper lobe (**Fig. 2.96**). Additionally, retroclavicular focal opacities were projected over the apical segment of the left upper lobe. Histologic analysis of bronchoscopic biopsies re-

vealed non–small-cell lung cancer in the right lung and scar tissue in the left lung. A right upper lobectomy was performed. The tumor was staged as pT2 R0 N0 M0. Difficulties were encountered with postoperative ventilation, so the patient was placed on positive end-expiratory pressure (PEEP) ventilation with a high oxygen concentration for several days. The patient was extubated on postoperative day 5. She continued to experience dyspnea. Her CRP was slightly elevated at 50 mg/L, WBC was in the high-normal range at 11 000 cells/µL, and she had a low-grade fever.

An immediate postoperative chest radiograph showed elevation of the right hemidiaphragm, an ipsilateral shift of the mediastinum, surgical clips projected over the superior pole of the right hilum, and emphysema in the right side of the chest wall (**Fig. 2.97 a**). During the next few days, focal opacities appeared in the lower and midzones of the right lung, which were interpreted as areas of dystelectasis or pneumonia (**Fig. 2.97 b–e**). When a chest radiograph was taken during a spontaneous breathing trial on postoperative day 5, carcinomatous lymphangitis was included in the differential diagnosis (**Fig. 2.97 c**). Chest radiographs on day 6 showed static infiltrates in the right lung and new linear opacities in the left lung (**Fig. 2.97 d, e**).

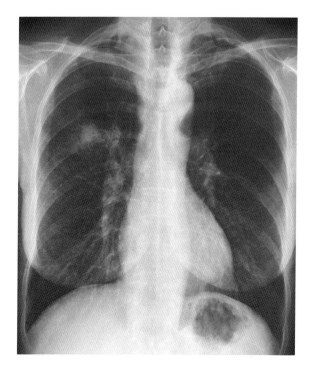

Fig. 2.96 Preoperative chest radiograph. The mass projected over the right upper lobe is consistent with a peripheral bronchial carcinoma.

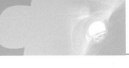

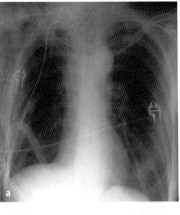
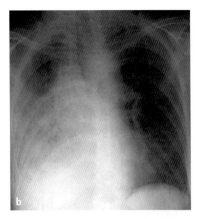
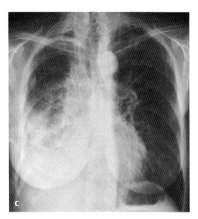

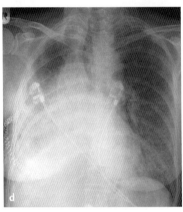
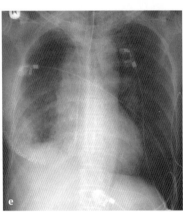

Fig. 2.97 a–e Postoperative follow-ups.

a Supine chest radiograph on the day of the operation. Radiology report noted decreased volume of the residual right lung, chest wall emphysema on the right side, surgical clips projected over the superior pole of the right hilum, two chest tubes on the right side, an endotracheal tube, and a jugular vein catheter on the right side.

b Supine chest radiograph on postoperative day 4. The report described confluent opacities projected over the right lower and mid zones, which were interpreted as dystelectasis or pneumonia.

c Postextubation upright chest radiograph on postoperative day 5. The report described confluent focal opacities projected over the right middle and lower lobes, decreased volume of the residual right lung, normal-appearing left lung, and regressive chest wall emphysema on the right side.

d Supine radiograph of nonintubated patient on postoperative day 6 after removal of the CVC. The report noted linear and reticular opacities in the left lung.

e Radiograph after reintubation on postoperative day 6 showed linear and reticular opacities in both lungs and confluent subpleural opacity in the right middle and lower lobe following placement of a right subclavian catheter.

Further Case Summary

Because of severe progressive dyspnea starting on postoperative day 6, bronchoscopy was scheduled for day 9 but was canceled due to poor pulmonary function. Clinical suspicion of pulmonary embolism was investigated by CT pulmonary angiography (**Fig. 2.98**), which showed a sharp cutoff of the right pulmonary artery close to the suture material that had been placed in the mediastinum. Intraluminal filling defects were not seen. Both lungs contained linear and reticular opacities, some confluent, which were more pronounced in the right lung. Patchy subpleural densities were also noted in the right lung. Findings indicated that the main trunk of the right pulmonary artery had been surgically ligated. Subsequent revision surgery confirmed the CT impression. The right lung

already showed dark discoloration and necrosis, necessitating a pneumonectomy. The patient subsequent developed clinically overt ARDS (adult respiratory distress syndrome) of the left lung.

Error Analysis and Strategy for Error Prevention

Prolonged PEEP ventilation with a high oxygen concentration, plus the ischemia caused by occlusion of the right pulmonary artery, apparently led to acute parenchymal injury. The "double insult" to the right lung caused greater damage on that side than on the left (**Tables 2.13, 2.14**). CT scans with a lung window showed the typical appearance of ARDS (see criteria below). This possibility was not con-

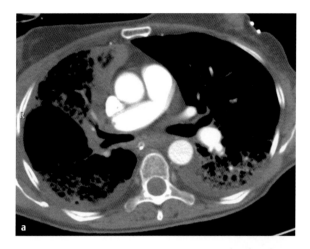

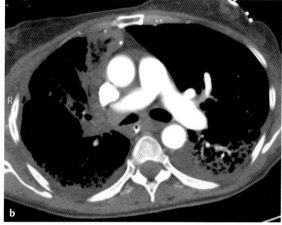

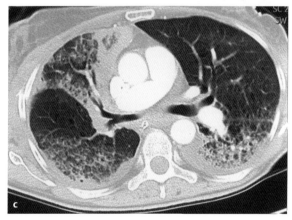

Fig. 2.98 a–c CT scans on postoperative day 9 show cutoff of the right pulmonary artery (**a, b**) with no evidence of a pulmonary embolism. Bilateral lung densities in ARDS are a result of prolonged PEEP ventilation with a high oxygen concentration (**c**). CT findings are more pronounced on the right side than on the left because the right lung was additionally compromised by pulmonary artery ligation.

sidered during interpretation of the chest radiographs taken the first few days after surgery, because the clinical ventilation problems were disregarded in the differential diagnosis. The term "atelectasis" refers to an area of non-ventilated lung, while "dystelectasis" means a hypoventilated lung area, regardless of the cause. The development of a bacterial or viral pneumonia was unlikely given the unimpressive laboratory findings. The previous surgery was sufficient to account for the mild CRP elevation and low-grade fever.

Table 2.13 Progression of radiographic findings in ARDS

Stage	Time of occurrence	Pathoanatomy	Radiography
I	First hour	Interstitial edema	Widening and unsharpness of the central vessels, bronchi and hila
II	First 24 hours	Progression to alveolar edema, microthrombi in the pulmonary capillaries	Diffuse opacities with widened vessels and bronchial walls, followed by focal confluent infiltrates
III	Days 2–7	Formation of microatelectases and hyaline membranes, incipient proliferation of fibroblasts	Combination of reticulostriate and focal or patchy opacities
IV	>1 week	Incipient fibrosis, progression to pulmonary fibrosis	Coarse reticular, linear, and patchy opacities with well-defined margins

ARDS

Clinical manifestations and pathophysiology. ARDS (adult respiratory distress syndrome, acute respiratory distress syndrome in adults, hyaline membrane syndrome in adults, shock lung) is a severe to life-threatening disturbance of pulmonary function that occurs acutely in adults with no prior history of lung disease. It is characterized by noncardiogenic edema, pulmonary inflammation, hypoxia, and decreased pulmonary compliance. ARDS begins suddenly with severe dyspnea, a restrictive ventilatory defect, hypoxia, and pulmonary infiltrates. Potential causes include shock of any etiology, toxic exposure, and sepsis. The pathophysiology of ARDS involves a stereotypic response of the lung tissue to a variety of injurious agents. The initial stage is marked by an increase of alveolar membrane permeability due to changes in the pneumocytes. Leukocytes and plasma enter the alveolar space, where hyaline membranes are formed. The changes eventually culminate in pulmonary fibrosis. The changes may regress or become static, but a fatal outcome is common.

Radiographic stages. ARDS typically has a latent period of 12–24 hours between the pulmonary insult and the appearance of initial radiographic changes. The following radiographic stages have been identified but do not always progress in classic fashion (**Table 2.13**):
- **Stage I:** Findings may be normal during the first few hours, or radiographs may show faint perihilar linear opacities due to incipient interstitial lung edema.
- **Stage II:** Radiographs during the first 24 hours show homogeneous opacities with a thickened peribronchovascular interstitium caused by alveolar lung edema.
- **Stage III:** Alveolar infiltrates are the dominant finding on days 2–7, later progressing to increased linear and reticular markings. Persistent coarse focal opacities are indistinguishable from foci of secondary bronchopneumonia.
- **Stage IV:** By approximately 1 week, coarse reticular and linear opacities occupy large areas of the lung. These changes signify progression to pulmonary fibrosis.

Pulmonary Embolism / Pulmonary Ischemia

In approximately 90% of cases, the chest radiograph shows no abnormalities during the first 24 hours after a pulmonary embolism. Radiographic findings may continue to be normal for some time thereafter. If changes appear, direct or indirect signs of pulmonary embolism will usually develop after 1–3 days. A characteristic feature is a discrepancy between normal-appearing radiographs and severe clinical complaints. This is explained by the interaction of various factors such as the degree of obstruction of the pulmonary vascular tree, the individual response of the organism to hypoxia, and preexisting diseases.

Pulmonary Embolism without Infarction
This condition is manifested by the following findings:
- **Local oligemia:** Occlusions of lobar and segmental arteries lead to a regional decrease of pulmonary vascularity and increased lucency of the dependent, still-aerated portion of the lung parenchyma.
- **Peripheral pruning of pulmonary arteries:** When a sufficient number of pulmonary arterial branches are obstructed, the preocclusive pulmonary arterial pressure rises, causing dilatation of the central arterial segments. The pulmonary

arteries distal to the occlusion are contracted due to oligemia and hypoxia (vascular pruning).
- **Platelike dystelectasis or atelectasis:** Elevation of the ipsilateral hemidiaphragm is usually present only during the first 24 hours after the embolism and occurs only in approximately one-third of patients. It may result from reflex guarding due to pleurisy or may be caused by slight ventilation defects not visible on radiographs.
- **Signs of right heart overload**, marked by enlargement of the right ventricle and widening of the pulmonary trunk.
- **Pleural effusions** also occur.

Pulmonary Infarction
Postinfarction pneumonia (superinfection of an ischemic area) appears radiographically as a patchy wedge-shaped opacity, typically occurring at a subpleural site. They are detectable no earlier than 12–24 hours after the embolism. Edema associated with more or less prominent hemorrhagic areas clears within 1–2 weeks. Larger areas of ischemic necrosis or postinfarction pneumonia, which may undergo central necrotic liquefaction, may take weeks or months to regress.

Table 2.14 Radiographic signs of pulmonary embolism

- Vascular pruning in the lung with dilated central vessels and hypoperfused peripheral vessels
- Elevation of the ipsilateral hemidiaphragm (decreased lung volume due to reflex bronchial constriction and pleural pain)
- Platelike areas of dystelectasis and atelectasis
- Pleural effusion
- Peripheral parenchymal opacities (pulmonary infarction and/or postinfarction pneumonia)
- Signs of right heart overload (acute cor pulmonale)

References and Further Reading

Lee WL, Slutsky AS. Hypoxemic respiratory failure, including acute respiratory distress syndrome. In: Mason RJ, Broaddus VC, Murray JF, Nadel JA, eds. Murray and Nadel's Textbook of Respiratory Medicine. 4th ed. Philadelphia: Elsevier Saunders; 2005: 2352–2378

Matthay MA, Martin TR. Pulmonary edema and acute lung injury. In: Mason RJ, Broaddus VC, Murray JF, Nadel JA, eds. Murray and Nadel's Textbook of Respiratory Medicine. 4th ed. Philadelphia: Elsevier Saunders; 2005: 1502–1543

Meningitis/Meningeal Granulomatosis/ Meningeal Tumor Spread/ Hemorrhage/CVC Malfunction/CVC Malposition

History and Clinical Findings

The patient, a 1-year-old prematurely born child, had been diagnosed at birth with bronchopulmonary dysplasia (BPD), pulmonary arterial hypertension secondary to the BPD, and a type II atrial septal defect (ASD). The latter had been repaired with an occluder at 6 months of age. The child had had repeated, lengthy hospitalizations for pulmonary problems, and for the past 5 months had been ventilated in a pediatric ICU for bronchiolitis mediated by the respiratory syncytial virus (RSV). The patient had been

successfully resuscitated 3 weeks before the current examination. An intrapulmonary hemorrhage had been suspected at that time due to copious blood suctioned from the endotracheal tube. Intra-abdominal hemorrhage had been diagnosed 5 days before the current examination.

On the basis the chest radiograph shown in **Fig. 2.99**, it was determined that the Broviac catheter introduced from the left side was projected over the right atrium and needed to be withdrawn by approximately 1 cm.

The child was clinically and radiographically stable for the next two days. Because increasingly high pressures were needed to deliver infusions through the central venous catheter (CVC), a chest radiograph was taken 2 days later, at which time 1 mL of an iodinated, low-osmolar contrast medium was injected into the CVC. According to the written radiography report, the film showed no change in the position of the CVC. No contrast extravasation was observed because of the small injected contrast volume.

Anisocoria was noted 3 days after placement of the CVC, accompanied by an absence of limb movements in response to painful stimuli. MRI of the skull and spinal column showed thickening and abnormal enhancement of the meninges (differential diagnosis: meningitis, meningeal granulomatosis, meningeal tumor spread) and dilatation of the inner and outer cerebrospinal fluid (CSF) spaces (**Fig. 2.100**).

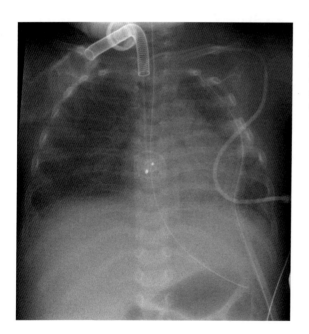

Fig. 2.99 Chest radiograph shows the status following closure of a type II ASD with an occluder. The report described predominantly interstitial and some alveolar fluid collections in both lungs with preexisting pulmonary emphysema and a correctly placed endotracheal tube. The tip of the CVC was projected over the right atrium, and the report stated that it needed to be withdrawn by approximately 1 cm.

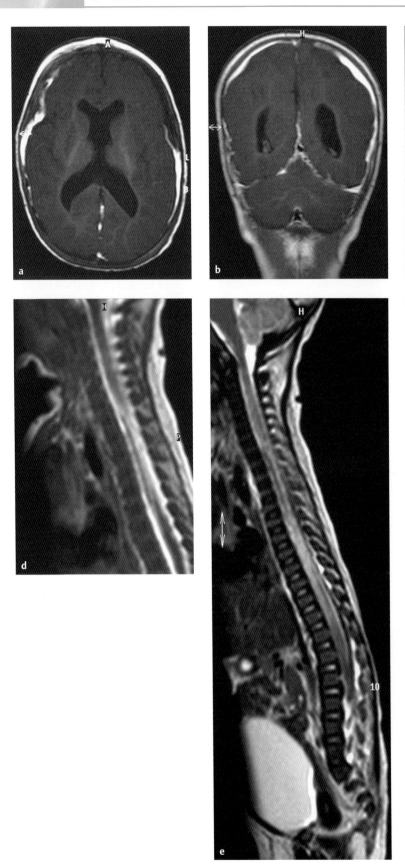

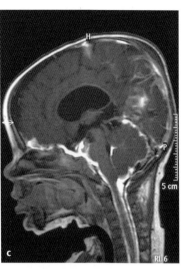

Fig. 2.100 a–e   Cranial and spinal MRI. T1-weighted images after IV contrast administration (**a–d**) and T2-weighted image without contrast medium (**e**) show diffuse thickening and enhancement of the meninges. The inner CSF spaces are dilated at the supratentorial level, with no signs of increased intracranial pressure.

Further Case Summary

After the MRI study, the ward physicians reported that there had never been sufficient aspiration of blood through the catheter. At that point the pediatrician requested radiographs of the chest and cervical spine in two planes following the injection of 20 mL of an iodinated, low-osmolar contrast medium through the CVC (**Fig. 2.101**). These films showed opacification of the subdural CSF spaces. When the intraspinal position of the CVC was known, it was clear in retrospect that even the previous examination with 1 mL of contrast medium on the same day had shown faint opacification of intraspinal structures. Most likely the catheter had been introduced at the wrong site or had been misdirected through an intervertebral foramen into the spinal canal.

The child died shortly after the last radiographic examination.

Error Analysis and Strategy for Error Prevention

A review of the first chest radiograph showed that the descending limb of the newly placed catheter did not follow the normal course of the superior vena cava but took an aberrant course along the midline. The inability to aspirate blood through the catheter was an important clue to the malposition of the CVC. A lateral chest radiograph could probably have clarified the situation as well.

The MRI findings are explained by the fact that solutions had been continuously infused through the CVC for 3 days. This incited a meningeal inflammation with consequent thickening and hypervascularization of the meninges. When the MRI images were interpreted, the intraspinal limb of the catheter was interpreted as a nonenhancing segment of the thickened meninges (**Fig. 2.102**).

To our knowledge, there have been no published reports on the intraspinal malposition of CVCs introduced via the subclavian vein. There have been isolated reports of CVCs advanced through lower-extremity veins and into the ascending lumbar vein rather than the common iliac vein, causing infused solutions to enter the epidural veins. Fratino et al. (2000) evaluated the outcomes of 418 central venous catheterizations in 386 children based on a total of 107012 catheter days. The complication rate per 1000 catheter days was 0.87 for catheter infection, 0.78 for catheter malfunction, 0.45 for mechanical complications, and 0.08 for CVC-related thromboembolism.

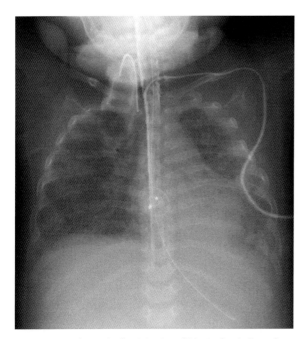

Fig. 2.101 Radiograph after injection of 20 mL of an iodinated, low-osmolarity contrast medium through the CVC. Opacification of the subdural CSF spaces confirms intraspinal malposition of the CVC. The descending catheter limb is projected over the right lateral portions of the opacified outer CSF spaces of the spinal canal from the C7/T1 to T7/T8 level. The nasogastric tube and endotracheal tube are also visible.

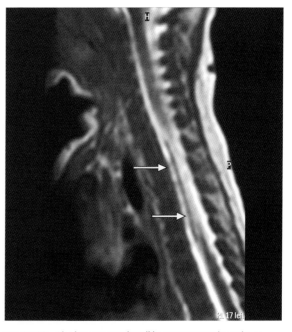

Fig. 2.102 The hypointense bandlike structure in the right anterolateral spinal canal of the upper and midthoracic spine represents the intraspinal limb of the CVC (arrows). Its upper limit marks the level at which the CVC enters the spinal canal.

Bronchopulmonary Dysplasia (BPD)

BPD is the most common chronic pulmonary complication in immature preterm infants. Numerous factors may cause damage to immature lungs. Various forms of lung damage may occur, depending on the nature of the disturbance and the timing and duration of its effect (prenatal: steroids, chorioamnionitis, intrauterine growth retardation, genetic factors; postnatal: mechanical ventilation, oxidative stress, inflammations, steroids, pulmonary edema, malnutrition, genetic factors). The "old" BPD originally affected newborns with IRDS (infant respiratory distress syndrome = hyaline membrane disease) that had received aggressive mechanical ventilation with high oxygen concentrations. This syndrome has become less common over time. The "new" form of BPD is interpreted as a developmental anomaly. In preterm infants with a birth weight < 1000 g or a gestational age < 28 weeks, even minimal injurious agents are sufficient to disrupt postnatal maturation of the pulmonary alveoli and capillaries. The main histopathologic correlates are alveolar spaces that are too large and have an insufficient surface area available for gas exchange. Recurrent inflammations also give rise to pulmonary fibrosis. BPD may cause protracted lung injury lasting into early adulthood or may lead to death.

Complications of Central Venous Catheterization

According to a review by McGee and Gould (2003), mechanical complications occur in 5–19% of all central venous catheterizations in adult patients. Inflammatory complications occur at a rate of 5–26%, and thrombotic complications at 2–26%. Mechanical complications are described in 6–10% of catheterizations via the subclavian vein (arterial puncture 3–5%, hematoma 1–2%, hemothorax < 1%, pneumothorax 2–3%), in 6–12% of catheterizations via the internal jugular vein (arterial puncture 3–5%, hematoma 1–2%, pneumothorax 2–3%), and in 13–19% of catheterizations via the femoral vein (arterial puncture 9–15%, hematoma 4–5%). Fratino et al. (2000) reported higher complication rates in children (see above).

References and Further Reading

Baraldi E, Filipone M. Current concepts: chronic lung disease after premature birth. N Engl J Med 2007; 357: 1946–1955

Filan PM, Salek-Haddadi Y, Nolan I, Sharma B, Rennie JM. An under-recognized malposition of neonatal long lines. Eur J Pediatr 2005; 164: 469–471

Fratino G, Molinari AC, Parodi S, et al. Central venous catheter-related complications in children with oncological/hematological disease: an observational study of 418 devices. Ann Oncol 2000; 16: 648–654

Kelley MA, Finer MM, Dunbar LG. Fatal neurologic complication of parenteral feeding through a central vein catheter. Am J Dis Child 1984; 138: 352–353

Khemani E, McElhinney DB, Rhein L, et al. Pulmonary artery hypertension in formerly premature infants with bronchopulmonary dysplasia: clinical features and outcomes in the surfactant era. Pediatrics 2007; 120: 1260–1269

McGee DC, Gould MK. Preventing complications of central venous catheterization. N Engl L Med 2003; 348: 1123–1133

Myocardial Contusion/ Myocardial Infarction

History and Clinical Findings

A 37-year-old roofer had fallen to the ground from a height of almost 20 feet (6 m). He was intubated by the emergency physician and taken to the emergency room. Because he had visible injuries to the head and trunk, the patient was immediately scanned by spiral CT from the cranial vault to the pelvic floor. The examination began with noncontrast scans of the skull and cervical spine. Then 30 mL of IV contrast medium was injected to opacify the ureters. The chest and abdomen were scanned during the parenchymal phase after the IV administration of 120 mL contrast medium. The principal findings were multiple craniofacial fractures, air in the outer CSF spaces,

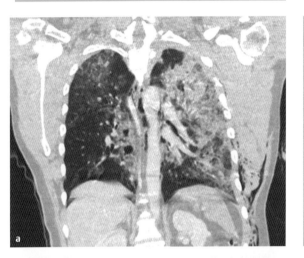

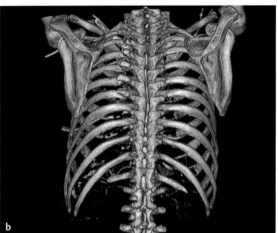

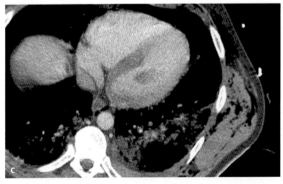

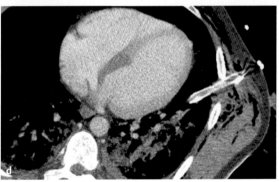

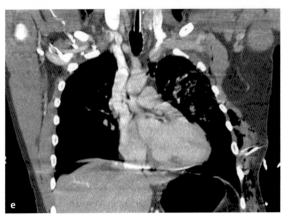

Fig. 2.103 a–e Thoracic spiral CT at 12:22. Data acquisition after IV contrast administration. The scans were described as showing predominantly left-sided pulmonary hemorrhages and contusions (**a**), fractures of the left clavicle, scapula, and posterior left ribs (**b**), and chest wall emphysema on the left side (**a, c–e**). The hypodense septum and posterior wall of the left ventricle were noted to be suspicious for myocardial ischemia (**c–e**).

a, e Coronal reformatted images.
b 3D volume-rendered image.
c, d Axial scans.

a fracture of the left scapula, fractures of the fourth through eighth ribs on the left side, hypodensity of the left ventricular myocardium (**Fig. 2.103**), parenchymal lacerations and contusions in both lungs, a left-sided pleural effusion, a bilateral peripheral pneumothorax, a circumscribed hypodensity in liver segment VI, and soft-tissue emphysema in the left thoracic and abdominal wall.

When clinical deterioration occurred, additional CT scans were taken 6 hours later. The findings were as follows (**Fig. 2.104**):

- A contusional hemorrhage in the left temporoparietal area, with extension to the basal ganglia

- A left frontal subdural hematoma
- Contusional hemorrhages in the right temporal area
- Signs of brain edema with nondelineation of the basal cisterns
- Increased blood in the pleural spaces
- Bilateral lung contusions, more pronounced on the left side
- No change in left-sided pneumothorax
- Increased emphysema in the left chest wall
- Lacerations of the hepatic parenchyma
- Perihepatic intraperitoneal fluid

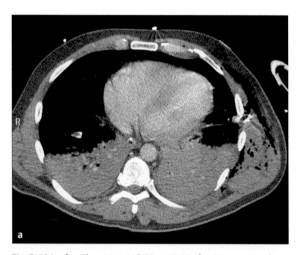 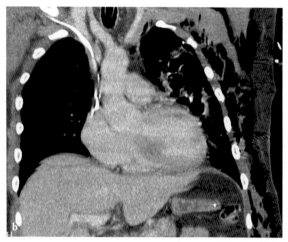

Fig. 2.104 a, b Thoracic spiral CT at 17:55 after IV contrast administration and placement of a left-sided thoracostomy tube. These images show increased pulmonary hemorrhages and left chest-wall emphysema relative to the previous examination. The bilateral lung contusions are unchanged.

a Portal venous phase after IV contrast administration.
b Coronal reformatted image.

Further Case Summary

The patient died 24 hours post injury as a result of cerebral trauma. An autopsy was performed and verified herniation of the cerebrum beneath the tentorium as the cause of death. It also confirmed the skeletal, pulmonary, and hepatic injuries demonstrated by CT. An intravital thrombus was excluded in coronary artery segments that were grossly visible at autopsy. Gross inspection revealed posterior contusions in the septal wall of the left ventricle. Since the CT cardiac findings were not known at autopsy and the cerebral injuries were the cause of death, the affected portion of the myocardium was not analyzed histologically.

Error Analysis and Strategy for Error Prevention

Ischemia of the ventricular septum and medial posterior wall of the left ventricle described at CT did not have an ischemic cause but resulted from myocardial contusion.

The trauma mechanism was reconstructed as follows: The patient struck the ground with the left anterior side of the body. This is evidenced by the left-sided skeletal fractures, left frontal brain injuries, and the greater severity of lung injuries on the left side. The force of the impact pushed the elastic anterior rib cage back toward the static spinal column, which also slung the heart against the vertebrae. Because of the cardiac position, the impact chiefly affected the posterior portion of the ventricular septum and the posteromedial wall of the left ventricle. Analogous to the contusions in the left lower lobe (**Fig. 2.103 a, c, d**), the blunt trauma presumably led to the rupture and obstruction of capillaries and to petechial

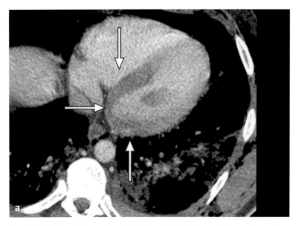
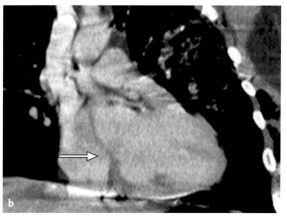

Fig. 2.105 a, b Thoracic spiral CT at 12:22 showed hypodense demarcation of the septum and posterior wall of the left ventricle (arrows) compared with the rest of the myocardium, which showed normal contrast enhancement.

a Axial scan.
b Coronal reformatted image.

Enhancement Kinetics

All blood vessels have endothelial gaps of variable size, depending on the particular organ region. Only the cerebral vessels are largely devoid of these gaps (blood–brain barrier). Most intravascular CT and MRI contrast agents are nonspecific, i.e., they are not targeted to a particular organ. The imaging atoms (CT: iodine, MRI: generally gadolinium) are bound in chelate complexes to prevent toxicity and improve biological tolerance. During the first pass of a micromolecular contrast bolus (molecular weight of Gd-based contrast agents = 0.5–0.6 kDa) injected into a peripheral vein, imaging atoms pass through the endothelial gaps by passive diffusion and enter the interstitium. This process depends on the diameter of the iodinated macromolecules (CT) or Gd-containing chelates, the size of the endothelial gaps, and the magnitude of the colloid osmotic pressure gradient. When the agent has completed several circulatory passes, its intravascular osmolarity is reduced. The colloid osmotic pressure gradient is reversed, causing the imaging atoms to diffuse back into the vascular space until they are finally excreted by the kidneys.

When the region of interest is scanned repetitively with a temporal resolution of 1–1.5 seconds before, during, and after passage of the contrast agent, a temporal analysis of the signals measured after IV contrast administration will yield pathognomonic information (the basis for quantitative permeability measurements and viability assessment with CT and MRI). In evaluating the diagnostic significance of increased signal intensity after IV contrast administration, a distinction is made between the first pass of the contrast agent (first-pass effects), an equilibrium phase between the intravascular space and interstitium (enhancement), and the late phase (late or delayed enhancement). In hypoperfused and ischemic tissues, few if any imaging atoms enter the interstitium during the first pass and equilibrium phase. In the late phase, imaging atoms can diffuse from peripheral areas into an ischemic area, causing delayed enhancement. Hypervascular tumors and inflamed tissues usually have larger-than-normal endothelial gaps, enabling a larger number of imaging atoms to diffuse into the intercellular space during the first bolus pass, causing interstitial enhancement.

hemorrhages and fluid collections in the affected myocardial areas. The healthy portions of the myocardium were better perfused than the contused areas, and so the myocardial contusions appeared as hypodense areas in the initial CT examination (**Fig. 2.105**). In the second CT examination, the interval between contrast administration and image acquisition was so long that collateral blood flow at the periphery of the contusion as well as diffusion had largely equalized the attenuation values of the affected and healthy myocardium by the time imaging was begun. At CT follow-up and also at autopsy, no further significance was ascribed to this finding, presumably due to the clinical predominance of noncardiac injuries.

References and Further Reading

Daldrup-Link HE, Brasch RC. Macromolecular contrast agents for MR mammography: current status. Eur Radiol 2003; 13: 354–365

Goßmann A, Okuhata Y, Shames DM, Helbich TH. Prostate cancer tumor grade differentiation by dynamic contrast-enhanced MR imaging: comparison of macromolecular and small-molecular contrast media. Radiology 1999; 213: 265–272

Ulcerating Histiocytic Lymphoma/ Malignant Melanoma

History and Clinical Findings

A 74-year-old man was referred from dermatology for staging of a suspected ulcerating histiocytic lymphoma. Thoracic CT showed enhancing nodular densities up to 1.5 cm in diameter in the subcutaneous fat of the lower axilla on both sides. These lesions were considered to be consistent with histiocytic lymphoma (**Fig. 2.106a**). Isolated lymph nodes, partially calcified and < 1 cm in size, were found in the mediastinum. Coarse pericardial calcifications were also noted (**Fig. 2.106c**).

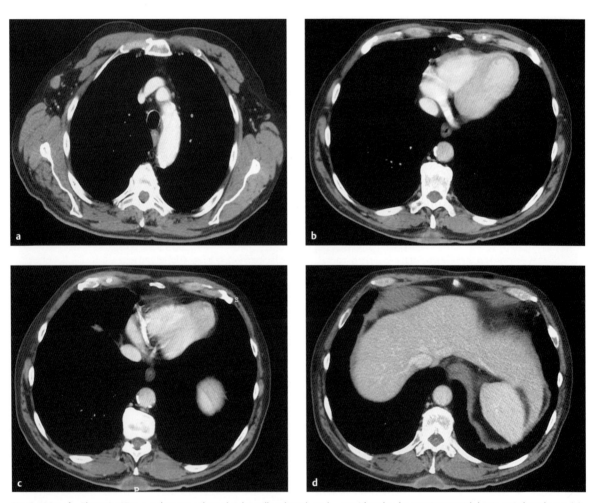

Fig. 2.106a–d Thoracic CT scans show an enlarged right axillary lymph node, considered to be consistent with histiocytic lymphoma (**a**), and coarse pericardial calcifications (**c**).

Further Case Summary

The ulcerating tumor, which was first classified histologically as histiocytic lymphoma and later as malignant melanoma, was located in the midline of the back (**Fig. 2.106 b–d**). It measured approximately 5 × 10 cm in its largest dimensions and extended to the spinous processes. The masses in both axillae were lymph node metastases (primary nodal stations for the median soft tissues of the back) and progressed rapidly over time.

Error Analysis and Strategy for Error Prevention

- Take a detailed history.
- Note the clinical findings: an ulcerating lesion must have infiltrated the skin or mucosa.
- "You see what you're looking for." Since advanced training tends to focus on issues in internal medicine and surgery, often too little attention is given to the skin and subcutaneous tissue except for the axilla and groin.

3

Breast

Breast

Normal Mammograms/ Breast Cancer

History and Clinical Findings

A 54-year-old woman noticed an approximately 1-cm, palpable, movable, nonpainful mass in her left breast. At mammography (**Fig. 3.1**) the radiographic density of the breast was classified as ACR 2, indicating a fibroglandular breast, based on the four-part classification of the American College of Radiology (**Table 3.1**). Although mammograms did not reveal a tumor, they were considered to warrant further evaluation (BI-RADS 0) when viewed within the context of clinical findings (**Table 3.2**).

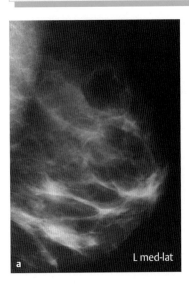 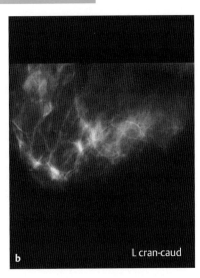

Fig. 3.1 a, b X-ray mammography of the left breast. Fibrocystic change is constant over time, with no evidence of malignancy.
a Mediolateral projection.
b Craniocaudal projection.

Table 3.1 Classification of parenchymal types based on American College of Radiology (ACR) criteria

ACR category	Description	Diagnostic confidence
1	The breast is almost entirely fat	Very high: > 95%
2	There are scattered fibroglandular densities	High: ≈ 90%
3	The breast is heterogeneously dense. This may lower the sensitivity of mammography	Moderate: ≈ 80%
4	The breast tissue is extremely dense, which could obscure a lesion in mammography	Low: ≈ 70%

Table 3.2 BI-RADS classification of the American College of Radiology (ACR) for x-ray mammography (BI-RADS R1–R6), breast ultrasound (BI-RADS S1–S6), and MR mammography (BI-RADS M1–M6). Stratified by increasing risk of malignancy, category 4 is further divided into subgroups 4a, 4b, and 4c

BI-RADS category	Description	Risk of malignancy
0	Assessment incomplete; need to review prior studies and/or complete additional imaging	
1	Negative; continue routine screening	0%
2	Benign finding; continue routine screening	0%
3	Probably benign finding; short-term follow-up mammogram at 6 months, then every 6 to 12 months for 1 to 2 years	< 2%
4	Suspicious abnormality; perform biopsy, preferably needle biopsy	≈ 30%
5	Highly suspicious of malignancy; appropriate action should be taken; biopsy and treatment, as necessary	≈ 95%
6	Known biopsy-proven malignancy, treatment pending; assure that treatment is completed	100%

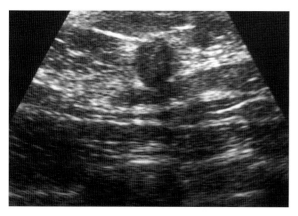

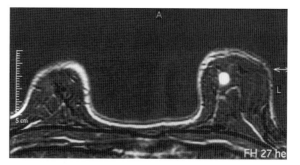

Fig. 3.3 MR mammography. T1-weighted sequence 2 minutes after IV contrast administration shows an intensely enhancing mass in the left breast at the site of the sonographic lesion.

Fig. 3.2 Ultrasound scan of the left breast shows an approximately 1-cm round, hypoechoic mass in the upper inner quadrant close to the midline.

Further Case Summary

At ultrasound, the palpable breast mass correlated with an approximately 1-cm, round, hypoechoic mass that was considered suspicious for malignancy (**Fig. 3.2**).

The lesion showed intense contrast enhancement on preoperative magnetic resonance (MR) mammography (**Fig. 3.3**). The ultrasound and MR findings were classified as highly suspicious for malignancy (BI-RADS categories S5 and M5, **Table 3.2**). The patient underwent a breast-conserving lumpectomy. Specimen histology identified the lesion as stage pT1b G2 N0 M0 invasive ductal carcinoma. At her latest follow-up visit the patient had been free of disease for 12 years.

Error Analysis and Strategy for Error Prevention

The risk of missing a tumor on mammograms increases with the size and density of the breast (ACR categories 3 and 4). Kolb et al. (2002) found that x-ray mammography had a sensitivity of 48% for detecting carcinoma in radiographically dense breasts. But even in women with smaller, nonfibrocystic breasts, the difference in density between a tumor and its surroundings may be so small that the contrast differences caused by x-ray attenuation in the tissue are not sufficient for visual perception of the tumor on mammograms.

Because x-ray mammography and ultrasound are based on different physical tissue parameters (radiographic density vs. acoustic impedance of the parenchyma), each of the two modalities effectively complements the other. In the study by Kolb et al., for example, x-ray mammography and ultrasound had a combined sensitivity of 97% in the detection of breast cancer. This means that breast ultrasound is an essential adjunct for investigating a palpable mass in a dense breast in cases where the lesion is either not visible on mammograms or has an equivocal radiographic appearance. MR mammography should also be added if necessary.

Definitions

Multifocality: The detection of one or more focal lesions located < 2 cm from the index tumor or confined to one quadrant. Therapeutic implication: a more extensive resection.

Multicentricity: The detection of one or more focal lesions located > 2 cm from the index tumor, generally occurring in multiple quadrants. Therapeutic implication: mastectomy in most cases.

References and Further Reading

American College of Radiology. BI-RADS®Atlas. http://www.acr.org/SecondaryMainMenuCategories/quality_safety/BIRADSAtlas/BIRADSAtlasexcerptedtext.aspx (accessed January 6, 2011)

Kolb TM, Lichy J, Newhouse JH. Comparison of the performance of screening mammography, physical examination, and breast US and evaluation of factors that influence them: an analysis of 27,825 patient evaluations. Radiology 2002; 225: 165–175

Moy L, Slanetz PJ, Moore R, et al. Specificity of mammography and US in the evaluation of a palpable abnormality: retrospective review. Radiology 2002; 225: 176–181

Tabár L, Tot T, Dean PB. Breast Cancer. The Art and Science of Early Detection with Mammography. Stuttgart: Thieme; 2005

Fibrocystic Change/ Breast Cancer

History and Clinical Findings

A 51-year-old woman was diagnosed with an osteolytic lesion in her left humerus. Mammograms taken elsewhere to search for a primary tumor showed a new, rounded, subareolar density located in the upper outer quadrant of the left breast (**Fig. 3.4**). The lesion was classified as suspicious for malignancy (BI-RADS 4, see **Table 3.2**). It was decided to proceed with local tumor excision following x-ray stereotactic localization of the lesion. When mammograms were taken in preparation for spring hookwire localization, there was no clear evidence for differentiating between fibrocystic change and a breast tumor. Also, ultrasound did not demonstrate a hypoechoic mass.

MR Mammography (MRM)

Indications

- Contradictory results of x-ray mammography and ultrasound
- Preoperative staging (multifocality, multicentricity) in patients with dense breasts (ACR 3 and 4)
- CUP syndrome in which axillary lymph node metastasis or skeletal metastasis from an unknown primary is histologically consistent with breast cancer
- Evaluating response to neoadjuvant chemotherapy (distinguishing responders from nonresponders by comparing MR mammograms before treatment and after the second and fourth chemotherapy cycles)
- Distinguishing between tumor recurrence and scar tissue in cases that are equivocal by x-ray mammography and ultrasound (interval between surgery and MR mammography should be >6 months to avoid false-positive findings)
- Prosthetic breast reconstruction after mastectomy
- Confirm or exclude a prosthetic defect: noncontrast examination
- Surveillance of high-risk patients (BRCA carriers), with MRM serving as an adjunct to x-ray mammograms and ultrasound

MRM should not be used to investigate indeterminate microcalcifications because it cannot reliably detect or exclude possible intraductal tumor growth. False-positive findings due to hormonal stimulation of the breast parenchyma can be avoided by imaging between days 7 and 17 of the menstrual cycle (premenopausal women), after 3 months' withdrawal from hormonal products (postmenopausal women), and in non-lactating breasts.

Tumor Neoangiogenesis

The tumor-induced formation of new blood vessels (tumor neoangiogenesis) influences the growth of a carcinoma and its potential for hematogenous and lymphogenous metastasis. The newly formed capillaries have larger interspaces (pores) between the intercellular junctions of the endothelial cells and a discontinuous basement membrane. These "endothelial gaps" allow proteins and contrast medium to diffuse from the vessels into the interstitium. They also make it easier for tumor cells to invade the newly formed capillaries than preexisting vessels, and therefore the likelihood of metastasis increases with vascular density. Because neoangiogenesis occurs in close proximity to the cancer cells owing to chemotactic factors that are secreted by the tumor cells, these cells must travel only a short distance to invade the newly formed capillaries. Several studies have shown a good correlation between the immunohistochemically determined vascular density of a tumor and the amplitude of the signal intensity increase detectable by MRM.

Analytical Criteria

The following parameters should be considered in the analysis and interpretation of MR mammograms:

- The *morphologic* analysis of MR mammograms (matrix, shape, margins) is like that for x-ray mammograms and sonograms except for the different tissue parameters that are used for imaging.
- *Enhancement kinetics* refers to the pattern of contrast enhancement over time. Three basic patterns are distinguished: centrifugal (probably benign), constant (indifferent), and centripetal (probably malignant).
- *Enhancement dynamics* refers to the change in signal intensity over time after contrast administration. Two main phases are distinguished: an initial phase (first 2 minutes after contrast injection) and a postinitial phase (minutes 3 through 8). The initial signal rise describes the peak enhancement that occurs during the first 2 minutes relative to the baseline value of the noncontrast examination. Little or no rise in signal intensity (50–100 % over baseline) is suggestive of benignancy, while a marked rise in signal intensity (>100 %) is suggestive of malignancy. A slow rise during the postinitial phase (minutes 3–8) and a plateau phase (± 10 %) are more characteristic of benign lesions, whereas a washout effect (>10 % fall of signal intensity) is more suggestive of malignancy.

Given the discrepancy between the mammograms taken 3 weeks apart and the negative findings at breast ultrasound, MR mammography was performed. The MR images showed an approximately 2-cm elliptical mass in the upper outer quadrant of the left breast near the chest wall. A time–intensity curve was plotted for the intensely en-

hancing lesion and showed an early, rapid rise of MR signal intensity followed by a plateau (**Fig. 3.5**). Two other lesions located in the anterior portion of the left breast were interpreted as fibrocystic changes due to their slow-rising time–intensity curve and the presence of similar enhancing zones in the right breast.

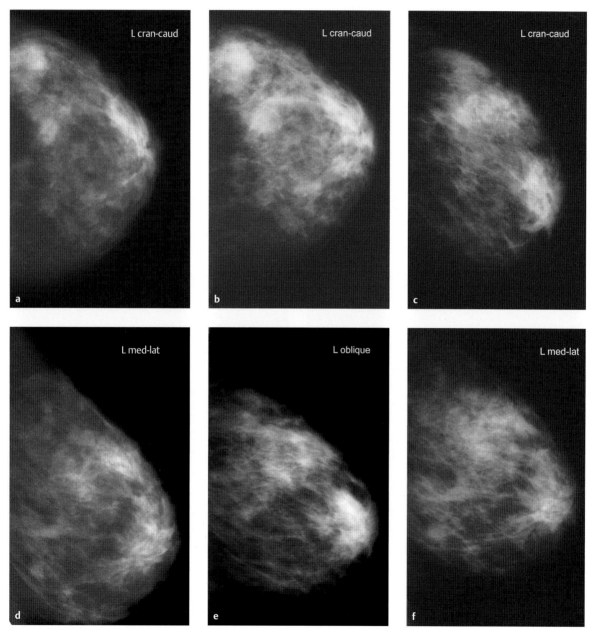

Fig. 3.4 a–f Serial mammograms. Mammograms were taken 3 weeks after the current examination to aid in planning preoperative x-ray stereotactic localization of the suspicious lesion described in images **b** and **e**. The later mammograms were unable to reproduce the suspicious finding. The parenchyma of both breasts is dense and shows fibrocystic changes (ACR 4).

a, d Previous examination 4 years ago.
b, e Current examination.
c, f Mammograms taken 3 weeks after **b** and **c**.

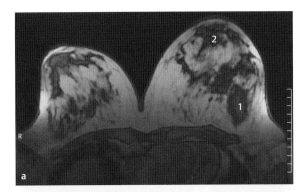

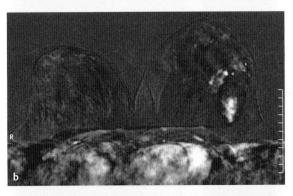

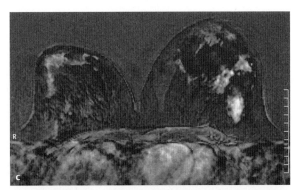

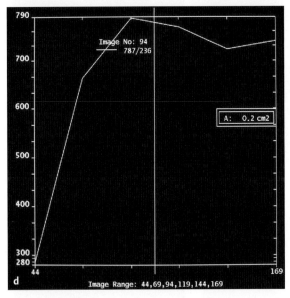

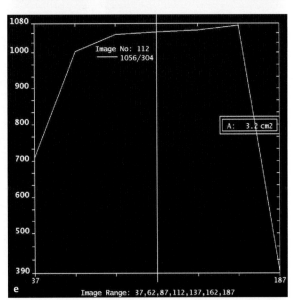

Fig. 3.5 a–e MR mammography. An elliptical mass located near the chest wall in the upper outer quadrant of the left breast (**a**) shows intense contrast enhancement in the early perfusion phase (**b**). The subareolar enhancing areas in the left breast were interpreted as fibrocystic changes due to their slow-rise enhancement pattern and the presence of enhancing zones in the right breast.

a T2-weighted sequence without contrast medium.
b T1-weighted subtraction sequence in the early perfusion phase.
c T1-weighted subtraction sequence in the late perfusion phase.

d Time–intensity curve after an IV contrast bolus, calculated for zone 1 in **a**. Abscissa: time in seconds. Ordinate: signal intensity in arbitrary units. A = area of the region of interest.
e Time–intensity curve after an IV contrast bolus, calculated for zone 2 in **a**.

Further Case Summary

Excisional biopsy was performed following MR mammographic localization of the lesion with a spring hookwire (**Fig. 3.6**). Specimen histology revealed invasive ductal carcinoma with positive margins. A complete left mastectomy was performed. Pathology identified a diffusely infiltrating tumor located predominantly in the upper outer quadrant that had permeated almost the entire breast.

Error Analysis and Strategy for Error Prevention

In retrospect, breast cancer was not clearly or fully detectable on the x-ray mammograms. There were several reasons for this:

- The readability of the mammograms was limited by the radiographic density and inhomogeneity of the breast parenchyma and tumor. Based on reports in the literature, mammography misses approximately 50% of all cancers in breasts with a radiographic density of ACR 4.
- The question of whether tumor tissue was already detectable in 4-year-old prior mammograms cannot be answered. It is conceivable that the asymmetry of the breast parenchyma in the initial examination was caused by neoplasia rather than fibrocystic change.
- The serial mammograms had been positioned somewhat differently, making them difficult to compare due to discrepancies in imaging geometry.
- The prior mediolateral mammogram (**Fig. 3.4d**) was inverted and mislabeled. This technical error added to the difficulty of interpretation.
- It is true that ultrasound is the most important adjunct to x-ray mammography, in many cases allowing for direct tumor detection owing to high contrast between the hypoechoic tumor tissue and hyperechoic mammary lobules. Nevertheless, even ultrasound may fail to detect smaller cancers. This results from the broad overlap in the sonographic appearances of benign and malignant changes.

- When the MR images were interpreted, the reader missed several morphologic tumor signs in the unenhanced sequence: asymmetry of the breast sizes, multiple hypointense foci with ill-defined margins in the left breast, and an inhomogeneous tumor matrix (**Fig. 3.5a**).
- Not only the tumor labeled "1" (**Fig. 3.5a**) but also two additional zones in the anterior part of the left breast, which were hypointense in the plain sequence, showed early, patchy enhancement after IV contrast administration (**Fig. 3.5b, c**).
- The time–intensity curves plotted for areas 1 and 2 (**Fig. 3.5a**) both displayed malignant-type enhancement kinetics. Area 1 showed an initial rise of 233% ($100 \times [787\,AU - 236\,AU]/236AU$, **Fig. 3.5d**) while area 2 showed an initial rise of 247% ($100 \times [1056\,AU - 304\,AU]/304\,AU$, **Fig. 3.5e**). The postinitial signal curve reached a plateau in area 1 and showed a 10% decline (washout) in area 2.

References and Further Reading

Kolb TM, Lichy J, Newhouse JH. Comparison of the performance of screening mammography, physical examination, and breast US and evaluation of factors that influence them: an analysis of 27,825 patient evaluations. Radiology 2002; 225: 165–175

Tabár L, Tot T, Dean PB. Breast Cancer. The Art and Science of Early Detection with Mammography. Stuttgart: Thieme; 2005

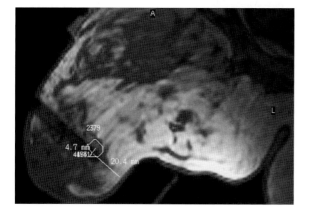

Fig. 3.6 MR mammographic tumor localization with a nonferromagnetic spring hookwire. The signal void caused by the hookwire is broader than the actual wire diameter (4.7 mm vs. 2.0 mm). Electronic markers indicate the tumor volume and the distance between the tumor center and the skin (20.4 mm).

Breast Cancer/Fibrocystic Change with Microcysts

History and Clinical Findings

A 52-year-old woman noticed a palpable nodule at the 3-o'clock position in her left breast. Mammograms showed an approximately 1.3-cm nodular density with irregular margins at the same location (**Fig. 3.7**). The breast parenchyma showed extensive involution and fatty replacement (ACR 1). Microcalcifications were not present. The mammographic lesion was classified as highly suspicious for malignancy (BI-RADS 5). It correlated with a 1.5-cm hypoechoic mass on initial breast ultrasound (**Fig. 3.8**), but the lesion was not reproducible on follow-up scans. Owing to the sharp contrast between the lesion and surrounding atrophic breast tissue on mammograms, an x-ray stereotactic vacuum biopsy was obtained for histologic analysis. The biopsy was performed using standard technique (**Fig. 3.9**). The pathology report indicated fibrocystic breast change with microcysts but no evidence of malignancy.

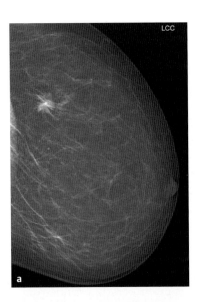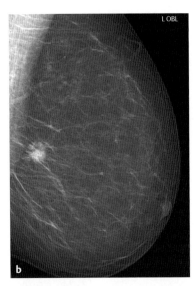

Fig. 3.7 a, b Mammograms of the left breast. The breast parenchyma is largely involuted (ACR 1). A rounded density with ill-defined margins is visible at the 3-o'clock position near the chest wall. The lesion was classified as highly suspicious for malignancy (BI-RADS 5).
a Craniocaudal projection.
b Mediolateral projection.

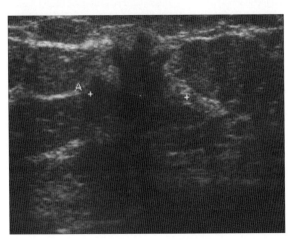

Fig. 3.8 High-resolution B-mode ultrasonography. Initial breast ultrasonogram showed a hypoechoic mass classified as highly suspicious for malignancy. The lesion was missed on follow-up scans.

Further Case Summary

Given the high index of mammographic suspicion, it was assumed, when all findings were reviewed, that the vacuum biopsy had missed the suspicious lesion. For this reason, an excisional biopsy was performed after x-ray stereotactic wire localization of the focal lesion. Mammography prior to wire localization showed a rounded density in the left breast (4-o'clock) that was new since the initial examination (**Fig. 3.10**). Both lesions were localized (**Fig. 3.11**).

Intraoperative frozen-section histology confirmed invasive ductal carcinoma in the primary lesion. Treatment consisted of a segmental mastectomy followed by local advancement of the remaining breast tissue and removal of the sentinel lymph nodes. Specimen histology finally indicated a poorly differentiated invasive lobular carcinoma 1.5 cm in diameter, staged as pT1c pN0 (sn 0/3) G3 R0, and a separate, older hemorrhagic area caused by the vacuum biopsy.

Chest radiography, abdominal ultrasound, and radionuclide bone scans were negative, confirming an M0 status. Adjuvant treatments consisted of chemotherapy with 5-fluorouracil, epirubicin and cyclophosphamide, radiotherapy, and endocrine therapy.

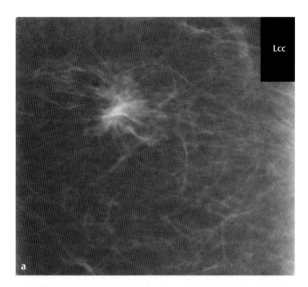

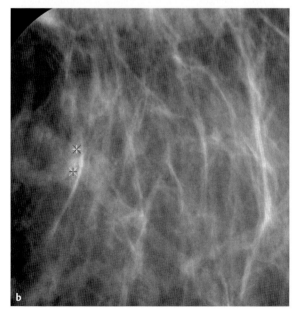

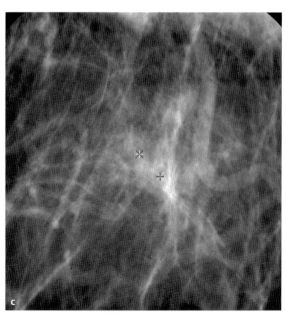

Fig. 3.9 a–c   X-ray stereotactic vacuum biopsy. The patient was positioned on the table of the prone digital stereotactic system, and the spot films in **b** and **c** were taken to locate the tumor. The lesion margins were manually tagged with cursors on the monitor, and the biopsy coordinates were automatically computed.
a Digital mammogram prior to biopsy.
b Stereotactic planning image with target points marked, angled +15° relative to the sagittal plane.
c Stereotactic planning image with target points marked, angled −15° relative to the sagittal plane.

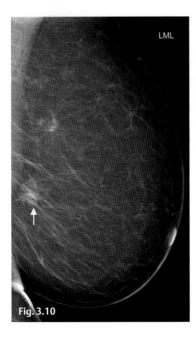

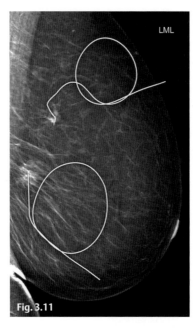

Fig. 3.10 Digital mammogram before preoperative x-ray stereotactic tumor localization. The new rounded density anterosuperior to the suspicious lesion (arrow) is a hematoma at the site of the previous unsuccessful vacuum biopsy.

Fig. 3.11 Preoperative x-ray stereotactic localization of the two main lesions.

Error Analysis and Strategy for Error Prevention

As evidenced by the hematoma on preoperative mammograms (**Fig. 3.10**), the target lesion was missed by x-ray stereotactic biopsy. This is explained by the difficult imaging conditions for planning the x-ray stereotactic biopsy of a mass that does not contain microcalcifications. Imaging conditions are altered by technical variations in the x-ray stereotactic spot films and digital survey films in the form of:

- Examination in the supine, standing, or sitting position
- Different compression conditions
- Acquisition matrix up to 512^2 or 1024^2 pixels for planning the stereotactic biopsy versus up to 4096×3328 pixels in digital mammography

- Spot films with a $5.5\,cm \times 5.5\,cm$ field of view versus survey films with an edge length of $18\,cm \times 24\,cm$ or $24\,cm \times 29\,cm$

(See **Table 3.3**, **Fig. 3.7**, **Fig. 3.9**, **Fig. 3.10**.) Because of the smaller field of view, it can be difficult to detect the target lesion in x-ray stereotactic spot films and distinguish it from other structures such as normal glandular breast tissue. This particularly applies to lesions without microcalcifications, in which case there is often very little difference in density between the target lesion and its surroundings.

Sometimes it is easier to detect invasive carcinoma on specimen radiographs than on survey mammograms because there is less scattering of the x-rays. For this reason, specimen radiographs are often obtained even after biopsies of masses that do not contain tumor-associated calcifications (**Fig. 3.12**).

Core-Needle and Vacuum Biopsies

False-positive findings, which are common due to the low specificity of x-ray mammography (range of 64–91% based on published reports), are a significant limiting factor in the pre- and postoperative management of breast cancer. The specificity of breast ultrasound, including color duplex scans, and of MRM is too low to permit a confident benign/malignant differentiation of BI-RADS category 3–5 lesions detected on x-ray mammograms. Unnecessary surgery imposes a physical and psychological burden on patients and incurs significant unnecessary costs for payors.

For these reasons, national and international guidelines dealing with early breast cancer detection and the diagnosis, treatment, and follow-up of breast cancer state that at least 90% of surgically treated breast tumors should be histologically confirmed by percutaneous core-needle biopsy or vacuum biopsy prior to operative treatment. False-negative rates of 1–15% have been reported for core and vacuum biopsies in the literature. On current guidelines, these rates should be lower than 5%. An interdisciplinary conference should be convened to coordinate clinical, radiologic, and histologic results with the goal of recognizing discrepant findings.

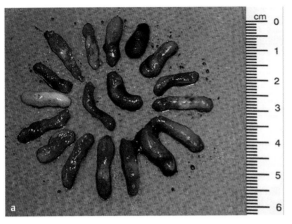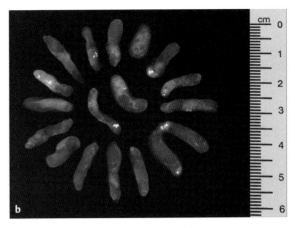

Fig. 3.12 a, b Specimen radiography in a different patient who underwent vacuum biopsy for suspicious microcalcifications.
a Biopsy cores.
b Specimen radiograph.

Table 3.3 Technical factors for digital mammograms and digital x-ray stereotactic spot films

Technical factors	Survey mammograms	X-ray stereotactic spot films
Body position	Standing or sitting	Prone
Compression	Semiautomatic	Manual
Degree of compression	Relatively high	Relatively low
Projection	Craniocaudal, oblique, or mediolateral	Spot films at +15° and –15° to the selected sagittal and coronal planes; transverse projection is geared toward target position and is variable over an approximately 360° range
Data acquisition matrix	Up to 4096 × 3328 pixels	512^2 or 1024^2 pixels
Field of view	18 cm × 24 cm, 24 cm × 29 cm	5.5 cm × 5.5 cm
Automatic exposure control	Yes	No (yes for scout views)
Voltage	25–34 kV	22–34 kV
Anode material	Molybdenum or tungsten	Molybdenum

References and Further Reading

Kreienberg R, Kopp I, Lorenz W, et al. Interdisciplinary S 3 Guidelines for the Diagnosis, Treatment and Follow-up Care of Breast Cancer. First updated version 2008; http://www.uni-duesseldorf.de/WWW/AWMF/ll/ (accessed November 10, 2010)

Perry N, Broeders M, de Wolf F, Törnberg S, Holland R, von Karsa L, eds. European Commission. European Guidelines for Quality Assurance in Breast Cancer Screening and Diagnosis. 4th ed. Cologne: Bundesanzeiger Verlag; 2006. www.euref.org/

Peter D, Grünhagen J, Wenke R, Schäfer FK, Schreer I. False-negative results after stereotactically guided vacuum biopsy. Eur Radiol 2008; 18: 177–182

Riedl CC, Pfarl G, Memarsadeghi M, et al. Lesion miss rates and false-negative rates for 1115 consecutive cases of stereotactically guided needle-localized open breast biopsy with long-term follow-up. Radiology 2005; 237: 847–853

Shah VI, Raju U, Chitale D, Deshpande V, Gregory N, Strand V. False-negative core needle biopsies of the breast. An analysis of clinical, radiologic, and pathologic findings in 27 consecutive cases of missed breast cancer. Cancer 2003; 97: 1824–1831

Breast Cancer?

History and Clinical Findings

A 63-year-old woman complaining of pain in her left breast of several weeks' duration was referred for curative mammography. Two weeks earlier she had felt a nodule in the upper outer quadrant of her left breast. Since then, however, she claimed that the mass was no longer palpable. Inspection and palpation of the breast revealed no abnormalities. Mammograms were described as showing fibrocystic changes with microcalcifications in both breasts (**Fig. 3.13**). Subsequent left breast ultrasound showed an approximately 2-cm elliptical hypoechoic mass at the junction of the upper outer quadrant and axillary soft tissues. It was noted that the lesion was most likely a lymph node or possibly a fibroadenoma. MRI was recommended for definitive exclusion of a malignant tumor.

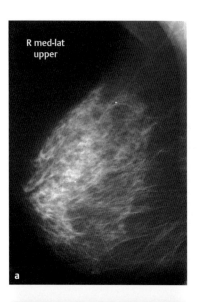
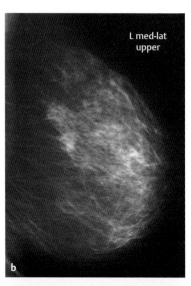
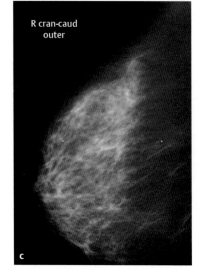
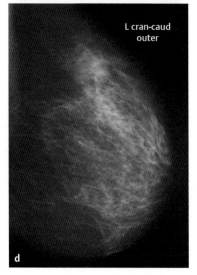

Fig. 3.13 a–d X-ray mammography. The report described fibrocystic breast changes with microcalcifications.

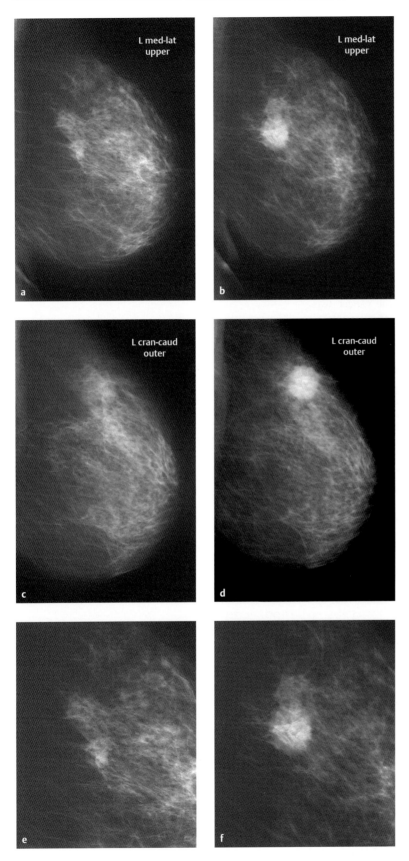

Fig. 3.14 a–f Mammographic follow-up of the left breast. The upper outer quadrant contains a rounded lesion that was already visible on initial mammograms. Since then it has increased in size and density.

a, c Initial examination.
b, d Follow-up at 1 year 9 months.
e Magnified view of the lesion in **a**.
f Magnified view of the lesion in **b**.

Further Case Summary

One year and 9 months later, the patient presented again for mammographic evaluation of an approximately 3-cm palpable mass in the upper outer quadrant of her left breast (**Fig. 3.14b, d**). It was unclear why previously recommended MR mammograms had been withheld (the patient did not have private health insurance). In addition to the movable nodule in the left breast, enlarged lymph nodes were palpable in the left axilla. Mammograms showed an approximately 3-cm rounded density with ill-defined margins and amorphous microcalcifications at the site of the palpable mass. In retrospect, the lesion was already visible on initial mammograms and had enlarged during the interval between examinations (**Fig. 3.14a, c**).

Excisional biopsy yielded a histologic diagnosis of invasive ductal carcinoma. Treatment consisted of a breast-conserving lumpectomy and axillary dissection. The tumor measured 3 cm in diameter, and metastases were present in five axillary lymph nodes. The cancer was staged as pT2 N1 M0 G3. Despite adjuvant chemoradiation, the patient died 1½ years later from disseminated disease.

Error Analysis and Strategy for Error Prevention

The following errors were made in interpreting the initial mammograms:

- The breasts were not analyzed for symmetry in the mediolateral and craniocaudal projections. Such a comparison would have revealed the increased density of the axillary tail on the left side.
- The regional density of the breast parenchyma was not systematically analyzed. Otherwise the rounded mass in the upper outer quadrant would have been detected.
- Even on initial mammograms, it was apparent that the tumor contained clustered, amorphous microcalcifications that were suspicious for malignancy and should have drawn attention to the surrounding density.
- Until proven otherwise, nonpainful enlarged axillary lymph nodes are suspicious for metastatic breast cancer in women without a personal cancer history.

Interval Cancers in Mammographic Screening

Estimates of the incidence of breast cancers that are missed due to the misinterpretation of x-ray mammograms are available based on data from national and international mammographic screening programs.

Interval cancers are defined as cancers that reach a volume between two examinations that is sufficient for tumor detection in the subsequent examination. In most screening programs the interval between screening rounds is 2 years.

The incidence of interval cancers is of fundamental importance for evaluating the efficacy of a screening program. For this reason, serial mammograms taken in patients who develop interval cancers undergo a retrospective analysis to distinguish between "true interval cancers" and "false-negative findings," or missed cancers.

Current guidelines state that the overall rate of interval cancers should be less than 50% of regularly diagnosed cancers and that "false-negative findings" should account for less than 20% of interval cancers. Data on the true incidence of false-negative findings in mammographic screening range from 3% to 56%, depending on the methodology of the retrospective analysis. The results vary according to whether the true cancer rate is known or unknown during the analysis, whether the mammograms are interpreted by one or more readers, and whether the series contained only interval cancers or also included normal findings. All analyses published to date have been based on 70–130 interval cancers, and the incidence of false-negative findings in all studies increased with the density of the breast parenchyma.

References and Further Reading

Albert U-S für die Mitglieder der Planungsgruppe und die Leiter der Arbeitsgruppen Konzertierte Aktion Brustkrebs-Früherkennung in Deutschland. Stufe-3-Leitlinie Brustkrebs-Früherkennung in Deutschland. 1. Aktualisierung 2008; http://www.uni-duesseldorf.de/WWW/AWMF/ll/ (accessed November 10, 2010)

Duncan AA, Wallis MG. Classifying interval cancers. Clin Radiol 1995; 50: 774–777

Ikeda DM, Andersson I, Wattsgard C, Janzon L, Linell F. Interval carcinomas in the Malmö mammographic screening trial: radiographic appearance and prognostic consideration. AJR 1992; 159: 287–294

Moberg K, Grundström H, Törnberg S, et al. Two models for radiological reviewing of interval cancers. J Med Screen 1999; 6: 35–39

Moberg K, Grundström H, Törnberg S, et al. Radiological review of interval breast cancers. J Med Screen 2000; 7: 117–183

Perry N, Broeders M, de Wolf F, Törnberg S, Holland R, von Karsa L, eds. European Commission. European Guidelines for Quality Assurance in Breast Cancer Screening and Diagnosis. 4th ed. Cologne: Bundesanzeiger Verlag; 2006. http://www.euref.org/

Breast Cancer?

History and Clinical Findings

A 48-year-old woman presented with a new palpable nodule in her left breast. The nodule was located 2 cm from the nipple at the 3-o'clock position and was described as "firm." Digital mammography showed involuted breasts with fibrocystic changes in the remaining glandular tissue, with findings unchanged relative to analog screen–film mammograms taken 2 years earlier (**Fig. 3.15**). A mammographic correlate for the palpable nodule could not be found. Given the discrepancy between palpable and mammographic findings, the case was classified as ACR 2 (**Table 3.1**) and BI-RADS 0 (**Table 3.2**).

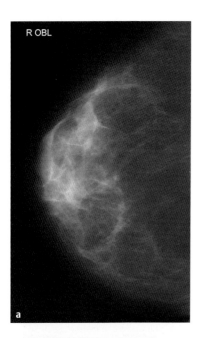

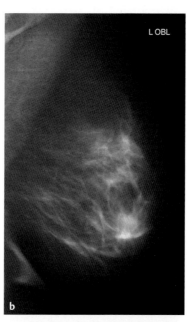

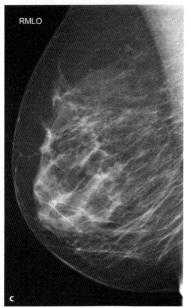

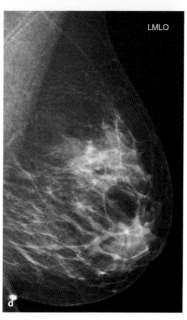

Fig. 3.15 a–h Prior screen–film mammograms (**a, b**) and digital images taken 2 years later (**c, d**). All mammograms were interpreted as negative. Due to the presence of a palpable nodule, the diagnosis was classified as BI-RADS 0.

a, b Prior examination.
c, d Current examination.

Fig. 3.15 e–h ▶

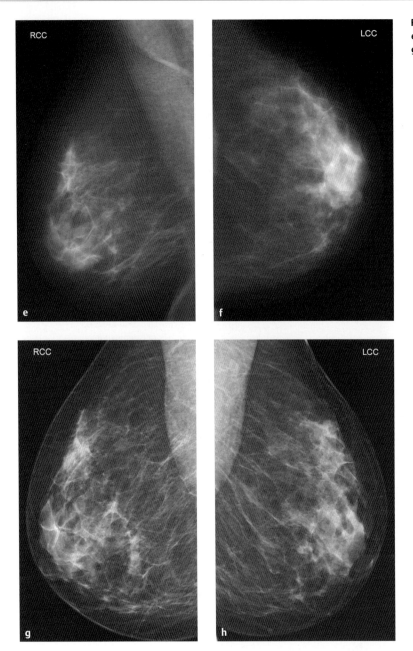

Fig. 3.15 e–h continued
e, f Prior examination.
g, h Current examination

Further Case Summary

Breast ultrasound with a high-resolution 13-MHz transducer demonstrated an approximately 2-cm hypoechoic, inhomogeneous mass with irregular margins and scattered calcifications at the site of the palpable nodule (**Fig. 3.16**). The mass was associated with posterior acoustic shadowing and acoustic enhancement. The ultrasound findings were classified as highly suspicious for malignancy (BI-RADS 5).

Ultrasound-guided biopsy identified the lesion as invasive ductal carcinoma. Treatment consisted of a breast-conserving segmental mastectomy with a reduction mammoplasty, axillary dissection, and a symmetrizing reduction mammoplasty of the right breast. Adjuvant chemotherapy, radiotherapy, and hormonal therapy were added. Specimen histopathology revealed invasive ductal carcinoma staged as pT1c (maximum diameter 1.8 cm) pN0 pM0 G2.

Error Analysis and Strategy for Error Prevention

Approximately 10% of newly diagnosed breast cancers are not visible on x-ray mammograms even when their presence is known. Most of these tumors are first detected by breast self-examination or during individual routine examinations (palpation, ultrasound). The detectability of a tumor depends on its contrast with surrounding tissues, regardless of breast size. Because this contrast varies in different imaging techniques, discrepant findings may be encountered in some cases. If the tumor resembles normal mammary lobules in its shape and if the lateral symmetry of the breasts is not altered by the mass, the cancer may elude detection on x-ray mammograms. Because the density distribution within the breasts (the physical basis of x-ray mammography) does not correlate with differences in acoustic impedance at tissue interfaces (the physical basis of ultrasonography), the two imaging modalities are complementary. Ultrasound or MRM is definitely indicated in patients who have a palpable breast mass and negative x-ray mammograms.

References and Further Reading

American College of Radiology. Breast Imaging and Interventions. http://www.acr.org/SecondaryMainMenuCategories/quality_safety/guidelines/breast.aspx (accessed November 10, 2010)

American College of Radiology. BI-RADS Atlas (excerpted text). http://www.acr.org/SecondaryMainMenuCategories/quality_safety/BIRADSAtlas/BIRADSAtlasexcerptedtext.aspx (accessed November 10, 2010)

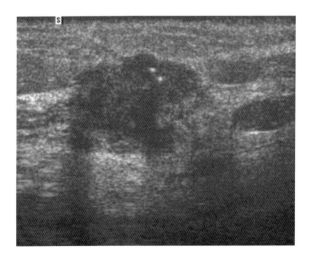

Fig. 3.16 Sonographic appearance of a carcinoma at the site of the palpable nodule. The mass has irregular scalloped margins, an inhomogeneous internal echo pattern, and a hypoechoic matrix. The margins and echo pattern of the mass are consistent with carcinoma. The acoustic shadows posterior to the lesion result from variable sound absorption within the tumor and relate to its varying tissue composition.

Correct Histopathology Report?

History and Clinical Findings

A 46-year-old woman with chronic lymphocytic leukemia (CLL) presented for mammography to exclude a second tumor. No visible or palpable breast abnormalities were found. Mammograms showed dense breasts (ACR 2, see **Table 3.1**) with fibrocystic changes. Two adjacent, dense, rounded or triangular clusters of pleomorphic microcalcifications were noted in the upper outer quadrant of the left breast (**Fig. 3.17**). The finding was classified as BI-RADS 4 due to suspicion of ductal carcinoma in situ (DCIS) or invasive ductal carcinoma (see **Table 3.2**), and it was decided to proceed with x-ray stereotactic vacuum biopsy. Tissue cores were first sampled from the smaller, pleomorphic microcalcification cluster as it was considered more suspicious for carcinoma.

Specimen radiography showed good representation of the microcalcifications in the biopsy cores (**Fig. 3.18 a**). Specimen histopathology indicated fibrocystic change with microcysts and no evidence of malignancy. At routine postinterventional radiology, the histopathologic and mammographic findings were considered to be concordant and the patient was scheduled for 6-month follow-up mammograms of the left breast.

When the patient returned 6 months later, the follow-up mammograms showed that some of the microcalcifications had been removed from the upper outer quadrant of the left breast (**Fig. 3.19**), but otherwise the findings were unchanged. Due to the residual cancer risk, it is was decided to take an x-ray stereotactic biopsy from the second microcalcification cluster located at a higher and more lateral site in the left breast.

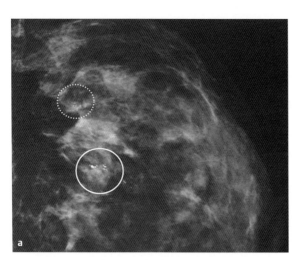

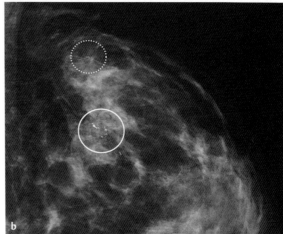

Fig. 3.17 a, b Initial findings. Magnified view of the upper outer quadrant of the left breast. The dotted circle indicates the microcalcification cluster that was biopsied first. The solid circle marks the cluster that was biopsied 6 months later.

a Craniocaudal projection.
b Mediolateral projection.

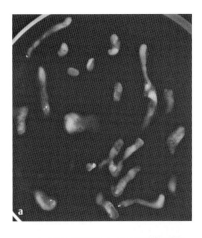

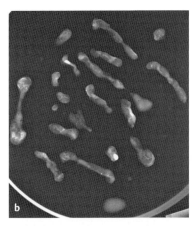

Fig. 3.18 a, b Specimen radiographs of tissue cores sampled during the first (a) and second (b) x-ray stereotactic vacuum biopsy. The tissue samples were assumed to be representative owing to the presence of microcalcifications.

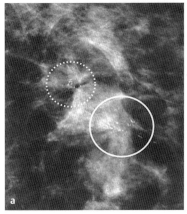

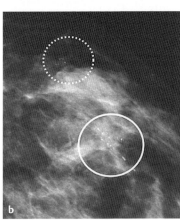

Fig. 3.19 a, b Follow-up mammograms 6 months later. Magnified views of the upper outer quadrant of the left breast show a reduction in the number of microcalcifications in the biopsied cluster (dotted circle). The appearance of the non-biopsied microcalcification cluster (solid circle) is unchanged.
a Craniocaudal projection.
b Mediolateral projection.

Further Case Summary

Histologic analysis of the tissue cores from the second vacuum biopsy yielded a diagnosis of moderately differentiated invasive ductal carcinoma, DCIS, and leukemic infiltrates in the setting of CLL. Chest radiographs, abdominal ultrasound, and radionuclide bone scans were negative (stage M0). Treatment consisted of a segmental mastectomy after sonographic tumor localization with a spring hookwire, followed by local advancement of the remaining breast tissue, mastopexy, and removal of the sentinel lymph nodes. Histology revealed invasive ductal carcinoma classified as stage pT1c (maximum diameter 1.6 cm) pTis pN0 (metastasis in 0 of 3 lymph nodes examined). The postoperative course was uneventful. Following adjuvant chemotherapy of the breast cancer, the patient was released for medical management of her CLL by an oncologist.

Error Analysis and Strategy for Error Prevention

The two microcalcification clusters were closely adjacent to each other and had a similar imaging appearance. For this reason alone, it was unlikely that the microcalcifica-

tions in the first cluster were due to fibrocystic change while those in the second cluster arose from a mixed histologic pattern of invasive ductal cancer and DCIS. This discrepancy was discussed with the pathologist. A new histopathologic work-up of the tissue blocks from the first vacuum biopsy revealed the presence of DCIS with a van Nuys score of 2. The histopathology error resulted from the fact that the biopsy cores had not been sliced deeply enough.

While DCIS does not always progress to invasive ductal breast cancer, the potential for malignant transformation cannot be accurately predicted in any given case, and therefore surgical resection is indicated in all patients with DCIS. Higher van Nuys scores (grades 2 and 3) correlate with a greater likelihood of malignant transformation.

Acceptance of the false-negative histopathology finding during final evaluation of the mammograms for the first vacuum biopsy caused a 6-month delay in the diagnosis and treatment of the invasive ductal cancer. The delay resulted from an overemphasis on the accuracy of the pathology report. Because errors do occur in histopathologic analysis, the European guidelines on mammographic screening (Perry) define rigorous quality criteria for the conduct and interpretation of these procedures. Concurrent biopsies of both microcalcification clusters were initially omitted because the smaller cluster was considered more suspicious and it was felt that both clusters would have required preoperative localization. Because the initial biopsy was interpreted as benign, that result was applied uncritically to the second lesion because of the similarity of the x-ray findings.

Ductal Carcinoma In Situ (DCIS) I

Microcalcifications. Mammograms can detect microcalcifications in approximately 90% of all histopathologically confirmed ductal carcinomas in situ. By contrast, only 20–40% of invasive ductal carcinomas are found to contain microcalcifications at mammography. Microcalcifications in the setting of DCIS and invasive ductal carcinoma represent calcified casts that have formed in the duct system. Typically they are arranged in clusters, are pleomorphic, and present a variety of sizes, shapes, and densities within any given cluster. They often show a linear or segmental arrangement due to their relationship to the mammary ducts. The microcalcifications that form in association with benign conditions (fibrocystic change) are generally scattered throughout the breast parenchyma and are homogeneous in their size, shape, and density. In one series of 190 histologically confirmed DCIS cases, microcalcifications were the most common indicator of malignancy (117/190, 62%). Masses of soft-tissue density were present in 43 of the 190 patients (23%), and 30 of the patients (16%) had normal mammographic findings.

Size. The extent of DCIS is often underestimated on mammograms. The likelihood of underestimating tumor volume increases with the size of the DCIS. The maximum diameter of low- and intermediate-grade DCIS (see below) is underestimated by 2 cm in up to 50% of cases, depending on the study design. Nevertheless, the size and location of mammographic lesions suspicious for DCIS should be determined as accurately as possible for the planning of breast-conserving surgery. Bilateral involvement by DCIS is described in approximately 20% of DCIS patients.

MR mammography and ultrasound. MR mammography and ultrasound are less useful for the diagnosis of DCIS due to their relatively poor spatial resolution, which is too low for assessing the configuration of microcalcifications. The imaging features of DCIS are nonspecific in both modalities. As a general rule, the shape of the MRM time–intensity curve plotted after IV contrast administration (enhancement kinetics, see p. 134) is also consistent with benign breast conditions such as fibrocystic change. By contrast, MRI sequences after IV contrast administration are very sensitive for the detection of invasive ductal carcinoma. MRM has also shown increasing success in the detection of DCIS, although its sensitivity and specificity are inferior to x-ray mammography. Because specificity is so limited, MR-guided percutaneous biopsy should be performed to confirm the diagnosis.

Mammography and histology. While mammographic findings can provide a high index of suspicion for DCIS, the definitive diagnosis relies on histopathology. On the one hand, there is no imaging modality that can detect penetration of the basement membrane, which is necessary in order to distinguish DCIS from invasive ductal carcinoma. On the other hand, inflammation and fibrosis in the tissues surrounding DCIS can produce malignant-type soft-tissue changes on mammograms even though the carcinoma has not penetrated the basement membrane or invaded the stroma. Percutaneous biopsies can at most investigate a sample—preferably a representative sample—of the tissue changes. This explains why histopathologic analysis of the surgical specimen can detect invasive ductal tumor elements in 10–20% of tumors classified preoperatively as DCIS.

Histopathologic classification. With the growing popularity of breast-conserving operations, histopathologic classifications have been developed with the goal of estimating the risk of DCIS progression to invasive ductal cancer and the likelihood of a recurrence. The van Nuys score is based on nuclear grade and the presence or absence of necrosis. Three groups are distinguished: low nuclear grade without necrosis (type 1), low nuclear grade with necrosis (type 2), and high nuclear grade with necrosis (type 3).

References and Further Reading

American College of Radiology. Practice Guideline for the Management of Ductal Carcinoma In-Situ of the Breast. http://www.acr.org/SecondaryMainMenuCategories/quality_saftey/guidelines/breast/mri_breast.aspx (accessed January 7, 2011)

Bazzocchi M, Zuiani C, Panizza P, et al. Contrast-enhanced breast MRI in patients with suspicious microcalcifications on mammography: results of a multicenter trial. AJR 2006; 186: 1723–1732

Kreienberg R, Kopp I, Lorenz W, et al. Interdisciplinary S3 Guidelines for the Diagnosis, Treatment and Follow-up care of Breast Cancer. First updated version 2008. http://www.uni-duesseldorf.de/WWW/AWMF/ll/ (accessed November 10, 2010)

Perry N, Broeders M, de Wolf F, Törnberg S, Holland R, von Karsa L, eds. European Commission. European Guidelines for Quality Assurance in Breast Cancer Screening and Diagnosis. 4th ed. Cologne: Bundesanzeiger Verlag; 2006. http://www.euref.org/

Vag T, Baltzer PA, Renz DM, et al. Diagnosis of ductal carcinoma in situ using contrast-enhanced magnetic resonance mammography compared with conventional mammography. Clin Imaging 2008; 32: 438–442

4

Abdomen

Liver, Pancreas, and Retroperitoneum

Gastrointestinal Tract

Urogenital Tract

Complications of IV Contrast Infusion

History and Clinical Presentation

A 51-year-old man with left-sided nephrolithiasis and a double-J ureteral catheter underwent abdominal CT scanning before and after the IV administration of 150 mL of a nonionic contrast agent (**Fig. 4.1**). Immediately after the examination the patient began coughing and had areas of skin redness. There was no evidence of respiratory complaints or tachycardia. His symptoms were interpreted as an allergic reaction to the IV contrast agent and were treated by IV administration of 4 mg dimethindene, 50 mg ranitidine, and 250 mg methylprednisolone. Symptoms improved after this therapy. During the next 15 minutes the documented images were analyzed on the CT console, and the findings were discussed with the patient. By that time the patient was free of complaints and returned to the ward.

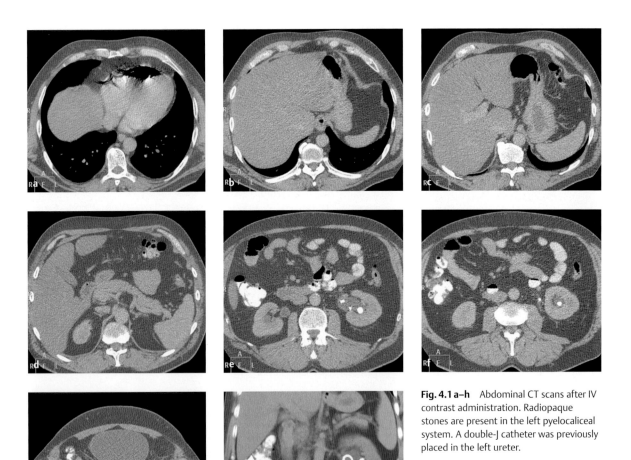

Fig. 4.1 a–h Abdominal CT scans after IV contrast administration. Radiopaque stones are present in the left pyelocaliceal system. A double-J catheter was previously placed in the left ureter.

Further Case Summary

The radiology report written immediately after the examination noted the presence of free air in the right ventricle (**Fig. 4.2**). This was immediately reported to the ward physician and patient. There was no mention of dyspnea, chest pain, or circulatory symptoms that would indicate clinically overt pulmonary embolism. The patient was closely monitored over the next few hours. Thoracic CT was performed 6 hours after the first examination and showed no air in the cardiac chambers or in pulmonary artery segments that were visible at CT (**Fig. 4.3**). The further clinical course was uneventful.

Error Analysis and Strategy for Error Prevention

The contrast dose of 150 mL was administered through an antecubital vein with a high-pressure injector at a flow rate of 3 mL/s. The high-pressure pump delivered the contrast agent from a sterile container through sterile tubing to a plastic IV catheter in the patient's arm. When the steps in the procedure were carefully reconstructed, it was concluded that the tubing had not been cleared of air before the injection was initiated, causing air to be injected into the patient's veins ahead of the contrast agent. The air passed through the veins of the shoulder girdle and the superior vena cava into the right heart. The resulting air embolism was responsible for the clinical symptoms (dyspnea, tachycardia). Small, asymptomatic air bubbles are occasionally observed after IV contrast injection. The intravascular air inclusions are distributed along the anterior vessel wall in a supine patient (**Fig. 4.4**).

References and Further Reading

Bundesinstitut für Arzneimittel und Medizinprodukte (BfArM). Luftembolien durch Kontrastmittelinjektoren. Referenz-Nr. 2198/04, Einstelldatum 18.09.2007. http://www.bfarm.de/cln_103/DE/Home/home_node.html (accessed November 10, 2010)

Mirski MA, Lele AV, Fitzsimmons L, Toung TJK. Diagnosis and treatment of vascular air embolism. Anesthesiology 2007; 106: 164–177

Palmon SC, Moore LE, Lundberg J, Toung T. Venous air embolism: a review. J Clin Anesth 1997; 9: 251–257

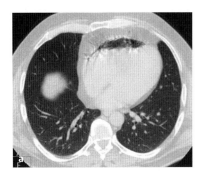
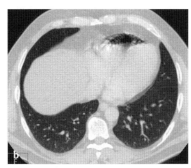
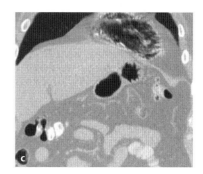

Fig. 4.2 a–c   Abnormal air in the right ventricle due to air embolism.

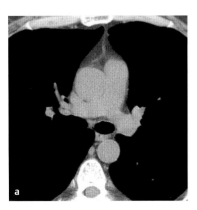
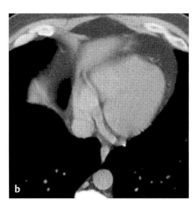

Fig. 4.3 a, b   Thoracic CT scans 6 hours after the first examination show normal appearance of the cardiac chambers and pulmonary artery with no air inclusions.

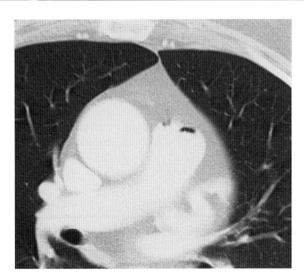

Fig. 4.4   Small air embolism in the main pulmonary artery of a different patient.

Venous Air Embolism

Venous air embolism is defined as the introduction of air into the right heart and pulmonary circulation, leading to systemic effects.

Causes. The most frequent causes are neurosurgical operations with the patient in a sitting position (pressure gradient between atmospheric pressure and the venous blood pressure in the heart) and the improper use or malfunction of venous infusion pumps. Two patients died in 2007 from the inadvertent injection of air with a high-pressure contrast injector (BfArM 2008). As far as the authors are aware, most high-pressure injectors available on the world market do not have adequate air-detection safeguards, making it imperative to test for air as described in the device operating instructions before proceeding with contrast injection.

Clinical manifestations. The morbidity and mortality of venous air embolism depend on the volume of air and its rate of entry into the venous circulation. Animal studies have shown that 0.5–0.8 mL of air per kg body weight (b.w.) is lethal in rabbits, while 7.5–15.0 mL of air/kg b.w. is lethal in dogs. Precise figures are unavailable in humans, but individual case reports indicate that the rapid venous injection of 200–300 mL of air, or 3–5 mL of air/kg b.w., is fatal to humans. The rate at which the air enters the venous circulation is important, as slow flow rates give the air time to disperse in the peripheral vasculature and become absorbed (see below). For example, dogs survived 1400 mL of air injected over a period of several hours.

There are two pathophysiologic mechanisms by which venous air embolism can lead to death:
- **Acute right heart failure.** When large amounts of air are inadvertently infused, an air bubble obstructs the right ventricular outflow tract, interrupting blood flow from the right ventricle into the pulmonary artery.
- **Respiratory failure.** The air may mix with blood, depending on the embolism volume and injection rate, causing air bubbles to enter the pulmonary circulation with the bloodstream. In the most favorable case these microemboli are absorbed in the periphery of the lung. In other cases, however, the bubbles may incite a clinically severe or fatal hypoxia. This results from a ventilation–perfusion mismatch caused by the induction of pulmonary arterial hypertension (vasoconstriction, peripheral circulatory obstruction by blood clots due to air-induced platelet aggregation), by diffusion abnormalities (pulmonary edema due to increased membrane permeability caused by release of toxic and inflammatory mediators), and by reactive bronchoconstriction.

Treatment. Air injection is discontinued at once. Asymptomatic patients should be monitored with ready access to resuscitation facilities, and symptomatic patients should receive adequate cardiovascular support (oxygen administration, resuscitation). Right heart catheterization and aspiration of air from the right ventricle may be advised in selected cases.

Thrombosis/Flow Effects

History and Clinical Findings

A 56-year-old woman underwent a hysterectomy for uterine cancer 3 years earlier. She was now diagnosed with a tumor on the right abdominal wall that was consistent with lymph node metastasis. Abdominal CT was requested for restaging. Besides the abdominal wall tumor, CT scans showed inhomogeneous opacification of the inferior vena cava, raising suspicion of thrombosis (**Fig. 4.5**).

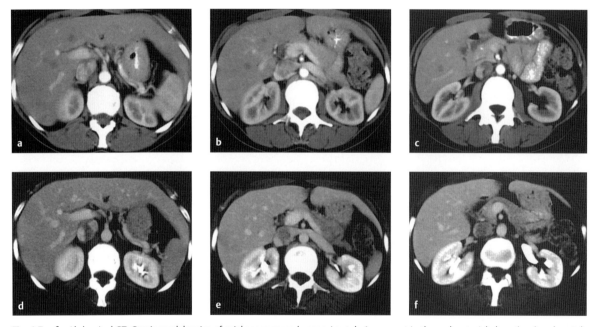

Fig. 4.5 a–f   Abdominal CT. Craniocaudal series of axial scans spaced approximately 1 cm apart in the early arterial phase (**a–c**) and portal venous phase (**d–f**) after IV contrast administration.

Further Case Summary

Duplex ultrasound scans proved that the inferior vena cava was clear and patent.

Error Analysis and Strategy for Error Prevention

The inhomogeneous densities in the immediate suprarenal portion of the inferior vena cava were caused by opacified blood from the renal veins (**Fig. 4.5 b, e**) mixing with nonopacified blood from the lower half of the body. A comparison of the images acquired in the early arterial phase and portal venous phase of hepatic perfusion shows a variability of densities in the same scan planes that would be inconsistent with filling defect caused by a solid thrombus.

To avoid diagnostic errors, it is important to note the time interval between contrast injection and image data acquisition as a function of cardiac output and flow velocity so that intravascular density changes can be correlated with specific phases of perfusion. In CT studies where data sets were acquired in different phases of enhancement, the imaging findings should be correlated with the physiology of organ and vascular perfusion.

Acute Cholecystitis/ Contraction of the Gallbladder

History and Clinical Findings

A 46-year-old man was hospitalized with pancytopenia, arthralgia, swollen lower limb joints, and fever spiking to 39 °C. His serum CRP had fallen from 77 mg/L to 55 mg/L in response to broad-spectrum antibiotics instituted by his family doctor. Serum AP, γGT, GOT, and LDH were elevated, while the haptoglobin level was low. GPT was normal. Paroxysmal hematuria had been excluded. The differential diagnosis included autoimmune hepatitis and possibly an infection or acute leukemia. Thoracic and abdominal CT scans mainly showed thickening and enhancement of the gallbladder wall (**Fig. 4.6a, b**) and fluid in the gallbladder bed (**Fig. 4.6a**). Both were interpreted as signs of acute cholecystitis. Additional findings were hepatosplenomegaly (**Fig. 4.6c**), splenic infarction, and bilateral nodular densities in the axillae, mediastinum, porta hepatis, hepatoduodenal ligament, and retroperitoneum, which were interpreted as lymphadenopathy due to an unknown cause.

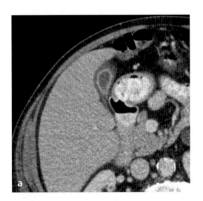
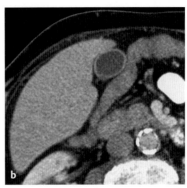
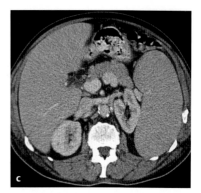

Fig. 4.6 a–c   Abdominal CT. Thickening and enhancement of the gallbladder wall and free fluid about the gallbladder prompted a diagnosis of acute cholecystitis (**a, b**). Hepatosplenomegaly is also present (**c**).

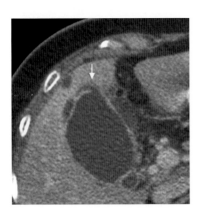

Fig. 4.7   CT appearance of perforated cholecystitis in a different patient. Note the thickening of the gallbladder wall, the defect in the wall of the fundus (arrow), and the presence of perivesicular fluid.

Further Case Summary

Histologic evaluation of tissue sampled from an axillary lymph node revealed T-cell non-Hodgkin lymphoma. Clinical findings were consistent with lymphomatous involvement of the liver, spleen, and axillary, mediastinal, retroperitoneal, and epigastric lymph nodes. The patient was placed on high-dose chemotherapy and underwent a splenectomy and stem-cell transplantation.

Error Analysis and Strategy for Error Prevention

The CT diagnosis of acute cholecystitis was wrong for several reasons:

- The patient had no history of gallstone disease and no clinical manifestations of acute cholecystitis (severe upper abdominal pain, Murphy sign). The clinical presentation (arthralgia, swollen leg joints, elevated liver transaminases, pancytopenia) and CT findings (hepatosplenomegaly, lymphadenopathy) were more consistent with an immune disorder or hematologic malignancy.

- The 3- to 4-mm thickness of the gallbladder wall was not a useful diagnostic criterion due to the minimal degree of gallbladder distension. Gallbladder hydrops was not present, and the gallbladder wall was not thickened. The apparent enhancement of the gallbladder wall was accentuated by the presence of hypoattenuating serous fluid around the gallbladder. Transudate in the perivesical peritoneal compartment may have various causes including hepatitis.

In a different patient 73 years of age, the clinical and CT findings were consistent with a diagnosis of cholecystitis (**Fig. 4.7**). Initial interpretation of the CT scans missed the discontinuity in the gallbladder wall indicating a perforated gallbladder. The diagnosis of acute cholecystitis with perforation of the gallbladder wall was finally confirmed at operation.

References and Further Reading

Zeman RK. Cholelithiasis and cholecystitis. In: Gore RM, Levine MS, Laufer I, eds. Textbook of Gastrointestinal Radiology. Volume II. Philadelphia: Saunders; 1994: 1636–1659

Acute Cholecystitis

Pathogenesis. In more than 95% of cases, acute cholecystitis develops as a complication of cholecystolithiasis. A gallstone may become impacted in the cystic duct, causing obstruction and stagnation of biliary flow. Intestinal bacteria such as *Escherichia coli*, enterococci, *Proteus mirabilis*, and *Klebsiella* species may migrate back through the bile ducts from the duodenum or via lymphatic pathways to reach the obstructed gallbladder. Less commonly, bacteria are excreted from the liver into the bile and reach the gallbladder by the antegrade route. The bacteria incite an inflammation of the gallbladder wall. Inflammatory wall edema further narrows the residual lumen of the cystic duct, resulting in gallbladder hydrops (maximum transverse diameter of the gallbladder >4 cm). Less frequent causes of acute cholecystitis are ischemia of the cystic artery, which may result from chemoembolization of the hepatic artery or toxic exposure, for example. Possible complications are ischemia and transmural necrosis of the gallbladder wall, inflammatory exudation and abscess formation in the perivesical peritoneal cavity, and hepatic abscess.

Clinical manifestations. Acute cholecystitis typically begins with severe abdominal pain in the right upper quadrant accompanied by nausea and vomiting. Extreme tenderness to pressure may be elicited below the right costal margin during inspiration as the inflamed gallbladder comes into contact with the examiner's fingers (Murphy sign).

Imaging. The imaging study of choice is ultrasound, which typically reveals gallstones, thickening of the gallbladder wall to >4 mm in fasted patients, stratification of the gallbladder wall, and fluid in the gallbladder bed. A Murphy sign can be elicited with the ultrasound transducer under visual control. The criteria for acute cholecystitis on CT scans are the same as in ultrasound.

Normal Findings/Zonal Fatty Infiltration of the Liver/Hepatic Metastasis

History and Clinical Findings

A 31-year-old man had had a superficial spreading melanoma removed from his right hand. The tumor was ulcerated. The Breslow thickness was 2.4 mm and the T stage was classified as IIb. Two years later a lymph node metastasis was surgically removed from the right axilla. Abdominal ultrasound during a routine follow-up visit 1 year later showed two hypoechoic masses with a maximum diameter of 1 cm located in the central portion of the right lobe of the liver (**Fig. 4.8**). The sonographic diagnosis was checked by ambulatory CT, which showed an ill-defined lesion at the center of the hepatic right lobe. This lesion was interpreted as benign (**Fig. 4.9**). Because of the discrepancy between sonographic and CT findings, ambulatory MRI was performed and was interpreted as normal (**Fig. 4.10**).

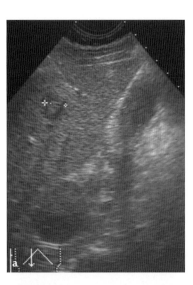
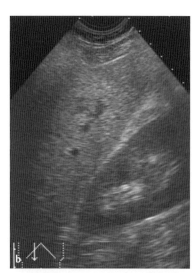

Fig. 4.8 a, b Abdominal ultrasound demonstrates two masses in the right lobe of the liver, which were interpreted as metastases.

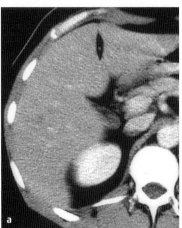
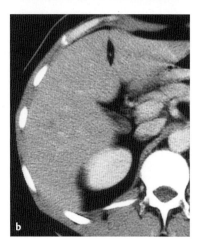

Fig. 4.9 a, b CT scans with a slice thickness of 10 mm. The images show an ill-defined central lesion in the right lobe of the liver, which was interpreted as benign.
a Early arterial phase after IV contrast administration.
b Portal venous phase after IV contrast administration.

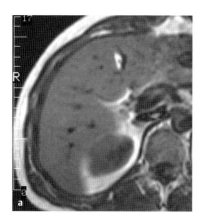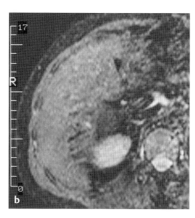

Fig. 4.10 a, b   MRI using a 10-mm slice thickness and the T1 sequences indicated below. Image documentation appeared to show that no postcontrast images were obtained. The report indicated no abnormalities.
a   T1-weighted sequence.
b   T1-weighted fat-suppressed STIR sequence.

Further Case Summary

Abdominal ultrasound was repeated approximately 4 weeks later (**Fig. 4.11**). These scans showed three hypoechoic masses in the right lobe of the liver. The two initial masses had doubled in diameter. The further course confirmed hematogenous metastasis. The patient died 1 year later from disseminated disease despite combination chemotherapy and chemoimmunotherapy.

Error Analysis and Strategy for Error Prevention

The following factors caused the two sonographically visible hepatic metastases to be missed or misinterpreted at CT and MRI:

- Ultrasound, CT, and MRI utilize different physical tissue properties to produce an image (ultrasound—acoustic impedance; CT—x-ray attenuation; MRI—proton density ϱ, T1 and T2 relaxation times, etc.). The detectability of a parenchymal lesion depends on its size and its contrast with surrounding structures. The smaller the lesion, the greater the contrast must be to obtain visualization. Because the various imaging modalities are based on different underlying physical principles, small masses may occasionally be demonstrated better by ultrasound than by CT or MRI, and vice versa.

- A slice thickness of 10 mm is unsuitable for defining a mass less than 15 mm in diameter (**Fig. 4.12**). It is unlikely that the lesion will be completely visualized in a single slice. More commonly, smaller masses are partially visualized in two adjacent slices. When the signals in two adjacent voxels are averaged together, they yield an altered signal value that does not correspond to reality (partial volume averaging), and the contrast with surrounding structures becomes too low for visual detection (**Fig. 4.13**).

- The MRI examination technique did not conform to medical requirements. Because MRI, unlike ultrasound and CT, is based on multiple tissue parameters, at least one T1-weighted and one T2-weighted sequence must

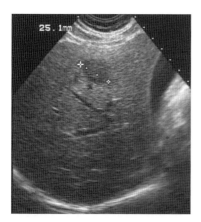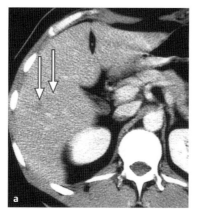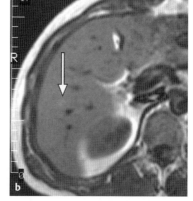

Fig. 4.11   Ultrasound follow-up 4 weeks after initial examination shows an enlarging hypoechoic mass, which proved to be a hepatic metastasis.

Fig. 4.12 a, b   Explanations for **Figs. 4.9 a** and **4.10 b**.
a   CT scan in the early arterial phase shows two hypodense masses with ill-defined margins in the right lobe of the liver (arrows). The large slice thickness made it more difficult to detect the two masses and hampered their benign/malignant differentiation.
b   MRI shows a rounded hyperintense feature in the right lobe of the liver (arrow). Metastatic melanomas may have high signal intensity on T1-weighted images, depending on their melanin content.

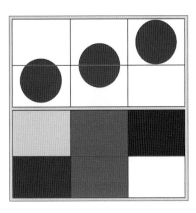

Fig. 4.13 Partial volume averaging. Top row: acquisition matrix; bottom row: display matrix. The processor determines the gray level of a pixel by averaging the densities of the structures within the pixel according to their relative volumes.

be obtained to exploit all contrast options and fully evaluate the region of interest. In the present case, a T2-weighted sequence was omitted. The fat-suppressed T1-weighted sequence could not be interpreted due to respiratory artifacts. Also, the documentation appears to indicate that images were not acquired after IV contrast administration.

■ Superficial spreading melanoma contains melanin. This accounts for the hyperintense appearance of the metastasis on T1-weighted MRI (**Fig. 4.12**), which is otherwise unusual for a tumor (differential diagnosis: hematoma, calcification).

References and Further Reading

American College of Radiology. ACR Practice Guidelines for Performing and Interpreting Diagnostic Computed Tomography (CT). http://www.acr.org/SecondaryMainMenuCategories/quality_safety/guidelines/dx/ctperforming_interpreting.aspx (accessed January 7, 2011)

American College of Radiology. ACR Practice Guidelines for Performing and Interpreting Diagnostic Magnetic Resonance Imaging (MRI). http://www.acr.org/SecondaryMainMenuCategories/quality_safety/guidelines/dx.aspx (accessed November 10, 2010)

American College of Radiology. ACR Appropriateness Criteria. Suspected Liver Metastases. http://www.acr.org/SecondaryMainMenuCategories/quality_safety/app_criteria/pdf/ExpertPanelonGastrointestinalImaging/SuspectedLiverMetastasesDoc14.aspx (accessed November 10, 2010)

Eisenhauer EA, Therasse P, Bogaerts J, et al. New response evaluation criteria in solid tumours: revised RECIST guideline (version 1.1). Eur J Cancer 2009; 45: 228–247

Therasse P, Arbuck SG, Eisenhauer EA, et al. New guidelines to evaluate the response to treatment in solid tumors. European Organization for Research and Treatment of Cancer, National Cancer Institute of the United States, National Cancer Institute of Canada. J Natl Cancer Inst 2000; 92: 205–216

Malignant Melanoma

The incidence of malignant melanoma in Central Europe is 10–12 new cases per 100 000 population per year. Various types of melanoma are distinguished clinically and histologically: superficial spreading melanoma (SSM), nodular melanoma, lentigo maligna melanoma, acral lentiginous melanoma. SSM tends to undergo early lymphogenous and hematogenous metastasis. Today approximately 90% of all melanomas are diagnosed as primary tumors without detectable metastasis.

Prognosis. The main prognostic factors in the initial diagnosis of malignant melanoma without metastasis are the Breslow vertical tumor thickness, the Clark level of invasion (**Table 4.1**), and the presence of histologically detectable ulceration (**Table 4.2**).

A tumor thickness > 1 mm, histologic ulceration, and a high Clark level are unfavorable prognostic signs. Malignant melanoma may undergo primary lymphogenous as well as primary hematogenous metastasis. Approximately two-thirds of all first metastases are confined initially to regional lymphatics. The prognosis becomes much worse when lymphogenous metastasis occurs (stage III disease). Hematogenous metastasis (stage IV disease) implies a grave prognosis even when the most modern surgical, immunochemotherapeutic, and radiotherapeutic options are employed. The scope and frequency of follow-up examinations depend on the tumor stage, clinical findings, and serum levels of the S100 tumor marker (see p. 221).

Table 4.1 Clark levels for describing the depth of skin invasion by melanoma

Clark level	Stage of invasion
1	Melanoma confined to the epidermis (melanoma in situ)
2	Invasion into the papillary dermis
3	Invasion to the junction of the papillary and reticular dermis
4	Invasion of the reticular dermis
5	Invasion into the subcutaneous fat

Table 4.2 Staging of malignant melanoma with pathologic criteria (adapted from American Joint Committee on Cancer [AJCC] criteria, 2002)

Stage	Primary tumor (pT)	Regional lymph node metastasis (N)	Distant metastasis (M)
0	In situ melanoma	None	None
IA	1.0 mm, no ulceration	None	None
IB	1.0 mm, with ulceration or Clark level 4/5	None	None
	1.01–2.0 mm without ulceration	None	None
IIA	1.01–2.0 mm with ulceration 2.01–4.0 mm without ulceration	None	None
IIB	2.01–4.0 mm with ulceration >4.0 mm without ulceration	None	None
IIC	>4.0 mm with ulceration	None	None
IIIA	Any tumor thickness without ulceration	Microscopic metastasis in one regional lymph node; microsopic nodal metastasis in two or three regional lymph nodes	None
IIIB	Any tumor thickness with ulceration	Microscopic metastasis in one regional lymph node; microsopic nodal metastasis in two or three regional lymph nodes; satellite or in-transit metastasis without regional nodal metastasis	None
	Any tumor thickness without ulceration	Macroscopic metastasis in one regional lymph node; macrosopic nodal metastasis in two or three regional lymph nodes; satellite or in-transit metastasis without regional nodal metastasis	None
IIIC	Any tumor thickness with ulceration; any	Macroscopic metastasis in one regional lymph node; macrosopic nodal metastasis in two or three regional lymph nodes	None
	Any tumor thickness ± ulceration	Metastasis in four or more regional lymph nodes	None
IV	Any tumor thickness ± ulceration	Any lymph node involvlement	Distant metastasis

RECIST 1.1 Criteria

According to the Response Evaluation Criteria in Solid Tumors (RECIST), the response of a tumor to treatment can be evaluated radiologically if the baseline CT and/or MRI examination is performed no more than 4 weeks before the start of treatment using a slice thickness no greater than 5 mm. At least one measurable lesion (target lesion, TL) must be present in the baseline evaluation. The longest extranodal diameter of the TL must be 10 mm or more, and the shortest nodal diameter must be 15 mm or more. TLs are defined as the largest lesions that can be reproducibly measured. Up to two TLs can be defined per organ region, and up to five TLs per patient. The basis for the evaluation is the sum of the diameters of all the TLs. Non-target lesions (NTLs) are defined as measurable lesions that were not defined as TLs, all lymph nodes from 10 to <15 mm in their short-axis diameter, and all nonmeasurable lesions (pleural carcinomatosis, peritoneal carcinomatosis, etc.). All NTLs should be included in the radiology report, and any size changes in these lesions should be noted during follow-ups.

The response criteria for target lesions are defined as follows:
- Complete response (CR) = disappearance of all TLs, maximum short-axis diameter of target lymph nodes <10 mm
- Partial response (PR) = at least a 30% decrease in the sum of the diameters of all the TLs
- Progressive disease (PD) = at least a 20% increase in the sum of the diameters of the TLs, at least a 5 mm increase in the sum of the diameters of the TLs
- Stable disease (SD) = neither more than a 30% decrease nor more than a 20% increase in the sum of the TL diameters

The following response criteria are used in the evaluation of non-target lesions:
- Complete response (CR) = disappearance of all NTLs (except lymph nodes)
- Stable disease (SD) = persistence of one or more NTLs
- Progressive disease (PD) = progression of NTLs or appearance of one or more new lesions on CT and/or MRI, new NTLs on FDG/PET compared with the baseline FDG/PET, and/or new NTLs on FDG/PET with a CT correlate when baseline FDG/PET is not available

Colon Cancer/Metastasis/ Inflammatory Pseudotumor

History and Clinical Findings

A 56-year-old man had undergone a bilobectomy 12 years earlier for a right-sided bronchial carcinoma (pT1 N0 M0). A chest radiograph on routine follow-up showed a new pulmonary nodule in the apical segment of the lower lobe of the right lung, which was scheduled for removal by segmentectomy (**Fig. 4.14**). The differential diagnosis included a pulmonary metastasis or a new, second bronchial carcinoma. Preoperative staging concluded with abdominal CT scans, which showed an area of increased tissue density near the right colic flexure with streaking of the surrounding mesenteric fat and perihepatic ascites (**Fig. 4.15**). Colonoscopy was incomplete due to a high-grade stenosis in the right transverse colon. A contrast enema 4 days later showed an eccentric stenosis of the right transverse colon and right flexure with wall rigidity arising from the mesocolic attachment and irregularity of the colon wall (**Fig. 4.16**). A review of the history, clinical findings, and radiologic findings yielded a preoperative diagnosis of colon cancer with local peritoneal carcinomatosis and a solitary pulmonary metastasis.

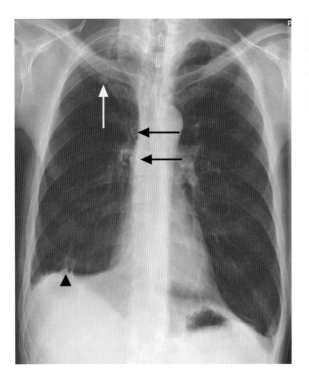

Fig. 4.14 Chest radiograph. The patient underwent a previous right upper bilobectomy for lung cancer. Current findings include elevation of the hemidiaphragm, pleural adhesions at the base of the residual lung (arrowhead), and suture material projected over the right hilum (black arrows). A nodule (white arrow) is projected over the apical segment of the right lower lobe, which occupies a right infraclavicular site following the bilobectomy.

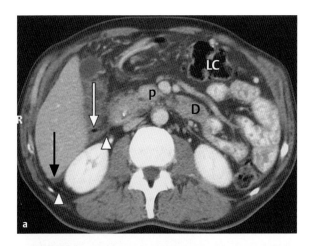

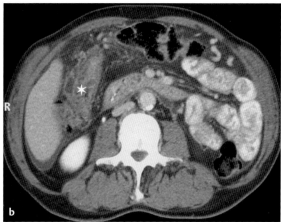

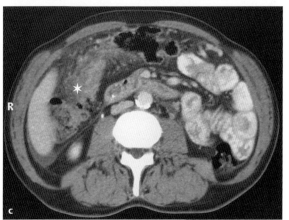

Fig. 4.15 a–c   Abdominal CT shows an area of increased tissue density near the right colic flexure with streaking of the surrounding mesenteric fat and pericolic air. Perihepatic ascites is also present.
Arrows = ascites; D = duodenum; LC = left colic flexure; P = pancreas; ✱ = inflammatory pseudotumor.

Further Case Summary

A right hemicolectomy was performed. Histologic evaluation showed a perforated inflammatory pseudotumor arising from chronic pancreatitis. A right pneumonectomy was subsequently performed. Histology indicated a stage pT1 N0 M0 bronchial carcinoma. Careful questioning of the patient revealed that he had suffered an episode of pancreatitis during the previous year. Serum pancreatic amylase at the time of the operation was 150 U/L (< 65 U/L is normal) and serum lipase was 338 U/L (< 190 U/L is normal).

Error Analysis and Strategy for Error Prevention

Given the patient's cancer history, an acute exacerbation of chronic pancreatitis was not considered during interpretation of the abdominal CT scans. Because a systematic analysis of all organs and organ regions was not performed, enlargement of the pancreatic head and thickening of the pararenal fascia went unnoticed (**Fig. 4.17**). Imbibition of the mesenteric fibrofatty tissue by inflammatory pancreatic exudate was misinterpreted as a solid mass, and the ascites was considered to have a neoplastic rather than inflammatory cause.

References and Further Reading

Schaefer-Prokop C. Pancreas. In: Prokop M, Galanski M, eds. Computed Tomography of the Body. Stuttgart: Thieme; 2003

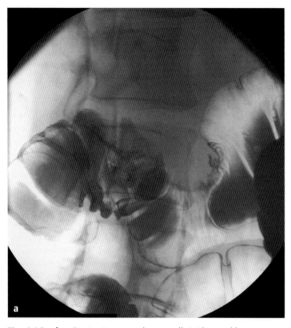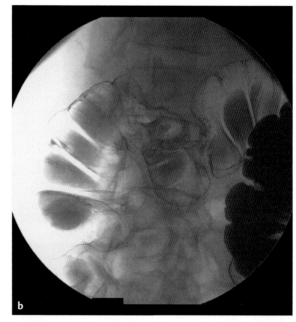

Fig. 4.16 a, b Contrast enema shows wall rigidity and long segmental narrowing of the colonic lumen with apparent spiculation of the colon wall in the area of the mesocolic attachment to the right flexure and right transverse colon.

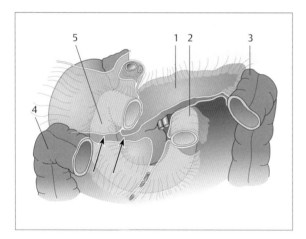

Fig. 4.17 Diagrammatic representation of the anatomic pathway (arrows) by which inflammatory exudate in pancreatitis can spread across the mesenteric root to the transverse colon and right colic flexure.
1 Pancreas
2 Jejunum
3 Left colic flexure
4 Right colic flexure
5 Duodenum

CT Signs of Acute Pancreatitis and an Acute Exacerbation of Chronic Pancreatitis

- Circumscribed or diffuse increase in pancreatic volume
- Indistinct organ margins
- Inhomogeneous parenchymal structure after IV contrast administration (demarcation of necrotic areas)
- Increased density of retroperitoneal and mesenteric fibrofatty tissue (imbibition by inflammatory pancreatic exudate)

- Retroperitoneal and mesenteric abscesses
- Thickening of the pararenal fascia
- Widening of adjacent bowel segments (inflammatory involvement)
- Ascites
- Parenchymal calcifications (chronic pancreatitis)

Cystic Pancreatic Carcinoma/Pancreatic Cystadenoma/ Inflammatory Pancreatic or Peripancreatic Pseudotumor

History and Clinical Findings

A 36-year-old woman complained of upper abdominal pain of recent onset. Ultrasound revealed a mass in the mid-upper abdomen. CT localized the mass to the junction of the head and body of the pancreas (**Fig. 4.18**). The mass showed peripheral contrast enhancement and central necrosis. It appeared to be continuous with the pancreatic head and body and extended anterolaterally into the peripancreatic fibrofatty tissue and along the hepatic artery into the porta hepatis. The mass was new relative to an examination that had been done 1 year earlier for the follow-up of pulmonary tuberculosis (**Fig. 4.19**). The overall impression was of a cystic pancreatic mass that could be carcinoma or an inflammatory pancreatic pseudotumor.

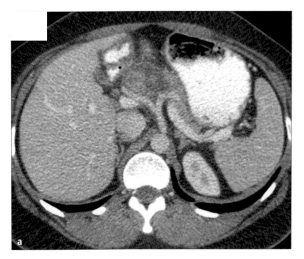
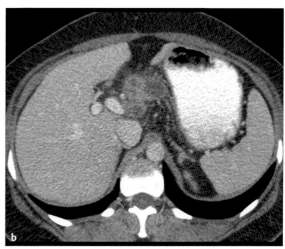

Fig. 4.18 a, b   Abdominal CT demonstrates a peripherally enhancing mass with central necrosis in the head of the pancreas.

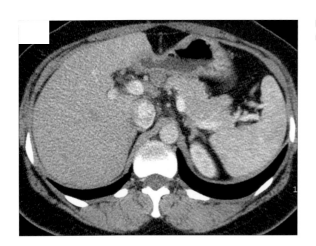

Fig. 4.19   Abdominal CT scan 1 year earlier was interpreted as normal.

Further Case Summary

Microbiologic analysis of an ultrasound-guided biopsy of the pancreatic mass yielded a diagnosis of tuberculosis. The CT examination was reevaluated in the light of this finding. Coronal and sagittal reformations of the image data showed that the inflammatory pseudotumor was abutting the outer surface of the pancreas (**Fig. 4.20**). A 2-year-old prior examination indicated cavitating pulmonary tuberculosis with axillary, mediastinal and peripancreatic lymph node involvement (**Fig. 4.21**). A review of past and present CT scans showed that all the features of peripancreatic tuberculous lymphadenitis had been present in the 2-year-old images and had largely resolved 1 year before the current examination, leaving an approximately 1-cm residual mass. This mass was located at the center of the inflammatory pseudotumor detected by current CT. Thus, reactivated peripancreatic tuberculous lymphadenitis was diagnosed by exclusion.

Error Analysis and Strategy for Error Prevention

The inflammatory pseudotumor was misinterpreted as a pancreatic tumor because:
- The CT image data had not been reformatted perpendicular to the axial scans (**Fig. 4.20**)
- The residual peripancreatic lymph node in the 1-year-old prior examination (**Fig. 4.19**) had been missed
- The 2-year-old prior examination (**Fig. 4.21**) had not been reviewed for comparison

Tuberculosis of peripancreatic lymph nodes can be diagnosed radiologically only by taking into account the history and clinical findings and any additional findings, and if necessary by comparison with prior examinations. Otherwise an enhancing peripancreatic mass with central necrosis will have a broad differential diagnosis based on imaging features alone. If doubt exists, a CT-guided or ultrasound-guided biopsy should be obtained for microbio-

Peripancreatic and Pancreatic Tuberculosis

Primary tuberculosis, which most commonly affects the lungs and occasionally the gastrointestinal tract, may be followed by postprimary tuberculosis that affects other organs due to hematogenous spread. Common sites of involvement are organs with a copious blood supply such as the kidneys, lymphatic system, liver, spleen, or meninges. Solitary organ involvement in the setting of postprimary tuberculosis is rare. Occasionally, postprimary tuberculosis can be difficult to distinguish from other conditions based on its imaging features alone.

Epidemiology. A total of 40612 cases of pancreatic cancer and 7359 cases of tuberculosis were reported in Germany in 2005. Based on WHO data for the year 2010, the incidence of tuberculosis was 29/100000 inhabitants in the Americas and 340/100000 inhabitants in Africa; the corresponding mortality rates 2/100000 inhabitants for the Americas and 50/100000 inhabit-

ants for Africa. In 2003–2007, the incidence of invasive pancreatic carcinoma was 13/100000 inhabitants in the USA. Accordingly, the majority of masses involving the pancreas are pancreatic carcinoma, with 60–70% of tumors occurring in the pancreatic head. Rare entities in the differential diagnosis of pancreatic masses are pseudotumors due to pancreatitis, cystadenomas, cystadenocarcinomas, neuroendocrine tumors, and hematogenous metastases. Hematogenous pancreatic tuberculosis and peripancreatic tuberculous lymphadenopathy are also rare. For example, no cases of pancreatic involvement were reported in an autopsy series of 300 patients with miliary tuberculosis in India. In a second autopsy series, only 3 of 112 patients with abdominal tuberculosis were found to have pancreatic involvement. In an overview of 1656 autopsies performed in tuberculosis patients, pancreatic tuberculosis was described in 5% of the cases.

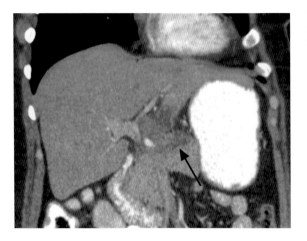

Fig. 4.20   Angled coronal reformation of the CT data set documents the peripancreatic location of the inflammatory pseudotumor (arrow).

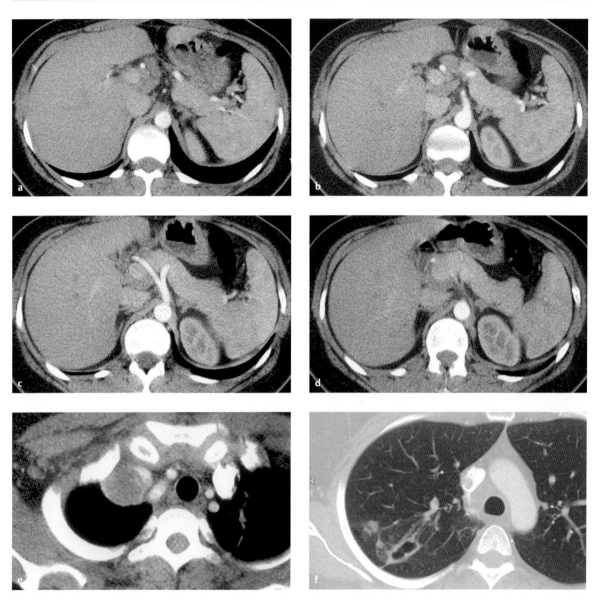

Fig. 4.21 a–f Two-year-old CT scans of the chest and abdomen show peripancreatic (**a–d**) and mediastinal (**e**) tuberculous lymphadenitis accompanied by exudative cavitating pulmonary tuberculosis (**f**).

References and Further Reading

CDC Centers of Disease Control and Prevention. Department of Health and Human Services. National program of Cancer Registries (NPCR). United States Cancer Statistics (USCS). http://apps.nccd.cdc.gov/uscs/cancersbyraceand-ethnicity.aspx (accessed January 16, 2011)

Cherian JV, Somasundaram A, Ponnusamy RP, Venkataraman J. Peripancreatic tuberculous lymphadenopathy. An impostor posing diagnostic difficulty. J Pancreas 2007; 8: 326–329

Itaba S, Yoshinaga S, Nakamura K, et al. Endoscopic ultrasound-guided fine-needle aspiration for the diagnosis of peripancreatic tuberculous lymphadenitis. J Gastroenterol 2007; 42: 83–86

Teo LLS, Venkatesh SK, Ho KY. Clinics in diagnostic imaging. Singapore Med J 2007; 48: 687–692

World Health Organization (WHO). Tuberculosis. Fact sheet No. 104, November 2010. http://www.who.int/mediacentre/factsheets/fs104/en/index.html (accessed January 16, 2011)

Retroperitoneal Lymph Node Metastases

History and Clinical Findings

A 33-year-old man was hospitalized in the urology department with right-sided flank pain of acute onset. Four days later an intravenous pyelogram (IVP) was obtained to exclude nephrolithiasis and was declared to be normal (**Fig. 4.22**).

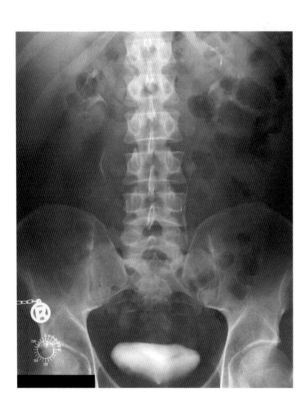

Fig. 4.22 Intravenous pyelogram, interpreted as normal.

Further Case Summary

Just 3 days before intravenous pyelography, abdominal CT was performed and showed a 3-cm precaval, infrarenal mass of soft-tissue density that was compressing the inferior vena cava (**Fig. 4.23**). Given the age and sex of the patient, the differential diagnosis of primary and secondary neoplasms included the lymphogenous metastasis of a malignant testicular tumor. The further course confirmed a metastatic seminoma.

Error Analysis and Strategy for Error Prevention

An IVP was not indicated in this case because all clinical questions could be answered much more accurately by CT.

Image interpretation. Displacement of the right ureter by a lymph node metastasis at the L4 level provided indirect evidence of the tumor on the pyelogram (**Fig. 4.24**). The clinical question (lithiasis) had directed attention away from that finding.

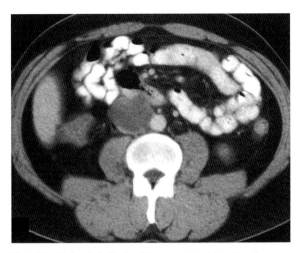

Fig. 4.23 Abdominal CT after IV contrast administration demonstrates a precaval lymph node metastasis from a testicular seminoma.

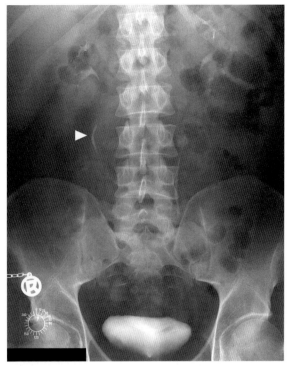

Fig. 4.24 Closer scrutiny of the IVP shows displacement of the right ureter by the lymph node metastasis at the level of the L4 vertebral body (arrowhead).

Organizational issues. The IVP was obtained without awareness of the CT scans taken 3 days earlier. This was due to organizational deficiencies:

- CT and intravenous pyelography were performed in different sections of the radiology department, which at that time did not have a radiology information system (RIS).
- Uncritical forwarding of the IVP request by the ward staff.

The following steps may help to avoid comparable diagnostic errors:

Systematic image analysis:

- Position, shape, and size of both kidneys, the pelvicaliceal system, the ureters, and the urinary bladder
- Inferior borders of the liver and spleen, psoas margins, the gallbladder, the major vessels, the lesser pelvis, and any calcifications projected over the excretory portion of the urinary tract
- Ribs, thoracic and lumbar spine, pelvic skeleton, femora, sacroiliac and hip joints

Organizational issues. An uncritical acceptance of clinical requests without studying the patient's medical record or talking with the patient or referring doctor carries the risk of unnecessary duplication of examinations. Before an im-

aging procedure is performed, it should be determined what clinical question is still unanswered and whether the selected procedure is capable of answering that question.

Lymphogenous Metastasis of Testicular Tumors

The lymphogenous metastasis of testicular tumors occurs along the testicular vein to the lymph nodes of the ipsilateral renal hilum (station 1, sentinel node) and continues through the aortointercaval lymph nodes to the lymph nodes of the contralateral renal hilum and the lymph nodes of the upper retroperitoneum, the mediastinum, and the retro- and supraclavicular nodes. Primary involvement of the aortointercaval and contralateral hilar lymph nodes via congenital collaterals is rare (approximately 8%). This pattern may be altered by previous inguinal or pelvic surgery.

Normal Findings/ Retroperitoneal Lymphomas

History and Clinical Findings

A 30-year-old woman experienced an unexplained weight loss of 12 kg over a 6-month period and presented with a body weight of 46 kg. Retroperitoneal lymphomas were diagnosed by ambulatory abdominal CT (**Fig. 4.25**).

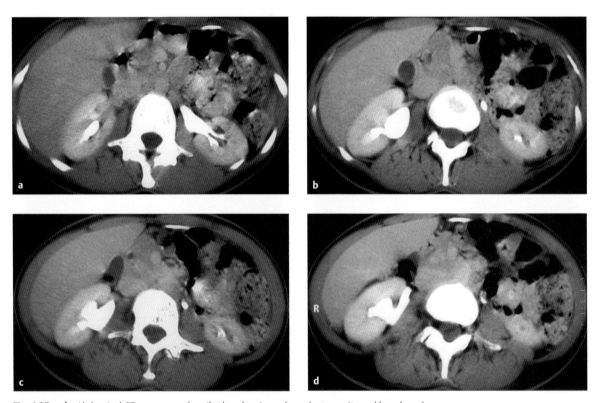

Fig. 4.25 a–d   Abdominal CT scans were described as showing enlarged retroperitoneal lymph nodes.

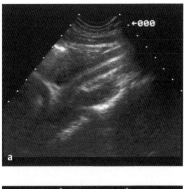

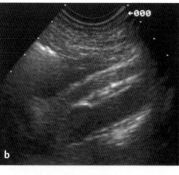

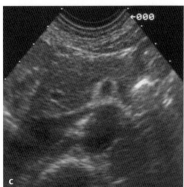

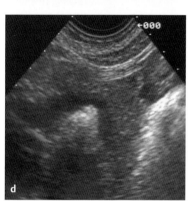

Fig. 4.26 a–d   Abdominal ultrasound shows no abnormalities.
a   Longitudinal scan through the suprarenal aorta.
b   Longitudinal scan through the infrarenal aorta.
c   Transverse scan of the pancreatic head and tail.
d   Transverse scan of the pancreatic tail.

Further Case Summary

The patient was hospitalized and underwent routine staging abdominal ultrasound, which was negative (**Fig. 4.26**). Since the scanning conditions were excellent (thin patient, no overlying bowel gas), MRI was not performed. All laboratory values were within normal limits. A somatic cause could not be found for the weight loss. Based on a psychological consultation into possible psychosomatic etiology, the weight loss was finally attributed to a self-imposed diet.

Error Analysis and Strategy for Error Prevention

The erroneous CT diagnosis resulted from the fact that fluid-filled bowel loops had not been opacified with contrast medium during the CT examination and were poorly delineated from one another due to a paucity of fat. This caused them to mimic the appearance of solid masses.

Complete bowel opacification with oral contrast is particularly useful in thin patients who have little retroperitoneal and mesenteric fat to provide intrinsic contrast for delineating anatomic structures. If necessary, the patient should drink additional contrast medium just before the examination or a second series of images should be acquired after a delay. In the interpretation of small, solid retroperitoneal masses, inadequate bowel opacification should be considered as a potential source of errors in image analysis, especially in very thin patients.

Hematoma/ Malignant Lymphoma/ Complicated Renal Cysts

History and Clinical Findings

A 58-year-old man experienced sudden, stabbing pain in the right upper quadrant of the abdomen. The character of the pain changed during the next two days. The patient was hospitalized with suspicion of kidney stones. Ultrasound showed a large, partially solid and partially liquid mass in the right upper abdomen. Complicated renal cysts were considered as an initial diagnosis. Subsequent CT showed a mesenteric mass of soft-tissue density located predominantly in the right upper quadrant (**Fig. 4.27**), raising suspicion of a malignant lymphoma. The patient was then referred to the surgery center for an excisional biopsy.

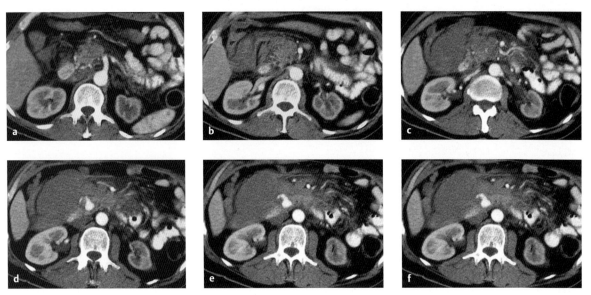

Fig. 4.27 a–f Abdominal CT shows a mesenteric mass that was initially interpreted as malignant lymphoma.

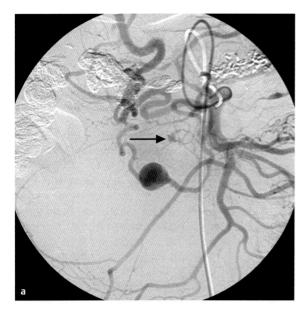
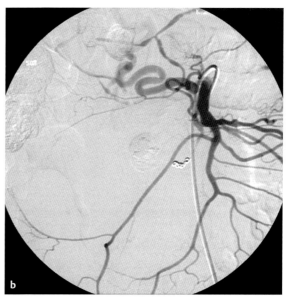

Fig. 4.28 a, b   Intra-arterial DSA demonstrates an approximately 2-cm aneurysm of the gastroduodenal artery and an approximately 5-mm aneurysm in the gastroduodenal arcade (**a**, arrow). The aneurysms were embolized with Ethibloc and microcoils (**b**).

a Preinterventional angiogram.
b Angiogram after embolization of both aneurysms.

Further Case Summary

When the CT images were reviewed during the preoperative surgical conference, the circumscribed dilatation of an artery with contrast extravasation was noted in the region of the gastroduodenal artery (**Fig. 4.27 e**), suggesting a hematoma arising from a perforated visceral artery aneurysm. Subsequent color duplex sonography confirmed this diagnosis. Intra-arterial digital subtraction angiography (DSA) revealed a larger aneurysm of the gastroduodenal artery and a smaller aneurysm of the gastroduodenal arcade as the source of the bleeding (**Fig. 4.28 a**). Both aneurysms were occluded with microcoils at interventional radiology (**Fig. 4.28 b**). The patient made a good recovery. He was clinically and radiologically stable at 5-year follow-up.

Error Analysis and Strategy for Error Prevention

The diagnosis of malignant lymphoma was not supported by the history, urologic ultrasound findings, the size of the mass detectable by CT, or the absence of lymph node enlargement in other body regions. Dilatation of the gastroduodenal artery was missed on initial interpretation of the CT scans.

References and Further Reading

Jörgensen M, Prokop M. Peritoneal cavity and retroperitonenum. In: Prokop M, Galanski M eds. Computed tomography of the body. Stuttgart: Thieme; 2003

Complication of Percutaneous Transhepatic Cholangiodrainage

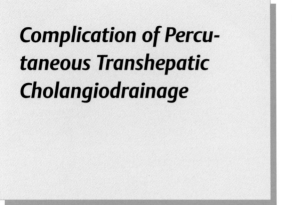

History and Clinical Findings

A 64-year-old woman was referred for endoscopic retrograde cholangiography (ERC) for the investigation of progressive extrahepatic cholestasis. The patient suffered from malignant B-cell lymphoma with thoracic and abdominal lymphomas and was in the terminal stage of that disease. Sectional imaging studies were not available. Endoscopy encountered an impassable duodenal stricture, and the examination had to be discontinued. It was then decided to proceed with percutaneous transhepatic cholangiodrainage (PTCD) so that the patient could be returned the next day with an internal biliary stent.

During PTCD, the dilated intrahepatic bile ducts in the right lobe were first opacified through a percutaneous fine needle (**Fig. 4.29**). Then a needle was inserted directly into a dilated bile duct in the right lobe. Contrast medium was injected, showing dilatation of the intrahepatic ducts (**Fig. 4.31**). A long segment of the common bile duct was found to be occluded. A guidewire and catheter were advanced through the obstruction (**Fig. 4.30**). The tip of the guidewire was placed within the duodenum, and three self-expanding stents were introduced over the guidewire. The lumen of the hepatic duct was expanded to 10 mm with a balloon-tipped catheter. Postinterventional imaging confirmed that contrast medium injected through the transhepatic catheter drained well through the recanalized hepatic duct and into the duodenum. There was no evidence of bleeding as the catheter was withdrawn. The percutaneous sheath was removed and the needle tract in the hepatic parenchyma was sealed with Gelfoam.

Approximately 4 hours later the patient developed the clinical manifestations of an acute abdomen.

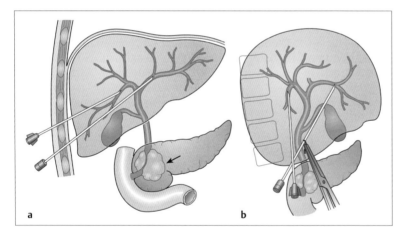

Fig. 4.29 a, b Principle of percutaneous transhepatic cholangiography.
a AP view. Arrow = tumor.
b Lateral view.

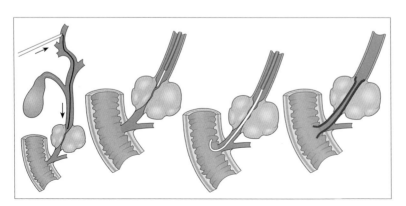

Fig. 4.30 Principle of percutaneous transhepatic cholangiodrainage (PTCD). Arrows = direction of catheterization.

Further Case Summary

Abdominal CT was indicated to investigate the cause of the acute abdomen (biliary peritonitis, internal bleeding, bowel ischemia due to an unknown cause, etc.). However, the patient's condition deteriorated so rapidly in the next hour that no additional tests could be performed. The patient died 7 hours after the end of the intervention with clinical signs of an acute abdomen and pulmonary edema. The family did not consent to autopsy.

Error Analysis and Strategy for Error Prevention

Since an autopsy was not performed, the cause of death remains speculative. The fulminating course is more consistent with a toxic process than a septic one. In retrospect, the fatal outcome of the intervention most likely resulted

from bile leakage into the perihepatic peritoneal cavity through the needle tract, inciting a toxic irritation that led to biliary peritonitis. It is reasonable to assume that when drainage had been restored by the interventional procedure, sludge in the intrahepatic bile ducts was flushed into the common hepatic duct and obstructed it. Since the liver is intraperitoneal except for its contact area with the diaphragm (bare area) and the insertion of the falciform ligament (**Fig. 4.32**), the resulting rise of intraluminal pressure pushed the bile back through the needle tract into the peritoneal cavity. It was a mistake to remove the sheath after the intervention. Left indwelling, it would have sealed the needle track during the critical postinterventional period and continued to provide access for further imaging and reintervention.

Contact with bile increased the permeability of the peritoneum, allowing fluid to diffuse from the interstitium into the peritoneal cavity and causing the clinical manifestations of an acute abdomen. The fluid shifted into the per-

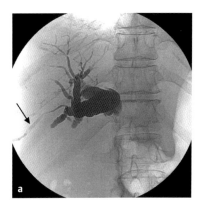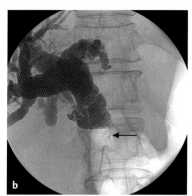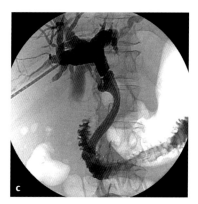

Fig. 4.31 a–c Percutaneous transhepatic cholangiodrainage. The bile ducts in the right lobe of the liver are dilated due to extrahepatic cholestasis. Contrast extravasation appears on the liver surface (arrow) after removal of the Chiba needle (**a**). The common bile duct is obstructed by surrounding enlarged lymph nodes in the setting of the underlying disease (arrow in **b**). Final angiogram after placement of a self-expanding stent across the distal duct obstruction (**c**).

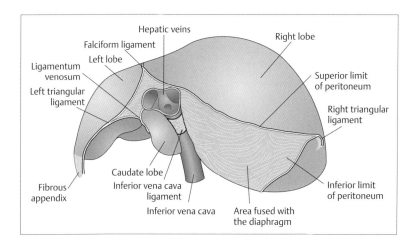

Fig. 4.32 Anatomy of the liver and perihepatic visceral peritoneum. The liver is completely surrounded by visceral peritoneum except for its contact area with the diaphragm (bare area) and the insertion of the falciform ligament, which subdivides the perihepatic peritoneal cavity into a right and left anterior compartment.

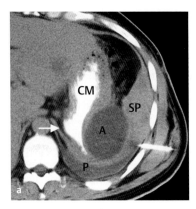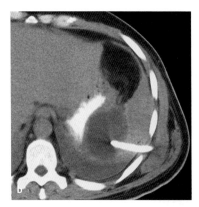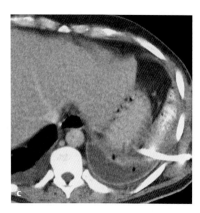

Fig. 4.33 a–c Pleural empyema (**c**) following CT-guided drainage of a subphrenic abscess (**a, b**). The needle track ran through the posterior costophrenic recess, leading to infection of the pleural space.

A, subphrenic abscess; P, pleural effusion; SP, spleen; CM, orally administered contrast medium in the stomach; arrow, left crus of diaphragm.

a CT-guided placement of a percutaneous abscess drain. Interim check.

b CT-guided placement of a percutaneous abscess drain. Final check.

c CT follow-up 5 days later shows development of a pleural empyema.

itoneal cavity (causing hypovolemia and electrolyte disturbances) and the increased abdominal pressure (causing a restrictive ventilatory defect due to decreased diaphragm motion) compromised gas exchange in the lung and contributed to respiratory failure. Given the patient's debilitated condition, the biliary intervention, and the acute abdomen, it is also reasonable to assume a preterminal failure of the heart and/or kidneys, leading to pulmonary venous congestive edema or excess lung water.

Even when the outcome is known, it is clear that PTCD was indicated for the palliative relief of cholestasis-related complaints (severe itching) and to prevent bacterial cholangitis (stasis of bacteria-laden bile) and coagulopathy (malabsorption of fat-soluble vitamin K, leading to decreased synthesis of prothrombin complex coagulation factors). Since ERC could not be performed due to duodenal stenosis and operative treatment was contraindicated by the stage of the disease and the lymphomas in the porta hepatis, PTCD was the only remaining palliative treatment option.

Most studies published during the early years of PTCD reported complication rates (bleeding, biliary peritonitis, sepsis, pneumothorax) of 5–15%. Today, these rates are almost certainly lower as a result of technical refinements. PTCD has become widely practiced, and palliative cases are likely to run a fateful course. The procedure has a reported procedural mortality rate of 0–4% and a 30-day mortality of 2–39%, depending on the underlying disease.

A different case also illustrates the sensitivity of serous-lined body cavities such as the pleural space and peritoneum to inflammatory complications of interventional procedures (**Fig. 4.33**). In this case the faulty placement of a percutaneous tube for the CT-guided drainage of a subphrenic abscess led to contamination of the pleura, resulting in the development of pleural empyema.

References and Further Reading

Keane PK, Belperio JA, Henson PM, et al. Inflammation, injury, and repair. In: Gore RM, Levine MS, Laufer I, eds. Textbook of Gastrointestinal Radiology. Volume II. Philadelphia: Saunders; 1994: 449–490

Rodriguez-Roisin R, Barber JA. Pulmonary complications of abdominal disease. In: Mason RJ, Broaddus VC, Murray JF, Nadel JA, eds. Murray and Nadel's Textbook of Respiratory Medicine. 4th ed. Philadelphia: Elsevier Saunders; 2005: 2223–2241

Teplick SK, Brandon JC, Harshfield DL. Transhepatic biliary drainage and interventional procedures. In: Gore RM, Levine MS, Laufer I, eds. Textbook of Gastrointestinal Radiology. Volume II. Philadelphia: Saunders; 1994: 1746–1761

Van Delden OM, Laméris JH. Percutaneous drainage and stenting for palliation of malignant bile duct obstruction. Eur Radiol 2008; 18: 448–456

Wagner HJ, Feeken T, Mutters R, Klose KJ. Bacteremia in intra-arterial angiography, percutaneous transluminal angioplasty and percutaneous transhepatic cholangiodrainage. RoFo 1998; 169: 402–407

Complication of Percutaneous Transhepatic Cholangiodrainage

History and Clinical Findings

A 67-year-old man underwent neoadjuvant chemotherapy for stomach cancer followed by gastrectomy with an esophagojejunostomy. Nine months after the operation, lymph node metastases were detected in the epigastrium and porta hepatis that were narrowing the common hepatic duct (CHD) and its bifurcation. The resulting extrahepatic cholestasis had to be relieved due to jaundice (itching, nonspecific debilitation), the risk of cholangitis (retrograde colonization of the bile ducts due to sphincter of Oddi dysfunction), and the risk of developing a coagulation disorder (decreased absorption of fat-soluble vitamin K, leading to decreased synthesis of prothrombin complex coagulation factors). Retrograde endoscopic therapy was not possible because of the patient's postoperative status. The only remaining option was PTCD, in which the stenosis in the CHD is dilated and stabilized by stent-assisted PTA (percutaneous transluminal angioplasty; see p. 174) (**Fig. 4.34**).

The postinterventional course was initially uneventful. Extrahepatic cholestasis recurred 5 months later as a result of progressive tumor growth. Cholangitis was diagnosed on the basis of new upper abdominal complaints, a CRP of 331 mg/L, a GOT of 316 U/L, a GPT of 179 U/L, and a γGT of 1802 U/L.

PTCD was repeated for the treatment of cholestasis and cholangitis (**Fig. 4.35**). Imaging confirmed the presumed stent occlusion by progressive tumor growth with secondary intrahepatic cholestasis. The left hepatic duct (LHD) and right hepatic duct (RHD) were punctured percutaneously at separate sites. Guidewires were then advanced through the RHD and LHD into the CHD and duodenum. A self-expanding stent was introduced into the CHD over the guidewire in the RHD and was extended with two additional self-expanding stents placed in the RHD and LHD. The vascular stents were molded to the bile ducts by balloon dilation. An imaging check confirmed good drainage. Next a pigtail catheter was introduced to secure the external and internal biliary drainage. Blood-tinged fluid collected in the drainage bag for the LHD.

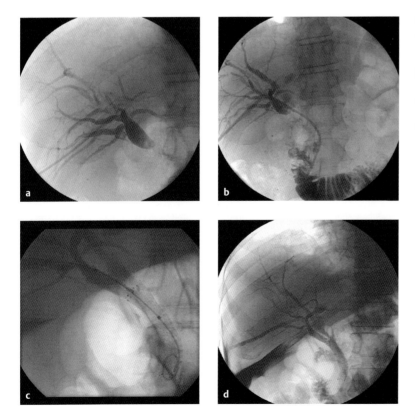

Fig. 4.34 a–d First PTCD.
a Initial findings: occlusion of the CHD and dilatation of the intrahepatic bile ducts.
b A catheter is advanced over the guidewire and into the duodenum.
c Status following placement of a self-expanding stent in the CHD.
d Final check confirms normal calibers of the intrahepatic bile ducts.

When contrast medium was instilled through the drain, it showed normal postinterventional findings.

Over the next few hours the patient's Hb fell from 10.6 g/dL to 9.5 g/dL and then to 4.5 g/dL. The source of the bleeding was investigated by plain CT followed by scans acquired during the arterial, portal-venous, and parenchymal phases after IV contrast administration (**Fig. 4.36**). The imaging report described hypoperfused areas in the hepatic parenchyma. The bile ducts and biliary tract were partially filled with contrast medium and air due to the previous PTCD. Active contrast extravasation was not observed. Ascites was noted in the area of the porta hepatis, in the gallbladder bed, and in the right paracolic gutter. The retroperitoneal tumor recurrence was also described.

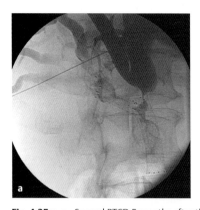
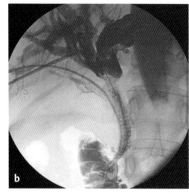
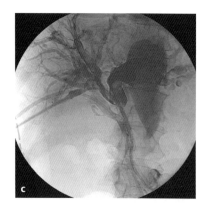

Fig. 4.35 a–c   Second PTCD 5 months after the first PTCD.
a The percutaneous needle is inserted into the right hepatic duct.
b Status following implantation of a new stent in the CHD and common bile duct and two additional stents for draining the right and left lobes of the liver.
c Final angiogram.

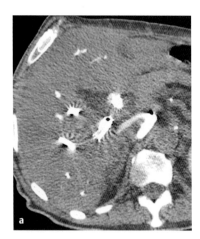
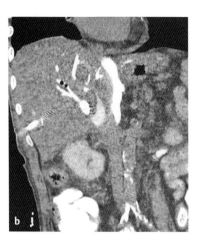
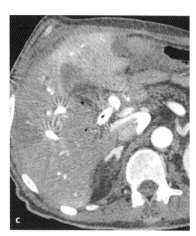

Fig. 4.36 a–c   CT examination following PTCD shows no evidence of a bleeding site. The report noted suspected hepatic infarctions and free intraperitoneal fluid.

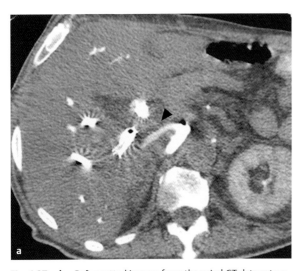 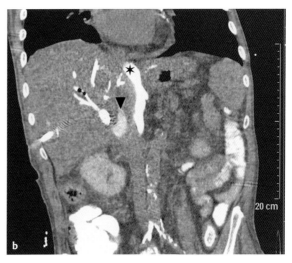

Fig. 4.37 a, b   Reformatted images from the spiral CT data set acquired 5 hours after the second PTCD (see also **Fig. 4.36 a, b**). Opacified fluid is visible in the porta hepatis (arrowhead in **a** and **b**) and in the peritoneal compartment bordering the medial aspect of the inferior vena cava (asterisk in **b**).

Further Case Summary

Disseminated intravascular coagulation with consumption coagulopathy developed during the next few hours. Despite maximum intensive care efforts, this culminated in the patient's death. The ward physician listed the cause of death as "natural causes" on the death certificate. The patient's family did not consent to autopsy.

Error Analysis and Strategy for Error Prevention

Without an autopsy, we can only speculate as to the cause of the fatal hemorrhage. The preponderance of evidence suggests an injury to the extrahepatic portion of the portal vein. The following observations support this conclusion:

- Noncontrast CT shows opacified fluid (bile, blood) in the porta hepatis spreading to the peritoneal compartment bordering medially on the inferior vena cava (**Figs. 4.36, 4.37**).
- The perfusion defects seen throughout the liver in the arterial and portal venous CT phases after IV contrast administration suggest a central vascular injury (**Fig. 4.36 c**).
- The contrast pool that spread superomedially from the porta hepatis in the second PTCD was an extravasation and did not represent the dilated LHD (**Figs. 4.35, 4.38**).
- The right and left hepatic ducts were both punctured at relatively central sites during the second PTCD (**Fig. 4.35 a**).

- Because of its shape, the hyperdense area seen in **Fig. 4.37** and **Fig. 4.38** was interpreted during the intervention as contrast medium in the gallbladder. Subsequent CT scans showed no trace of contrast medium in the gallbladder lumen but did show contrast in the biliary tract and retroperitoneum, and so the structure must be interpreted as an extravasated contrast pool in the peritoneal compartment just medial to the inferior vena cava.
- The filling defects projected over the dilated bile ducts on the left side are most likely blood clots (**Fig. 4.38**).
- The final check of the first PTCD showed opacified liquid (bile, blood) in the needle tract and in the perihepatic peritoneal cavity about the insertion site.

The second PTCD was appropriate for the treatment of cholangitis, even when the outcome is known. Because ERC could not be performed after the gastrectomy and esophagojejunostomy and metastases in the porta hepatis precluded open surgery, PTCD was the only way to establish vitally important biliary drainage. Sepsis resulting from cholangitis has a reported mortality rate of 10–14%, even in the absence of associated diseases and when appropriate treatment is given (biliary tract decompression, antibiotic therapy). The patient's life expectancy was limited due to metastatic cancer. Given the advanced stage of the disease and the damage to the liver parenchyma from the cholangitis and ischemia, it is doubtful that localization of the bleeding site and appropriate treatment would have significantly prolonged the patient's life.

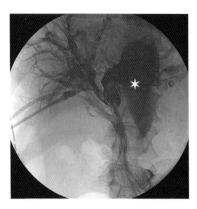

Fig. 4.38 Second PTCD (see **Fig. 4.35 d**) shows contrast extravasation in the peritoneal recess medial to the inferior vena cava (asterisk). Blood clots appear as filling defects in the dilated bile ducts on the left side.

Medical examiners and medical legal experts advise that the cause of death be listed as "uncertain" in comparable situations. The district attorney's office will usually order a forensic evaluation and even a postmortem examination if needed to establish the cause of death. Family consent is unnecessary due to the overriding importance of legal certitude in situations of this kind. The goal of this process is to establish a concrete chain of events leading to the death and protect against any unwarranted accusations that may follow.

References and Further Reading

Keane PK, Belperio JA, Henson PM, et al. Inflammation, injury, and repair. In: Gore RM, Levine MS, Laufer I, eds. Textbook of Gastrointestinal Radiology. Volume II. Philadelphia: Saunders; 1994: 449–490

Melzer M, Toner R, Lacey S, Bettany E, Rait G. Biliary tract infection and bacteremia: presentation, structural abnormalities, causative organisms and clinical outcomes. Postgrad Med J 2007; 83: 773–775

Rodriguez-Roisin R, Barber JA. Pulmonary complications of abdominal disease. In: Mason RJ, Broaddus VC, Murray JF, Nadel JA, eds. Murray and Nadel's Textbook of Respiratory Medicine. 4th ed. Philadelphia: Elsevier Saunders; 2005: 2223–2241

Rosing DK, De Virgilio C, Nguyen AT, El Masry M, Kaki AH, Stabile BE. Cholangitis: analysis of admission prognostic indicators and outcomes. Am Surg 2007; 73: 949–954

Teplick SK, Brandon JC, Harshfield DL. Transhepatic biliary drainage and interventional procedures. In: Gore RM, Levine MS, Laufer I, eds. Textbook of Gastrointestinal Radiology. Volume II. Philadelphia: Saunders; 1994: 1746–1761

Wagner HJ, Feeken T, Mutters R, Klose KJ. Bacteremia in intra-arterial angiography, percutaneous transluminal angioplasty and percutaneous transhepatic cholangio-drainage. RoFo 1998; 169: 402–407

Complication of CT-Guided Biopsy?

History and Clinical Findings

Two years and 3 months before his current presentation, a 57-year-old man was diagnosed with grade I, stage IIIA follicular B-cell non-Hodgkin lymphoma (B-NHL) with cervical, mediastinal, and retroperitoneal lymphomas and bulky left iliac disease. The patient underwent six cycles of combination chemotherapy with R-CHOP, cyclophosphamide, and doxorubicin and two cycles of rituximab monotherapy. Six months after the initial diagnosis, this regimen brought about a partial remission with a residual left iliac mass. The rituximab therapy was continued in a maintenance dose. Restaging 9 months after the initial diagnosis documented a complete remission. As for the iliac mass, it was concluded that the bulky lym-

phoma had healed, leaving a residual scar tissue mass in the left lesser pelvis (**Fig. 4.39**). CT performed 1 year after the initial diagnosis showed an increase in the volume of the residual left iliac mass, and the maintenance therapy was discontinued. Clinical and laboratory findings were still normal. Hematooncology requested histopathologic confirmation based on suspicion of recurrent lymphoma. Three months after the CT detection of recurrence, the patient was referred to radiology for CT-guided biopsy.

Informed outpatient consent for the biopsy included disclosure that the procedure could cause vascular injury requiring interventional treatment or open surgery. The patient's blood pressure and coagulation values were normal. Preinterventional planning included the acquisition of a spiral CT data set with the patient supine and a planning grid placed over the skin of the left lower abdomen. Intravenous contrast administration was withheld. Scans confirmed a soft-tissue mass measuring 8.8 cm × 3.2 cm located in the left iliac neurovascular sheath (**Fig. 4.40**). Aided by the CT image data set, the needle biopsy path was planned on the CT control console. Next, 5 mL of mepivacaine was injected subcutaneously at the proposed entry site, and the skin was sterile-draped. The mass was biopsied using a 10-cm long 18-gauge biopsy system (Gallini Medical Devices) with standard coaxial technique. Placement of the needle cutting chamber within the target volume was confirmed (**Fig. 4.41**), and a solid, whitish tissue core was sampled. When the biopsy needle was removed from the outer guide needle for specimen retrieval, pulsating arterial blood spurted from the still-indwelling hollow needle.

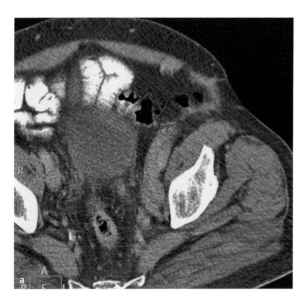
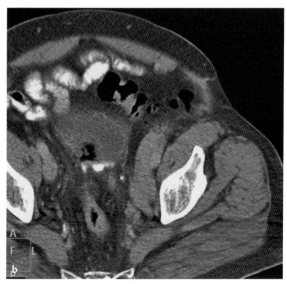

Fig. 4.39 a, b CT follow-ups 9 months (**a**) and 12 months (**b**) after the initial diagnosis of follicular B-NHL. The residual left iliac mass, apparently unchanged relative to a previous examination elsewhere, was classified as healed scar tissue 9 months after the initial diagnosis (**a**). Findings 12 months after the initial diagnosis were suspicious for recurrent lymphoma (**b**).

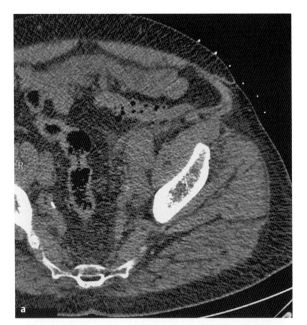

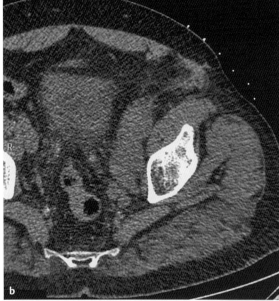

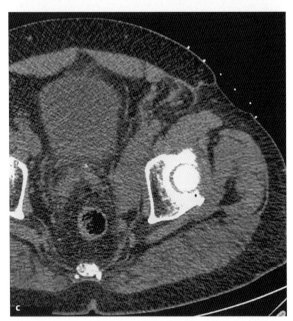

Fig. 4.40 a–c The plain spiral CT data acquisition for interventional planning showed enlargement of the left iliac mass relative to **Fig. 4.39**. Due to their comparable densities and the absence of intervening fat planes, portions of the iliac vessels are visually indistinguishable from the iliac mass. A planning grid was placed on the skin of the left lower abdomen.

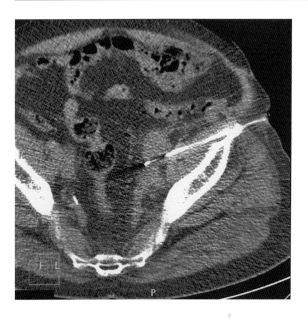

Fig. 4.41 Confirming correct placement of the cutting chamber of the biopsy needle within the target volume.

Further Case Summary

It was feared that an injury to the external iliac artery was responsible for the bleeding. For this reason, the stylet of the biopsy system was inserted into the hollow needle to tamponade the hemorrhage. With the hollow needle still in the same position, the pelvis was imaged immediately and 9 min after the IV bolus injection of 120 mL iohexol (Accupaque 350, GE Healthcare) at a flow rate of 3 mL/s (**Fig. 4.42**). This study confirmed the close proximity of the hollow needle tip to the external iliac artery. A distance of 2 mm was measured between the needle tip and lateral artery wall. There was no evidence of a hematoma and no visible extravasation of opacified blood.

The patient remained hemodynamically stable. With the hollow needle still in place, the patient was moved to the adjacent angiography suite for the proposed insertion of a coated stent (see "Vascular perforation during subintimal PTA and stenting," p. 339). During subsequent selective visualization of the left common iliac artery, left external iliac artery, and left internal iliac artery through an ipsilateral femoral approach, all of the left iliac arteries appeared normal. At that point the hollow needle was withdrawn under fluoroscopic guidance. Repeat selective visualization of the left external iliac artery and left internal iliac artery (**Fig. 4.43**) showed normal angiographic findings with no evidence of active contrast extravasation.

Fig. 4.42 CT scan 9 minutes after IV contrast administration with the biopsy needle in place shows absence of extravasation.

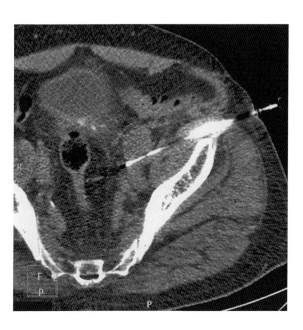

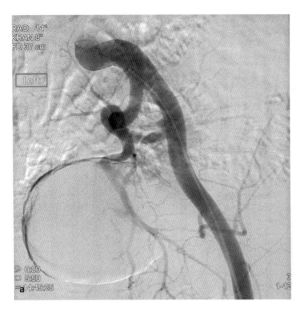

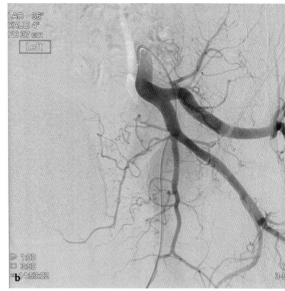

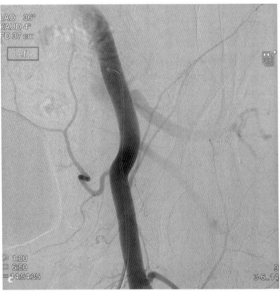

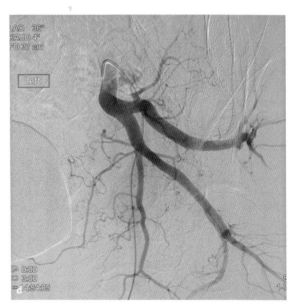

Fig. 4.43 a–d   Selective angiography of the left common and external iliac arteries (**a, c**) and the left internal iliac artery (**b, d**) before (**a, b**) and after (**c, d**) the hollow needle of the biopsy system was removed.

The patient was hospitalized for 24-hour observation. Eight hours after the intervention, noncontrast CT of the pelvis confirmed the absence of a retroperitoneal hematoma. Blood pressure and hemoglobin levels were stable in serial measurements.

Histopathology identified the mass as grade I follicular B-NHL. In retrospect, it is clear that the diagnosis of a complete remission 9 months after initial diagnosis was wrong (**Fig. 4.39 a**). Instead, there was still a significant volume of residual tumor tissue, whose growth had been suppressed by the rituximab maintenance therapy, causing the CT findings to appear constant over time.

Error Analysis and Strategy for Error Prevention

Bleeding after a CT-guided needle biopsy constituted an inherent risk in an extremely complex disease situation. Studies have shown that CT-guided biopsies rarely cause arterial bleeding. The few cases of clinically significant bleeding published to date generally occurred in patients with coagulation disorders, who had undergone liver biopsy.

As for the arterial bleeding in the present case, it was most likely caused by an injury to the external iliac artery due to the documented proximity of the biopsy needle tip to the lateral wall of that vessel. The leakage was tamponaded by the hollow needle with stylet, which remained in place until the completion of angiography. The following errors were made in planning and carrying out the intervention:

- The biopsy needle was directed almost perpendicularly to the iliac vascular axis, allowing the needle to cross and perhaps injure the iliac artery and vein if it were inadvertently advanced too far (**Figs. 4.41, 4.42**). Directing the needle parallel to the iliac wing would have greatly reduced this risk.

- Due to the interference of the selected needle path with the sigmoidal colon, it would have been better to take the biopsy from the lower portion of the tumor (**Fig. 4.40 c**) rather than from the central portion (**Fig. 4.40 b**). This would also have allowed for a more sterile biopsy track that did not cross the blood vessels.

- CT scanning with IV opacification of the vessels was omitted before the biopsy. The most recent prior CT examination was 3 months old. Because the vessels and the tumor had comparable unenhanced densities and there was no fatty tissue between the vessels and tumor at the targeted site (**Fig. 4.40 b**), the exact position of the iliac vessels in relation to the proposed biopsy site was unknown.

- The exact position of the needle tip could not be determined with millimeter accuracy due to beam-hardening artifact arising from the needle. Because of this, a 5–10 mm safety margin should have been maintained relative to the vessel axis.

References and Further Reading

Chojniak R, Isberner RK, Viana LM, Yu LS, Aita AA, Soares FA. Computed tomography-guided needle biopsy: experience from 1,300 procedures. Sao Paulo Med J 2006; 124: 10

Hatfield MK, Beres A, Sane SS, Zaleski GX. Percutaneous imaging-guided solid organ core needle biopsy: coaxial versus noncoaxial method. AJR 2008; 190: 413

Hesselmann V, Zähringer M, Krug B, et al. Computed tomography-guided percutaneous core needle biopsies of malignant lymphomas: impact of biopsy, lesion and patient parameters on diagnostic yield. Acta Radiol 2004; 45: 641

Terjung B, Lemnitz I, Dumoulin FL, et al. Bleeding complications after percutaneous liver biopsy. An analysis of risk factors. Digestion 2002; 67: 138

Abdomen

Gastrointestinal Tract

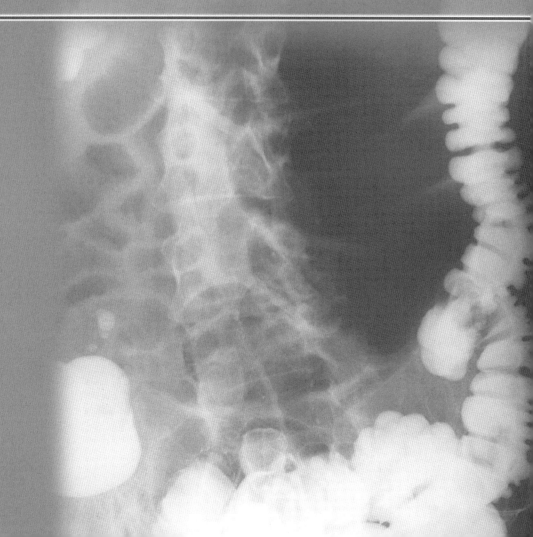

Iodinated Oral Contrast vs. Barium Sulfate

History and Clinical Findings

A 56-year-old man suffered from hyperthyroidism due to autonomous thyroid nodules. After a euthyroid state had been achieved with antithyroid medication, the patient was scheduled for definitive radioiodine ablation of the thyroid. Because β-emissions from the iodine-131 (range of 0.5–2.0 mm) can exacerbate tracheal stenosis and may even cause life-threatening stridor, the patient was referred for tracheal spot films before treatment was initiated.

The x-ray report stated that the trachea was indented and displaced to the right by the retrosternal extension of a goiter on the left side (**Fig. 4.44 a, b**). This narrowed the tracheal diameter by approximately 10% below normal in the AP projection and by approximately 30% in the lateral projection, but the tracheal diameter changed very little in response to Mueller and Valsalva maneuvers (not shown). Imaging after iodinated oral contrast ingestion showed that the esophagus was slightly displaced toward the right side and was fully patent (**Fig. 4.44 c**). The report concluded that the patient had no significant tracheal stenosis or instability.

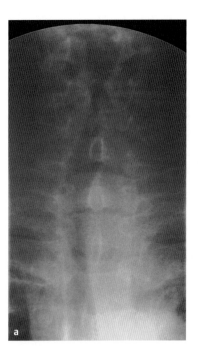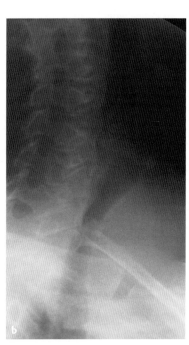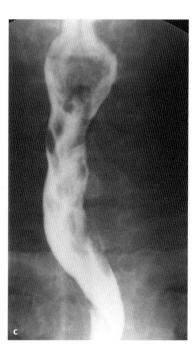

Fig. 4.44 a–c Spot radiographs of the trachea (**a, b**) and oral contrast examination of the esophagus (**c**).

Further Case Summary

The following day, the iodine-131 dose necessary for radioiodine therapy was determined by radioiodine testing (scintigraphic detection and quantification of the gamma-radiation component emitted by the decay of iodine-131.) Maximum radionuclide uptake by the thyroid gland was less than 3%. Consequently, radioiodine therapy had to be postponed by 4 weeks due to the thyroid blockade.

Error Analysis and Strategy for Error Prevention

The upper portion of the esophagus was included in the radiographic examination of the trachea because of its proximity to the gland. The patient was given iodinated oral contrast medium (Gastrografin), consistent with the standard work-up applied in visceral surgery. This agent contains inorganic stable iodine-127, which was absorbed in the small bowel and carried by the bloodstream to the thyroid gland, where it was actively transported into the parenchymal cells. On the following day the high intracellular concentration of iodine-127 competitively inhibited the uptake of iodine-131 administered by the same route.

Oral contrast examination of the esophagus with iodinated medium (**Fig. 4.44 c**) should have been withheld because it lacked a clinical and therapeutic rationale. An alternative oral agent is barium sulfate, which may have therapeutic relevance in preoperative planning. With all iodinated contrast media, clinically significant amounts of iodine atoms are released and metabolized following oral administration. The effect of free, dissociated iodine atoms in the blood is similar to that of perchlorate (Irenat), which is used to block iodine uptake by the thyroid gland in patients with thyroid autonomy. For this reason, iodinated contrast media should not be administered by either the oral or intravenous route prior to thyroid scanning with the iodine analog [^{99m}Tc]pertechnetate.

Radiographic Examination of the Trachea before Radioiodine Therapy

- Tracheal stenosis relevant to radioiodine therapy is assumed to be present when the tracheal diameter at the level of the goiter is reduced to 4–5 mm in one projection.
- Tracheomalacia is present when the trachea collapses in response to a Mueller maneuver (which creates a negative intrathoracic pressure) and/or a Valsalva maneuver (which creates a positive intrathoracic pressure).

Iodinated Ionic/Nonionic Contrast Medium

History and Clinical Findings

A 61-year-old man with stage pT3 N1 M0 G3 esophageal cancer had undergone a thoracoabdominal en bloc esophagectomy with continuity restored by gastric transposition through the posterior mediastinum and an intrathoracic anastomosis. Six months later the patient was diagnosed with histologically confirmed pleural and peritoneal carcinomatosis and anastomotic stricture of unknown cause (differential diagnosis: scar, tumor). When adequate oral food intake could not be maintained and a feeding tube could not be successfully inserted on the ward, the patient was referred to radiology for the fluoroscopically guided placement of a feeding tube. Before the procedure (**Fig. 4.45**), the patient denied having swallowing difficulties when ingesting fluids. Even with fluoroscopic guidance, an initial attempt to pass the guidewire into the transposed stomach was unsuccessful. The patient was then asked to take a swallow of oral ionic contrast medium for visualization of postoperative anatomy. Most of the contrast bolus was aspirated, but the medium still produced slight opacification of the anastomotic region, which was sufficient for advancing the catheter into the duodenum. The images were not documented due to the therapeutic nature of the procedure.

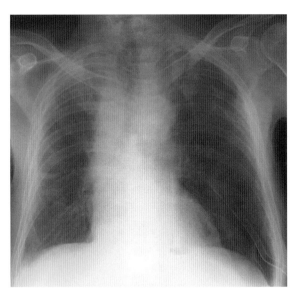

Fig. 4.45 Chest radiograph one day before the procedure shows mediastinal widening, an effusion in the right costophrenic angle, and a left-sided chest tube for draining a preexisting pleural effusion.

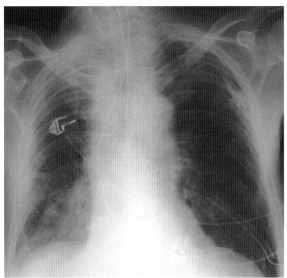

Fig. 4.46 Chest radiograph approximately 4 hours after the intervention documents correct placement of the stomach tube. New infiltrate is visible in the right lower lobe due to aspiration. The patient is still intubated.

Further Case Summary

Immediately after the intervention the patient was dyspneic and expectorated watery mucus. Intravenous cortisone was administered at once as a safety precaution. The patient's respiratory status continued to deteriorate rapidly during the next few hours, and he was transferred to the ICU, where he was intubated and mechanically ventilated because of respiratory failure. The chest radiograph in the ICU showed contrast aspiration in the lower lobe of the right lung (**Fig. 4.46**). Two days later the patient was diagnosed with nosocomial pneumonia and expired 8 days later.

Error Analysis and Strategy for Error Prevention

It was correct to use iodinated medium rather than barium sulfate for oral contrast imaging because aspirated barium sulfate may incite potentially fatal toxic inflammatory reactions. But iodinated contrast media may also produce adverse effects when aspirated. This is particularly true in debilitated patients or patients with preexisting lung disease. Pathophysiologically, the effects are due primarily to the high osmolarity of iodinated contrast media, which causes a fluid shift from the interstitium into the alveoli along with complex intra- and intercellular fluid shifts in the adjacent supportive tissues of the lung (alveolar pulmonary edema). Toxic inflammatory reactions are an additional mechanism by which some agents can produce adverse effects. Experimental animal studies have shown that ionic oral and parenteral contrast media may cause more pronounced side-effects due to their higher osmolarity than nonionic media administered by the parenteral route. For this reason, it would have been best either to use a nonionic parenteral contrast agent or switch to feeding by parenteral infusions. Given the patient's initial clinical status, however, it is doubtful whether these measures would have significantly influenced the further clinical course.

References and Further Reading

D'Agostino HR, Liebig RJ, McGovern M, Weinshelbaum A, Reich SB. Effects of iopamidol and iohexol in rat lungs following experimental aspiration. Invest Radiol 1989; 24: 899–902

Ginai AZ, ten Kate FJ, ten Berg RG, Hoornstra K. Experimental evaluation of various available contrast agents for the use in the upper gastrointestinal tract in case of suspected leakage. Effects on lungs. Br J Radiol 1984; 57: 895–901

McAllister WH, Askin FB. The effect of some contrast agents in the lung: an experimental study in the rat and dog. AJR 1983; 140: 245–251

Miyazawa T, Sho C, Nakagawa H, Oshino N. Effect of water-soluble contrast medium on the lung in rats. Comparison of iotrolan, iopamidol, and diatrizoate. Invest Radiol 1990; 25: 999–1003

Moore DE, Carroll FE, Dutt PL, Redd GW, Holburn GE. Comparison of nonionic and ionic contrast agents in the rabbit lung. Invest Radiol 1991; 26: 134–142

Gastrointestinal Perforation/ Functional Duodenal Stenosis

History and Clinical Findings

A 36-year-old paraplegic woman underwent abdominal radiography for investigation of midabdominal pain and vomiting (**Fig. 4.47**). The radiographs showed distention of the stomach and duodenum extending to the horizontal part of the duodenum, suggesting transient compression of the duodenum between the mesenteric root and spinal column (mesenteric compression syndrome) as the cause of the complaints in this thin patient. There was no evidence of intraperitoneal air that would suggest a gastrointestinal perforation.

Abdominal CT scans (**Fig. 4.48**) and an upper GI series with a water-soluble medium (**Fig. 4.49**) strengthened the presumptive diagnosis.

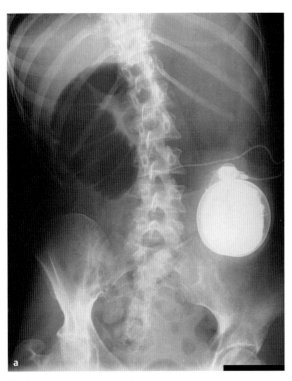

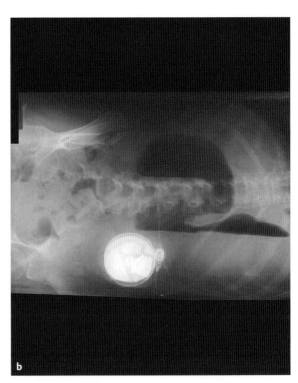

Fig. 4.47 a, b Abdominal plain films were described as showing distention of the stomach and duodenum extending to the horizontal part of the duodenum, suggesting transient duodenal compression between the mesenteric root and spinal column as the source of the complaints. There is no evidence of a pneumoperi-

toneum. An epidural electrode was previously implanted for pain relief.
a Supine radiograph.
b Left lateral radiograph.

Fig. 4.48 a–h Abdominal CT scans raised suspicion of functional ▶ duodenal stenosis due to compression of the duodenum between the mesenteric root and spinal column at the level of the Treitz ligament.

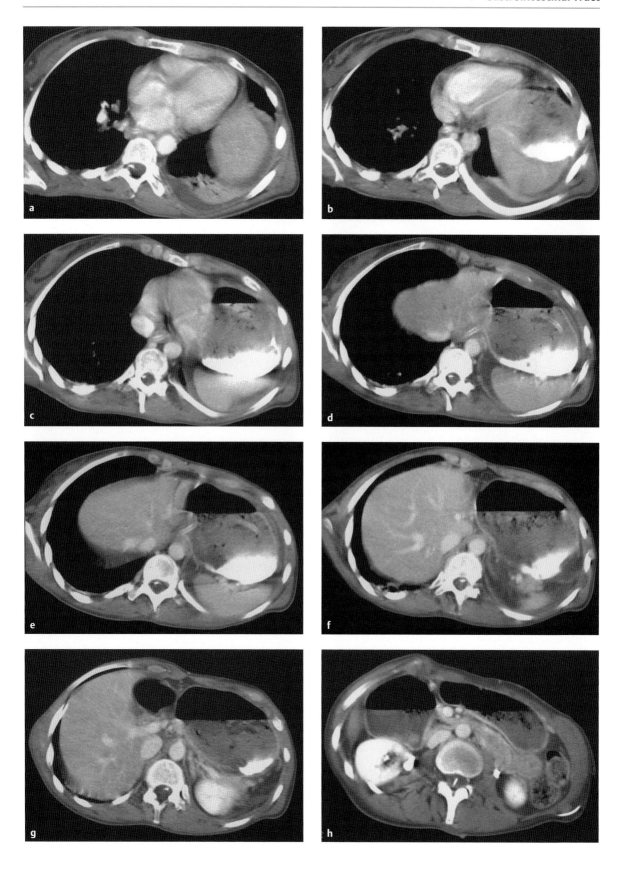

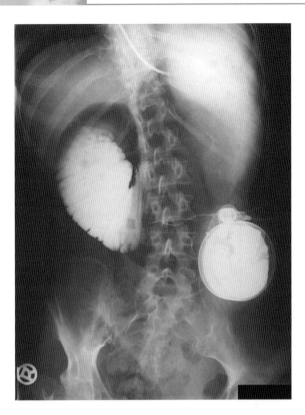

Fig. 4.49 Upper GI series with Gastrografin. Contrast medium injected via gastric tube collects in the distended stomach and duodenum. The small bowel and colon show a normal air content distal to the duodenojejunal flexure. The series confirmed the CT impression of functional duodenal stenosis.

Further Case Summary

Due to the discrepancy between radiologic and clinical findings, a double-contrast upper GI series was performed one day later (**Fig. 4.50**). Fluoroscopic control showed a confined perforation of the stomach arising from the posterior wall of the gastric fundus.

Error Analysis and Strategy for Error Prevention

The confined gastric perforation was missed on CT scans for the following reasons:

- The defect in the wall of the gastric fundus was overlooked (**Fig. 4.48 d**).
- Contrast extravasation beneath the diaphragm was cut at a tangential angle in the CT scan, causing it to be misinterpreted.
- Sagittal reformatted images were not obtained.

The confined perforation was not visible in the first GI series (**Fig. 4.49**) because it was mainly located behind the gastric fundus and therefore difficult to detect in the AP projection.

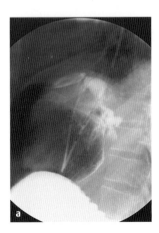
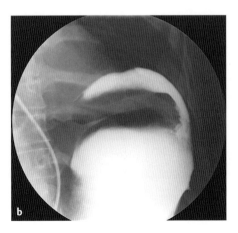

Fig. 4.50 a, b Upper GI series the next day shows a confined perforation of the stomach arising from the posterolateral wall of the gastric fundus. The tip of the stomach tube is curled back into the distal esophagus.

Dissecting Abdominal Aortic Aneurysm/ Bowel Obstruction and Enteritis

History and Clinical Findings

A 68-year-old man presented to his family doctor with diffuse abdominal pain. His doctor diagnosed "meconium ileus" at ultrasound and noted "expansion" of the aorta, which was interpreted as an abdominal aortic aneurysm (AAA). The patient was hospitalized for the suspected bowel obstruction, and in-patient ultrasound confirmed the diagnosis of a dissecting AAA. The patient was sent to vascular surgery for repair of the aneurysm. Images from the two examinations did not accompany the patient.

CT angiography was performed for preoperative planning. These images showed a normal appearance of the aorta and the major vessels arising from it (**Fig. 4.51**). All small-bowel loops were uniformly distended with fluid having approximately the same density as water. There was no evidence of bowel wall thickening (target pattern), solid obstructive bowel contents, or abnormal intra- or extraluminal air collections. A review of the clinical and radiological findings yielded a diagnosis of enteritis.

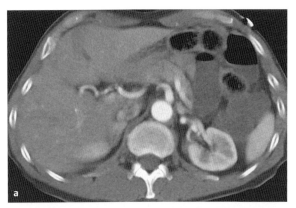
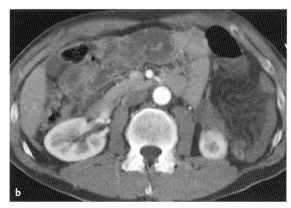
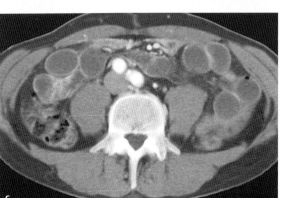

Fig. 4.51 a–c   CT angiography

Further Case Summary

The further clinical course confirmed the diagnosis of enteritis.

Error Analysis and Strategy for Error Prevention

The clinical symptoms were consistent with enteritis, which is marked by diffuse or colicky abdominal pain, vomiting, and diarrhea (may be mucus- or blood-tinged), depending on the underlying cause. The symptoms were not typical of a mechanical bowel obstruction or dissecting AAA, whose clinical manifestations range from minimal findings or pain due to decreased blood flow (progressive thrombosis of the aortic lumen, obstruction of vessels arising from the aorta) to the compression of surrounding structures or an acute abdomen.

The typical imaging findings of enteritis include the distention of all small-bowel loops, which are filled with fluid of near-water density or signal intensity. This finding is easily demonstrated by ultrasound. By contrast, ultrasound cannot detect or exclude a bowel obstruction because all incident sound waves are reflected at the interface of the intestinal air–fluid levels that result from the obstruction. All intestinal air–fluid levels are abnormal. They form when a cessation of normal peristalsis no longer keeps the bowel contents mixed, allowing material with a higher specific gravity (fluid, food constituents, stool) to gravitate downward while the air collects above it.

The misdiagnosis of a dissecting AAA may have resulted from confusion of fluid-filled bowel loops with the aorta.

References and Further Reading

Fernbach SK. Neonatal gastrointestinal radiology. In: Gore RM, Levine MS, Laufer I, eds. Textbook of Gastrointestinal Radiology. Philadelphia: Saunders; 1994: 1387–1423

Veccioli A, De Franco A, Maresca G, et al. Small bowel: cross-sectional imaging. In: Gore RM, Levine MS, Laufer I, eds. Textbook of Gastrointestinal Radiology. Philadelphia: Saunders; 1994: 789–801

Mechanical Bowel Obstruction and Ileus

Definition

Mechanical bowel obstruction is distinguished from functional (paralytic) ileus. Both conditions may cause a life-threatening interruption of gastrointestinal transit due to narrowing or obstruction of the bowel lumen or paralysis of the bowel.

Clinical Manifestations

The symptoms may have an acute onset or may progress gradually (partial obstruction) and consist of nausea and vomiting, meteorism with retention of stool and flatus, colicky pains, eructation, and peritonism (irritation of the peritoneum with tenderness, even in the absence of systemic inflammatory signs). Some cases may progress to fecal vomiting. The (reflex) inhibition of intestinal tonus and peristalsis, accompanied by increasing stasis of bowel contents and stretching of the bowel wall, results in local compromise of blood flow, bowel wall edema, and intestinal fluid and protein losses that produce systemic signs such as hypovolemia, hemoconcentration, decreased cardiac output, and possible shock.

Pathogenetic Classification

Mechanical Bowel Obstruction

- Obstruction of bowel transit due to narrowing of the bowel lumen (inflammatory or neoplastic stricture, scarring, luminal obstruction by polyps, scybala, meconium, gallstones, ingested foreign bodies, etc.; compression of the bowel by adhesions, bowel wall tumors, or adjacent organs, kinking of the bowel due to adhesions)
- Strangulation with decreased mesenteric blood flow due to an incarcerated hernia, intussusception, or volvulus

Ileus

- Paralytic ileus
  - *Inflammatory* cause due to pancreatitis, appendicitis, cholecystitis, peritonitis, etc.
  - *Metabolic* cause due to diabetic acidosis, uremia, hypokalemia, etc.
  - *Hormonal* cause (pregnancy)
  - *Reflex* cause (biliary and renal colic, early complication of abdominal surgery, overdistended bladder, vertebral body fractures, etc.)
  - *Vascular* cause (mesenteric arterial occlusion, mesenteric vein thrombosis)
  - *Pharmacologic* cause (opiates, antidepressants, etc.)
- Spastic ileus (lead poisoning, porphyria, ascariasis)

Special Form: Meconium Ileus

Meconium is the stool of an infant that forms during intrauterine development. Greenish-black in color due to its high biliverdin content, this material is normally passed completely during the postnatal period. Obstruction of the terminal ileum by this sticky, viscous material may cause a mechanical bowel obstruction in newborns. This has a reported incidence of 1:20 000 neonates. Meconium ileus is commonly associated with cystic fibrosis.

Paralytic Ileus/ Mechanical Bowel Obstruction/ Perforation

History and Clinical Findings

A 34-year-old woman was hospitalized with colicky abdominal pains of sudden onset. Gastroscopy revealed a gastric ulcer. Due to clinical suspicion of a perforated ulcer, the staff on duty obtained the abdominal radiograph shown in **Fig. 4.52**. The film was interpreted as showing distended small-bowel loops consistent with intestinal obstruction. Free intraperitoneal air was excluded.

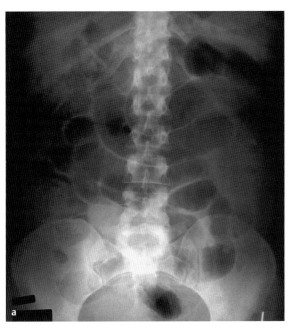
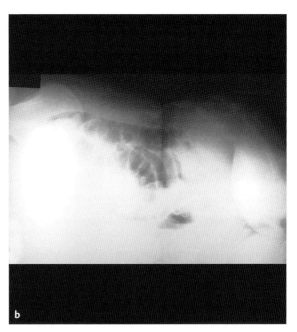

Fig. 4.52 a, b Abdominal radiographs show distention of small-bowel loops consistent with an obstruction. There is no evidence of free intraperitoneal air.

Table 4.3 Principal signs and symptoms in various types of bowel obstruction

	Pain	Vomiting	Meteorism	Peristalsis	Radiology
Mechanical obstruction					
High small-bowel obstruction	Usually slight	Immediate	Absent	Normal	Distention of duodenum and jejunum proximal to the obstruction, little or no air in the ileum and colon
Low small-bowel obstruction	Colicky	Present	Present	High-pitched, tinkling, squirting sounds	Small bowel distended proximal to the obstruction, little or no air in the colon
Colon obstruction	Cramping	Late	Present	High-pitched, tinkling, squirting sounds	Colon distended proximal to the obstruction, little or no air in the distal colon
Strangulation	Sudden onset	Often present initially	Increasing	Increased initially, absent later	Distention of small bowel proximal to the strangulation, little or no air in the colon
Paralytic ileus	Absent	Present	Present	Absent	Distention of the small and large bowel

Further Case Summary

Two days after admission the patient's clinical condition had deteriorated further and additional abdominal radiographs were obtained. High-pitched, tinkling bowel sounds were heard on auscultation (**Table 4.3**). A mechanical bowel obstruction was diagnosed based on the greatly distended small-bowel loops, fluid levels in the small bowel, and absence of air in the colon except for the rectosigmoid (**Fig. 4.53**). Surgery confirmed an adhesive bowel obstruction, which resulted from the appendectomy performed 12 years earlier.

Error Analysis and Strategy for Error Prevention

Both examinations showed the features of a mechanical small-bowel obstruction. The discrepancy between the distended small-bowel loops with air–fluid levels in left lateral body position (LLBP) and the almost airless colon suggested the correct diagnosis. The air that was visible in the right hemicolon during the first examination (**Fig. 4.54**) had passed through the ileocecal valve into the cecum and ascending colon in the antegrade direction before the acute obstruction supervened. By the second examination, the air had reached the rectosigmoid, while the small-bowel obstruction prevented any additional air from entering the large bowel. Because adhesions are the most frequent cause of mechanical small-bowel obstruction, information on the patient's post-appendectomy status would have narrowed the differential diagnosis. Given the different therapeutic implications of a mechanical bowel obstruction versus paralytic ileus, the radiology report should always state whether the obstruction is mechanical or nonmechanical (paralytic).

Upper GI Series

An upper GI series with water-soluble contrast medium is often performed in the investigation of bowel obstruction and seeks to determine whether the obstruction is complete or incomplete. It can also reveal the cause of the bowel obstruction in some cases. Additionally, the fluid shift induced by the hyperosmolar contrast medium will often improve gastrointestinal transit and reduce the severity of symptoms.

Intussusception

Intussusception refers to the prolapse of one bowel segment and its mesentery into the lumen of an adjacent aboral bowel segment. Children in the first two years of life are predominantly affected. Most intussusceptions have an ileocolic location. Colocolic and ileoileal intussusceptions are less common. In most cases, a specific cause cannot be established for the intussusception. Rare causes are Meckel diverticula, polyps, duplication cysts, lymphomas, and postoperative adhesions. Intussusception may present clinically with recurring, colicky abdominal pain, the anal passage of blood and mucus, vomiting, and a cylindrical abdominal mass. Recurrent intussusceptions are not uncommon. At ultrasound, the thickened edematous bowel involved by the intussusception may present a typical "double target" pattern. A contrast enema can confirm the diagnosis of an ileocolic or colocolic intussusception and aid in its reduction. The intussusception appears as a rounded filling defect in the colon. The contrast medium should consist of a water-soluble, isotonic solution and/or air. Pressure in excess of 120 mm Hg should not be used to reduce the intussusception. The complete reduction of a colocolic or ileocolic intussusception is indicated by the reflux of contrast medium into the terminal ileum.

References and Further Reading

Gore RM, Levine MS. Textbook of Gastrointestinal Radiology. 3rd ed. Philadelphia: WB Saunders; 2008

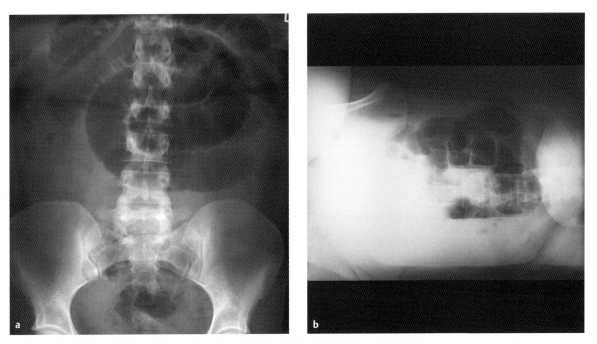

Fig. 4.53 a, b   Abdominal radiographs two days after admission. Mechanical small-bowel obstruction.

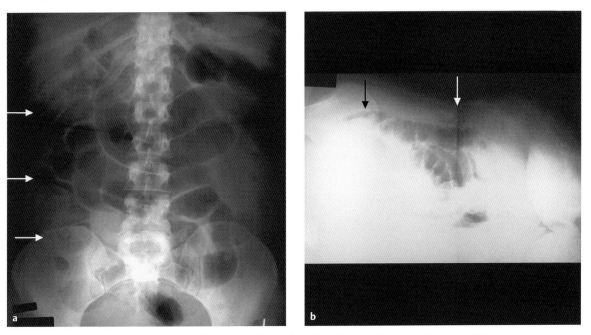

Fig. 4.54 a, b   Abdominal radiographs display the features of a mechanical small-bowel obstruction (compare with **Fig. 4.52**). Arrows indicate air in the cecum and ascending colon, which had passed through the ileocecal valve prior to the obstruction.

Distended Small-bowel loop/Mechanical Bowel Obstruction/Paralytic Ileus/Sigmoid Diverticulitis/Abscess

History and Clinical Findings

A 79-year-old man was hospitalized on a Tuesday with unexplained abdominal pain of increasing intensity. The pain was localized to the mid and upper abdomen. Laboratory inflammatory markers were elevated (WBC 15 900/µL, CRP 220 mg/L). The patient had a fever of 38 °C.

Five years earlier the patient had undergone a right hemicolectomy for colon cancer and had a disease-free history since then. He had been known for several years to have Wegener granulomatosis, which had been treated with a single dose of cyclophosphamide (Endoxan, Baxter Oncology) and steroids. Compensated renal failure (serum creatinine 1.9 mg/L) was present due to renal involvement.

On the following Friday during the night shift, the patient was sent for abdominal CT scans due to clinical suspicion of sigmoid diverticulitis. CT was performed after IV, oral, and transrectal contrast administration. The scans demonstrated a right-lower-quadrant mass with a transverse diameter of approximately 10 cm and an air–fluid level, which was interpreted as a markedly distended loop of small bowel (**Fig. 4.55**). CT also showed diffuse edema of the adjacent mesentery. There was no evidence of bowel wall thickening or abnormal enhancement, and there were no signs of diverticulitis. The report additionally described an infrarenal aortic aneurysm rimmed by thrombosis and atherosclerosis of the large abdominal and iliac arteries. The vessels arising from the aorta showed normal perfusion.

Fig. 4.55 a–h   Abdominal CT scans following IV, oral, and transrectal contrast administration. The report described a liquid mass in the mid-abdomen with an air–fluid level, interpreted as a distended small-bowel loop. Other findings were an infrarenal abdominal aortic aneurysm and atherosclerosis of the abdominal and iliac arteries.

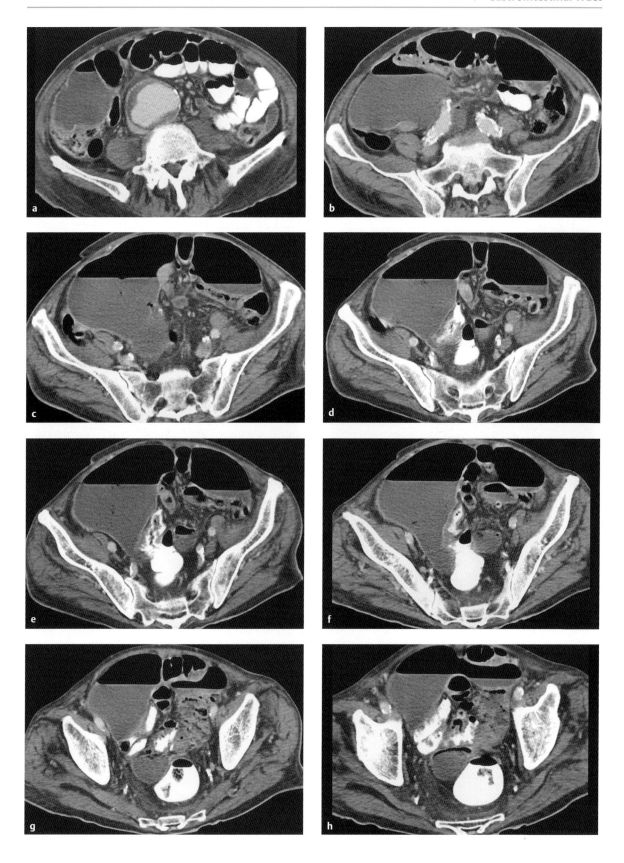

Further Case Summary

The patient's clinical condition deteriorated so markedly over the weekend that laparotomy was performed on Monday for a suspected mechanical bowel obstruction. Surgery revealed a perforated sigmoid diverticulitis that had led to an intraperitoneal abscess. Approximately 2 liters of pus was drained from the abscess. The patient required intensive care after the operation. He developed renal failure requiring dialysis and sepsis, from which the patient died on the sixth postoperative day.

Error Analysis and Strategy for Error Prevention

The air- and fluid-containing mass demonstrated by CT was not a distended small-bowel loop but a large intraperitoneal abscess that developed secondarily to perforated diverticulitis. The thickened and inflamed parietal peritoneum was mistaken for a thickened area of bowel wall. The following observations suggest the correct diagnosis:

- The air–fluid collection is not in continuity with the small bowel.
- The air–fluid collection is in direct contact with a narrowed, wall-thickened segment of sigmoid colon (**Figs. 4.55 e–g, 4.56**).
- Contrast extravasation can be seen issuing from the wall-thickened segment of sigmoid colon (**Figs. 4.55 d–f** and **4.56 a**).
- Individual diverticula can be seen in the distal part of the sigmoid colon (**Figs. 4.55 f, h, 4.56**). This supports the suspicion of sigmoid diverticulitis.

The correct diagnosis could have been made through proper analysis of the imaging findings and the distribution of rectally administered contrast medium. Any remaining doubts could have been resolved by diagnostic CT-guided fine-needle aspiration of the fluid.

References and Further Reading

Dunn DL. Intraabdominel Infection. In: Cameron JL, ed. Current Surgical Therapy. 7th ed. St. Louis: Mosby; 2001: 1283–1286

Gore RM, Levine MS. Textbook of Gastrointestinal Radiology. 3rd ed. Philadelphia: WB Saunders; 2008

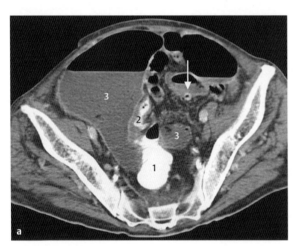
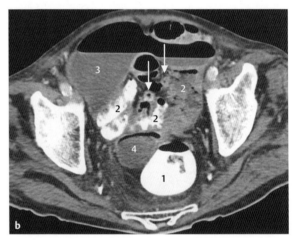

Fig. 4.56 a, b Topographic analysis of the CT findings. Arrows indicate wall-thickened sigmoid diverticula.

a Explanation for **Fig. 4.55 f**. 1 = Rectosigmoid; 2 = perforation; 3 = intraperitoneal fluid with an air–fluid level.

b Explanation for **Fig. 4.55 h**. 1 = Rectum; 2 = sigmoid colon; 3 = intraperitoneal fluid with an air–fluid level; 4 = fluid in the rectovesical pouch of the peritoneum with an air–fluid level.

Peritoneal Inflammations

Diffuse inflammation of the peritoneal cavity is called peritonitis. This condition may give rise to localized abscess formation. Approximately 85% of patients who develop peritonitis secondarily to a gastrointestinal perforation (the most frequent cause of intra-abdominal infections in surgery) can be cured by prompt surgery and appropriate antibiotic therapy. The mortality rate is 5–10%.

The peritoneal cavity is a closed, sterile space lined by mesothelial cells (parietal and visceral peritoneum). The peritoneal cavity encloses the small bowel, spleen, and liver along with approximately 50 mL of serous fluid. Intraperitoneal bacteria are phagocytosed by local macrophages or transported via transdiaphragmatic channels to the thoracic lymphatics, thoracic duct, and bloodstream, where they are eliminated by host defenses. The invasion of the peritoneal cavity by bacteria and their proliferation lead to peritonitis (results: intraperitoneal exudate, inflammatory thickening of the parietal and visceral peritoneum, septa formation). Several forms of peritonitis are distinguished.

Primary Peritonitis

Primary peritonitis is caused by an organism that gains access to the peritoneal cavity without perforating a hollow viscus. It most commonly occurs in association with ascites or in patients on peritoneal dialysis. The etiology may relate to hematogenous spread or direct inoculation of the peritoneum. The most frequent causative organisms of primary peritonitis are *Escherichia coli* and other Gram-negative bacteria, *Staphylococcus aureus*, *Enterococcus faecium* and *E. faecalis*, and occasionally *Candida* species. Generally only one causative organism is identified.

Secondary Peritonitis

Secondary peritonitis results from the perforation of a hollow viscus, allowing microflora to enter the peritoneal cavity from the perforated bowel. The number and spectrum of causative organisms increase with gastrointestinal transit. One milliliter of gastric juice normally contains 10^2–10^3 bacteria, while 1 g of feces contains 10^{11}–10^{12} bacteria. When small-bowel transit is impaired, the local organisms proliferate until the microflora in the small bowel increasingly resembles that in the colon. Because of the different growth characteristics of the various microorganisms, synergistic interactions of the organisms among themselves, and the effect of host defenses during the initial inflammatory phase, the broad spectrum of organisms that normally make up the intestinal flora is reduced to two or three dominant pathogens (most notably *Escherichia coli*, *Klebsiella pneumonia*, *Enterococcus faecium* and *E. faecalis*, *Bacteroides fragilis*, *Fusobacterium*, *Peptococcus*, and *Peptostreptococcus*).

Tertiary Peritonitis

Tertiary peritonitis develops as a complication of secondary peritonitis when the bacterial contamination persists—despite standard antibiotic therapy directed against the most common Gram-negative aerobic and anaerobic bacteria—and the inflammatory fluid collections and pus are not drained from the peritoneal cavity. Elderly patients with underlying debilitating diseases are predominantly affected. Even less-virulent bacterial strains may proliferate under these conditions (e.g., *Staphylococcus epidermidis*, *Candida albicans*, *Pseudomonas aeruginosa*).

Appropriate Work-up/ Underdiagnosis/ Overdiagnosis

History and Clinical Findings

A 46-year-old man had been suffering from a CDC stage C3 HIV infection for some years. He was admitted now with suspicion of HIV encephalopathy and progressive multifocal leukoencephalopathy (PML). He also had a history of microsporidial enteritis, perianal herpes zoster, tuberculous lymphadenitis, cerebral toxoplasmosis, exogenous depression, peripheral polyneuropathy, and CMV retinitis.

The prognosis was grave, and the patient was discharged home at his own request and that of his family. At that time he had no gastrointestinal complaints. His only pharmacologic treatment was morphine therapy prescribed by his family doctor.

Four days later the patient was admitted to the ER with the clinical presentation of an acute abdomen. An abdominal radiograph taken at 11:50 showed gaseous distention of the small and large bowel, continuous aeration of the gastrointestinal tract as far as the rectum, and scattered air–fluid levels in the small bowel and colon (**Fig. 4.57**).

Further management was discussed by telephone between the radiological and medical residents handling the case. Suspecting paralytic ileus, they agreed that the next step was an upper GI series with iodinated contrast (**Fig. 4.58**). Following oral contrast administration, abdominal radiographs were taken at 13:04, 14:13, and 18:15. The final radiology report stated that paralytic ileus was the most likely diagnosis, and laxative medication was recommended.

Further Case Summary

The patient died 2 hours after the last radiograph.

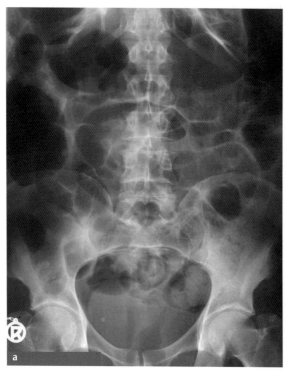

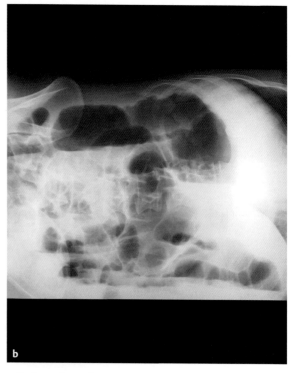

Fig. 4.57 a, b   Radiographs taken at 11:50. The report described fluid levels in the small and large bowel with no free air.

a Supine radiograph.
b LLBP radiograph.

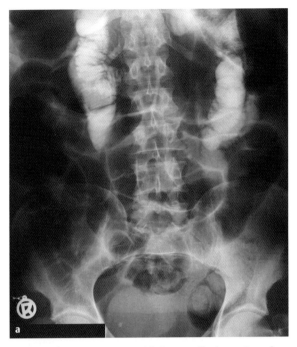
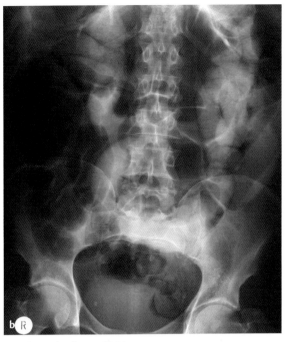

Fig. 4.58 a, b   Upper GI series with Gastrografin shows signs of paralytic ileus.

a   Radiograph taken at 13:04.
b   Radiograph taken at 18:15.

Error Analysis and Strategy for Error Prevention

The patient suffered from paralytic ileus brought on by morphine therapy without concomitant stimulation of peristalsis (**Table 4.4**). The abdomen plain film had already shown the classic features of paralytic ileus with continuous aeration of the gastrointestinal tract as far as the rectum, distention of the small and large bowel, and intestinal air–fluid levels. An upper GI series with iodinated contrast was not indicated, and the work-up was excessive because the initial radiographic examination was already diagnostic. Under other circumstances, the oral administration of an iodinated contrast medium such as Gastrografin may be clinically justified on therapeutic grounds since the hyperosmolarity of the medium will stimulate peristalsis by shifting fluid from the interstitium into the bowel lumen. While the use of Gastrografin would have been reasonable in a standard radiographic algorithm (p. 198), the work-up was not appropriate in this case because the patient had to endure multiple transfers to a central radiology unit during the last hours of his life.

References and Further Reading

Gore RM, Levine MS. Textbook of Gastrointestinal Radiology. 3rd ed. Philadelphia: WB Saunders; 2008

Table 4.4   Possible causes of paralytic ileus

Type	Cause
Functional	Inflammatory-toxic cause ■ Peritonitis ■ Abscess ■ Toxic exposure Metabolic cause ■ Electrolyte disorders ■ Protein deficiency Reflex cause ■ Abnormal ureteral peristalsis ■ Spinal fracture ■ Retroperitoneal hemorrhage Neurologic cause Pharmacologic cause ■ Morphine, etc.
Vascular	Arterial obstruction ■ Embolism ■ Thrombosis Venous obstruction ■ Superior mesenteric vein thrombosis ■ Portal vein thrombosis ■ Obstruction by a tumor Chronic arterial obstruction ■ Nonocclusive mesenteric ischemia ■ Vasculitis ■ Connective-tissue diseases

Mechanical Obstruction of the Small Bowel/ Large Bowel

History and Clinical Findings

The patient was a 52-year-old woman who came to the ER complaining of abdominal pain, vomiting, and retention of stool for the past 3 days. Her prior history included surgery for a bowel obstruction 10 years earlier, and she had undergone a left hemipelvectomy for osteosarcoma 8 years earlier. Abdominal ultrasound showed no abnormalities other than markedly distended bowel loops filled with air and fluid. A mechanical small-bowel obstruction was diagnosed on the basis of plain abdominal radiographs (**Fig. 4.59**).

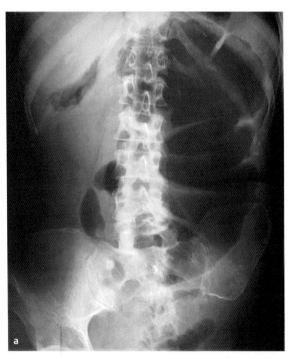
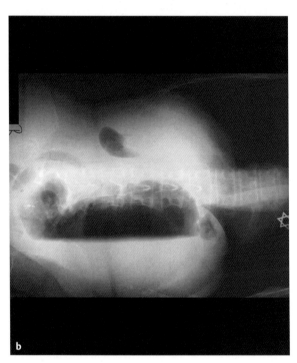

Fig. 4.59 a, b Abdominal radiographs in two planes demonstrate features of a mechanical small-bowel obstruction.

Further Case Summary

In preparation for operative treatment, the surgeon requested a contrast enema with water-soluble iodinated contrast medium (**Fig. 4.60**). This study revealed a mechanical obstruction of the small bowel. An adhesive bowel obstruction was found at operation. An ileocecal resection was performed, and continuity was restored. The patient had a normal postoperative course.

Error Analysis and Strategy for Error Prevention

It was difficult to localize the dilated, air-filled bowel loops to the ileum because the identifying valvulae conniventes were largely effaced by the distention and advanced edema of the bowel wall. The following signs still suggested the correct diagnosis, however:

- The valvulae conniventes were still identifiable in some bowel loops (**Fig. 4.61 a**).
- The left lateral decubitus abdominal radiograph showed dilated small-bowel loops in the left hemiabdomen (**Fig. 4.61 b**). These dilated loops were not visible in the supine film. The small-bowel loops in the

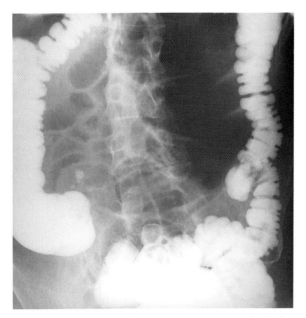

Fig. 4.60 Contrast enema shows a normal-appearing colon in the presence of a mechanical small-bowel obstruction.

right hemiabdomen affected by the mechanical obstruction were so fluid-distended that there was no significant absorption difference between the fluid-filled bowel loops and the surrounding soft tissues.

Incidental findings included a lumbosacral transitional vertebra, a previous laminectomy at L6–S1, and oily contrast residues from a previous myelogram, which typically are not absorbed.

References and Further Reading

Gore RM, Levine MS. Textbook of Gastrointestinal Radiology. 3rd ed. Philadelphia: WB Saunders; 2008

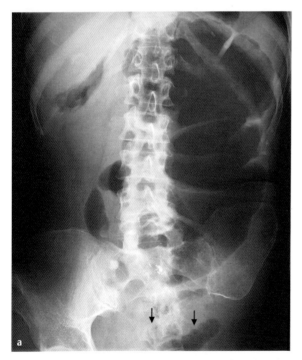

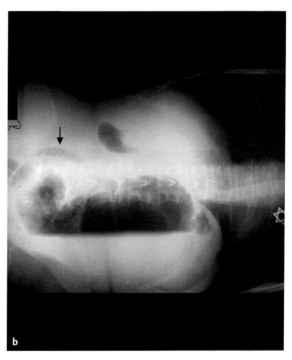

Fig. 4.61 a, b Plain abdominal radiographs in two planes (see also Fig. 4.59 a, b) show signs of mechanical small-bowel obstruction with marked distention of the small bowel and scant air in the colon. Incidental findings: lumbosacral transitional vertebra, prior laminectomy at L6-S1, left hemipelvectomy, and oily contrast residues from a previous myelogram.

a Supine abdominal radiograph. Valvulae conniventes (arrows).
b LLBP abdominal radiograph shows gravitational dependence of bowel structures (arrow) and their contents.

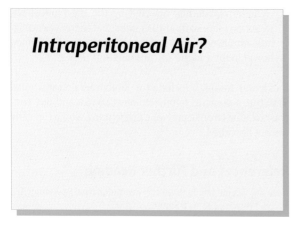

Intraperitoneal Air?

History and Clinical Findings

A 50-year-old man was hospitalized with the clinical presentation of an acute abdomen. The pain was localized to the mid-abdomen. Laboratory inflammatory markers were elevated (WBC 14 700/μL, CRP 230 mg/L). Body temperature was 38 °C. The patient had previously undergone a colectomy with ileostomy for ulcerative colitis. He had also suffered for years from Child C hepatic cirrhosis caused by chronic hepatitis C.

Abdominal radiographs were obtained to detect or exclude a gastrointestinal perforation (**Fig. 4.62**). The radiology report described fluid levels in the right upper quadrant of the abdomen.

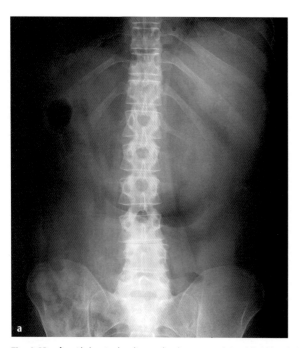
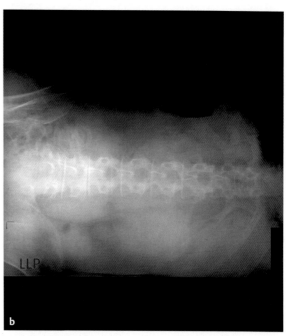

Fig. 4.62 a, b   Abdominal radiographs show unexplained fluid levels in the upper right quadrant with no distended bowel loops.

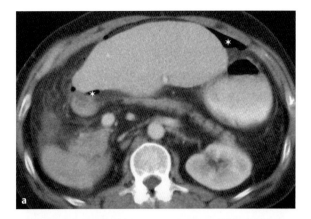

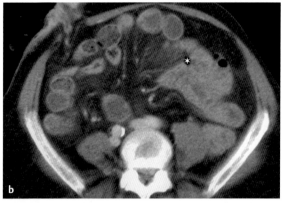

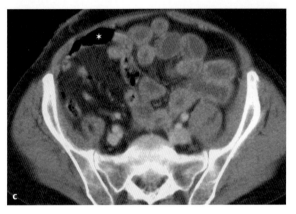

Fig. 4.63 a–c Abdominal CT scans after IV and oral contrast administration. Encapsulated intraperitoneal air collections (★) originate from a perforated gastric ulcer. The scans show evidence of peritonitis with wall thickening and abnormal contrast enhancement of all small-bowel loops, which are fluid-distended due to paralysis, along with diffuse fluid uptake in the mesentery. The patient had a previous colectomy with an ileostomy in the lower right quadrant.

Further Case Summary

Given the clinical severity of the patient's condition, abdominal CT was performed on the same day (**Fig. 4.63**). The scans showed circumscribed air collections throughout the peritoneal cavity. All the small-bowel loops were almost completely filled with fluid. The walls of the jejunum and ileum were thickened and showed increased contrast enhancement. The scans also showed diffuse mesenteric edema that varied markedly in different regions. The findings were interpreted as a gastrointestinal perforation with peritonitis. Other incidental findings were status post colectomy with an ileostomy and hepatic cirrhosis.

Subsequent surgery confirmed a perforated gastric ulcer resulting in diffuse peritonitis.

Error Analysis and Strategy for Error Prevention

Because of the adhesions that formed after the colectomy, the air that had entered the abdominal cavity through the gastric perforation was not distributed freely in the peritoneal cavity but collected within walled-off spaces in the right side of the abdominal cavity in the supine position (**Figs. 4.62a, 4.63**) and in the prone and LLBP positions (**Fig. 4.62b**). When the abdominal plain films were interpreted, it should have been noted that air and air–fluid levels projected over the liver are abnormal in a colectomized patient (**Fig. 4.64**). None of the air collections were associated with detectable valvulae conniventes because the air was not located in the jejunum or ileum. In retrospect, the distention of the gastric body and antrum was a manifestation of reflex paralysis.

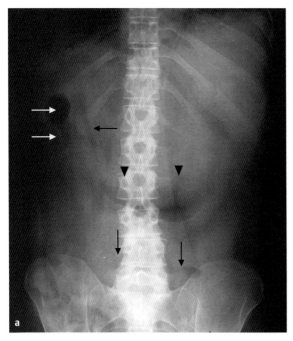
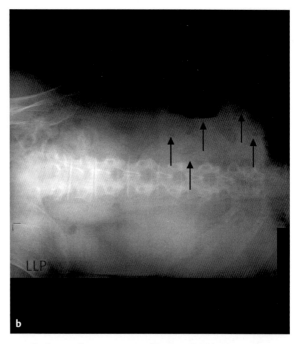

Fig. 4.64 a, b   Air collections on abdominal radiographs (arrows) are not consistent with air in the gastrointestinal tract in this colectomized patient. This particularly applies to air pockets projected over the liver and epigastrium. Isolated air–fluid levels are also seen. Distention of the gastric antrum and body are a result of paralysis (arrowheads).

Table 4.5   Frequent causes of perforation of an intra- or retroperitoneal hollow viscus and their radiologic differential diagnosis

Causes of pneumoperitoneum	Causes of pseudo-pneumoperitoneum
■ Perforated gastric or duodenal ulcer	■ Chilaiditi syndrome (right flexure interposed between the liver and diaphragm)
■ Perforated appendicitis	
■ Perforated sigmoid diverticulitis	■ Subdiaphragmatic fat
■ Perforated Meckel diverticulum	■ Basal pneumothorax
■ Perforated toxic megacolon	■ Distention of a hollow viscus
■ Perforated gallbladder (empyema, hydrops)	■ Omental fat between the liver and diaphragm
■ Perforated small-bowel ulcer	■ Subphrenic abscess
■ Uterine perforation or rupture	
■ Tubal rupture (pyosalpinx, ectopic pregnancy)	
■ Perforation of the pelvicaliceal system	
■ Necrotizing small-bowel ischemia	
■ Traumatic hollow viscus rupture	
■ Iatrogenic perforation	
■ Perforating foreign body	
■ Peritoneal dialysis	
■ Pneumothorax (congenital transdiaphragmatic pleuroperitoneal connections)	

Perforation of an Abdominal Hollow Viscus

The radiologic hallmark of a gastrointestinal perforation is the detection of extraluminal air. A perforated intraperitoneal viscus (jejunum, ileum, transverse colon, sigmoid colon) produces "free" air that can spread throughout the peritoneal cavity. Retroperitoneal perforations (duodenum, ascending and descending colon) lead to air collections in the corresponding compartments of the retroperitoneal space. If the leak includes fluid as well as air, air–fluid levels will be visible in horizontal projections and CT scans. This is a relatively infrequent cause of air–fluid levels and should not be mistaken for a bowel obstruction. Pneumoperitoneum is found in only 75–80% of surgically confirmed perforations. False-negative findings may result from confined perforations with early closure of the perforation site, an absence of air in the perforated bowel segment, the presence of adhesions, or technical flaws in the examination itself (overexposure, absent or incomplete imaging of the flank).

Plain abdominal radiographs. A horizontal projection (generally standing or in LLBP) is necessary for the detection of free air. The patient should remain in the imaging position for at least 10 min before filming to allow time for the intraperitoneal redistribution of air. Reportedly, the minimum detectable volume of free intraperitoneal air is 1–2 cm^3. A correctly exposed plain abdominal radiograph in LLBP can detect free intraperitoneal air in up to 90% of cases, whereas an upright film can detect free air in only about 55% of perforations.

Computed tomography. CT is more sensitive and specific than conventional plain films in the detection of free intraperitoneal air as well as intra- or retroperitoneal air collections that are encapsulated by adhesions. CT is also useful for evaluating the walls of the stomach and bowel and their surroundings to determine the perforation site, the cause of the perforation (**Table 4.5**), and associated diseases. Spiral CT can demonstrate the perforation site more frequently than incremental scans.

References and Further Reading

Earls JP, Dachmann AH, Colon E, Garrett MG, Molloy M. Prevalence and duration of postoperative pneumoperitoneum: sensitivity of CT vs. left lateral decubitus radiography. Am J Radiol 1993; 161: 781–785

Ghekiere O, Lesnik A, Hoa D, Laffargue G, Uriot C, Taourel P. Value of computed tomography in the diagnosis of the cause of nontraumatic gastrointestinal perforation. J Comput Assist Tomogr 2007; 31: 169–176

Grassi R, Romano S, Pinto A, et al. Conventional plain film, ultrasonography and CT in jejuno-ileal perforations. Acta Radiol 1998; 38: 52–56

Grassi R, Pinto A, Rossi G, et al. Gastroduodenal perforations: conventional plain film, US and CT findings in 166 consecutive patients. Eur J Radiol 2004; 50: 30–36

Hainaux B, Agneessens E, Bertinotti R, et al. Accuracy of MDCT in predicting site of gastrointestinal tract perforation. Am J Radiol 2006; 187: 1179–1183

Stapakis JC, Thickman D. Diagnosis of pneumoperitoneum: abdominal CT vs. upright chest film. J Comput Assist Tomogr 1992; 16: 713–716

Normal Postgastrectomy Findings/ Colon Perforation/ Postoperative Abscess/ Bowel Obstruction

History and Clinical Findings

A 65-year-old woman had undergone a gastrectomy with esophagojenunostomy and a Roux-en-Y anastomosis for cancer of the gastric cardia. She was referred for abdominal CT on a Sunday for investigation of an acute abdomen. The written report by the physician on duty described a small amount of ascites about the liver and in the gallbladder bed, a previous gastrectomy with a Roux-en-Y anastomosis, and a partial bowel obstruction (**Fig. 4.65**).

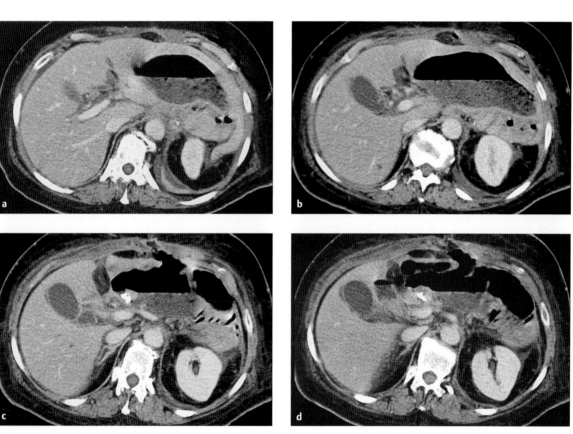

Fig. 4.65 a–d Abdominal CT scans were described as showing dysontogenetic liver cysts (differential diagnosis: metastases); no collections other than a small amount of ascites about the liver and in the gallbladder bed; a previous gastrectomy with a Roux-en-Y anastomosis; and a partial bowel obstruction.

Further Case Summary

On Monday, a routine review of the CT scans taken during the weekend revealed an extraluminal air–fluid collection arising from the transverse colon and extending anteriorly into the muscular portion of the median laparotomy, cephalad into the left anterior compartment of the peritoneal cavity, and posteriorly into the former lesser sac. Air was also present in the right anterior compartment. A perforation of the transverse colon was suspected, and a contrast enema confirmed the diagnosis (**Fig. 4.66**). Surgery was performed the same day, at which time the perforation in the transverse colon was oversewn and a protective ileostomy was created.

The definitive cause of the perforation was not determined. The most likely explanation is ischemic necrosis at the junction of the superior and inferior mesenteric artery territories rather than an iatrogenic bowel injury during the gastrectomy.

Error Analysis and Strategy for Error Prevention

The misdiagnosis was based on a deficient analysis of topographic anatomy (**Figs. 4.67, 4.68**). The broad, abnormal air track arising from the transverse colon should have been detected. Even after gastrectomy, the broad air–fluid level in the former lesser sac was unphysiologic and was suspicious for a complication. Similarly, free air in the right anterior peritoneal compartment was not a normal postoperative finding after gastrectomy. The flawed primary image interpretation delayed operative treatment. The further course was uneventful.

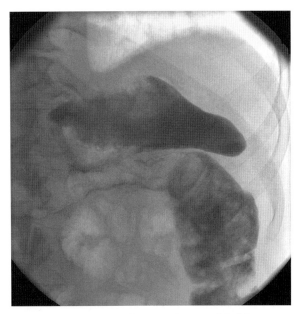

Fig. 4.66 Contrast enema shows a perforation of the left transverse colon proximal to the left flexure with contrast extravasation cranial to the transverse colon.

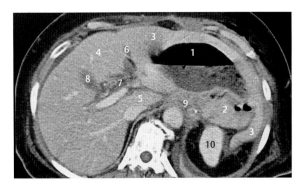

Fig. 4.67 Pathoanatomic analysis of the CT findings (**Fig. 4.65 a**). 1 = Air–fluid level in the former lesser sac; 2 = left colic flexure; 3 = left lobe of liver; 4 = right lobe of liver; 5 = caudate lobe; 6 = falciform ligament; 7 = porta hepatis; 8 = superior pole of gallbladder; 9 = esophagus with gastric tube; 10 = superior pole of left kidney.

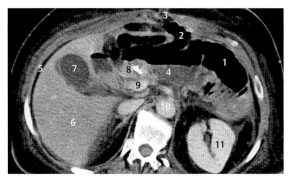

Fig. 4.68 Pathoanatomic analysis of **Fig. 4.65 d**. 1 = Transverse colon; 2 = perforation; 3 = medial laparotomy; 4 = air–fluid level in the former lesser sac; 5 = air in the right anterior compartment of the peritoneal cavity; 6 = right lobe of liver; 7 = gallbladder; 8 = transposed jejunum with gastric tube; 9 = portal vein; 10 = aorta with origin of celiac trunk; 11 = left kidney.

Free Intraperitoneal Air/ Intestinal Malrotation/ Normal Findings

History and Clinical Findings

A newborn infant was referred for a supine chest radiograph on the first day of life to check the position of a gastric tube. The radiograph showed air projected over the liver (**Fig. 4.69**). The differential diagnosis of this finding included free intraperitoneal air and malrotation of the bowel. A supine radiograph of the chest and abdomen documented normal aeration of the gastrointestinal tract. That projection could not be evaluated for the presence of a pneumoperitoneum. Given the normal clinical findings and to avoid unnecessary stress on the newborn, a cross-table radiograph with an upright cassette was not obtained. Three days later, clinical findings were still normal and a supine plain abdominal radiograph was taken in the early evening for follow-up. That film was interpreted as normal (**Fig. 4.70**).

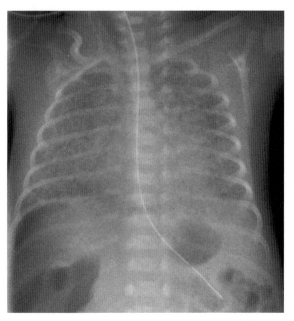

Fig. 4.69 Supine chest radiograph shows free air projected over the liver: pneumoperitoneum or intestinal malrotation. The gastric tube is correctly positioned.

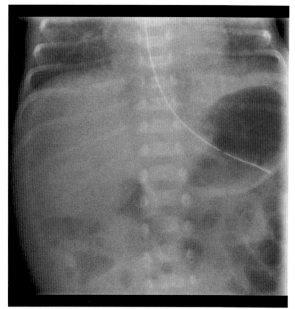

Fig. 4.70 Supine abdominal radiograph 3 days later shows normal findings with no evidence of free intraperitoneal air.

Further Case Summary

In a routine review of the images taken the night before, the findings were revised. A cross-table supine abdominal radiograph with an upright cassette confirmed the presence of free intraperitoneal air (**Fig. 4.71**), indicating a gastrointestinal perforation. A perforation of the small bowel approximately 30 cm proximal to the ileocecal valve was diagnosed intraoperatively and oversewn. A retrospective review of the clinical course and radiologic findings suggested that the perforation had occurred in utero or during the delivery.

Error Analysis and Strategy for Error Prevention

Air in the peritoneal cavity rises when the patient lies in a supine position. On radiographs taken in the AP projection, free air can be seen when it is present in a sufficient volume, appearing as a rounded or oval lucency superimposed over parenchymal and intestinal structures (**Fig. 4.69**). A supine radiograph taken in the cross-table projection with an upright cassette will provide a largely nonsuperimposed view of the free air, which collects beneath the anterior abdominal wall. Thus, the diagnosis in this case should have been confirmed on the first day of life by obtaining an abdominal plain film in the second projection.

The supine abdominal radiograph taken on the third day of life showed a faint lucent area projected over the right upper quadrant of the abdomen, consistent with free air. That finding was either missed or misinterpreted (**Fig. 4.72**).

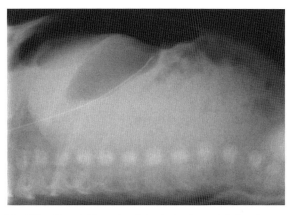

Fig. 4.71 Cross-table supine abdominal radiograph 1 day after that shown in **Fig. 4.70** demonstrates a pneumoperitoneum.

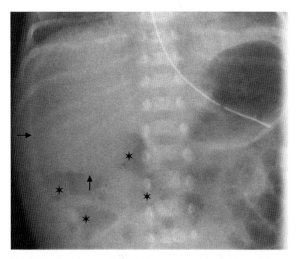

Fig. 4.72 Free intraperitoneal air appears as a lucent area with smooth lateral and inferior margins projected over the liver (arrows). Asterisks indicate the right flexure and transverse colon.

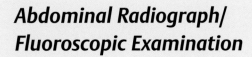

Abdominal Radiograph/ Fluoroscopic Examination

History and Clinical Findings

A 61-year-old man underwent an esophagectomy with gastric pull-up and gastrostomy. Afterward the visceral surgeon referred him for radiologic assessment of the duodenal tube. The radiology technician took the plain abdominal radiograph shown in **Fig. 4.73**.

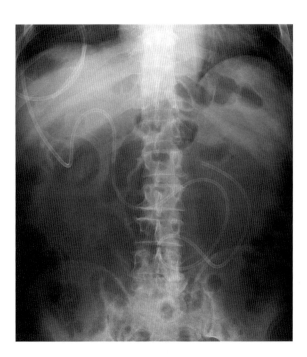

Fig. 4.73 Plain abdominal radiograph displays the duodenal feeding tube.

Further Case Summary

The patient had undergone a gastric pull-up esophagectomy for distal esophageal cancer. It was felt that postoperative necrosis at the anastomotic site would heal by scarring if oral intake were withheld for several weeks. The examination was indicated for the detection or exclusion of residual extravasation. Subsequent contrast injection into the feeding tube under fluoroscopic control showed normal postoperative findings.

Error Analysis and Strategy for Error Prevention

The indication and examination technique should have been checked by a competent physician (in this case the attending radiologist) as prescribed by law. From a radiation safety standpoint and given the clinical context, there was no sound rationale for plain abdominal radiography. Fluoroscopic images during the contrast examination should have been documented.

References and Further Reading

American College of Radiology (ACR). ACR Practice Guideline for Diagnostic Reference Levels in Medical X-ray Imaging. http://www.acr.org/SecondaryMainMenuCategories/quality_safety/RadSafety/RadiationSafety/guideline-diagnostic-reference.aspx (accessed November 10, 2010)

Amis ES, Butler PF, Applegate KE, et al. American College of Radiology White Paper on Radiation Dose in Medicine. J Am Coll Radiol 2007; 4: 272–284. http://www.acr.org/SecondaryMainMenuCategories/quality_safety/white_paper_dose.aspx (accessed November 10, 2010)

Council Directive 96/29/EURATOM of 13, May 1996 laying down basic safety standards for the protection of the health of workers and the general public against the danger arising from ionizing radiation. http://ec.europa.eu/energy/nuclear/radioprotection/doc/legislation/9629_en.pdf. (accessed January 10, 2011)

Council Directive 97/43/EURATOM of 30 June 1997 on health protection in individuals against the dangers of ionizing radiation in relation to medical exposure, and repealing Directive 84/466/Euratom. http://ec.europa.eu/energy/nuclear/radioprotection/doc/legislation/9743_en.pdf (accessed January 10, 2011)

Sonnek C, Bauer B. Die neue Röntgenverordnung. Berlin: H. Hoffmann; 2002

Example of How Directive 97/43/EURATOM Issued by the Council of the European Union Became National Law

"Justified Indication" as Defined in the German X-Ray Ordinance (RöV)

Article 2 of the RöV states that a medical doctor or dentist with the necessary expertise in radiation safety shall decide whether and in what manner humans will be exposed to x-rays in the practice of medicine or dentistry.

Article 23, paragraph 1 of the RöV states that the direct exposure of humans to x-rays in the practice of medicine or dentistry is permissible only if a qualified person as defined in article 24, paragraph 1, number 1 or 2 has established a justified indication for it, i.e., has determined that the health benefits of the x-ray exposure outweigh the risks of the exposure. Other procedures with a comparable health benefit that involve little or no x-ray exposure should be considered when this determination is made. A justified indication as defined in paragraph 1 may also be established by a referring physician....

Article 24, paragraph 1 of the RöV states that x-rays may be used in medicine or dentistry only by:

1. Persons who are accredited medical doctors, or are authorized to practice as such, and have the requisite expertise in radiation safety in the general diagnostic or therapeutic use of x-rays (full radiologists).
2. Persons who are accredited medical doctors or dentists, or are authorized to practice as such, and have the requisite expertise in radiation safety within their limited area of x-ray use (physicians without board certification in radiology).
3. Persons who are accredited medical doctors or dentists, or are authorized to practice as such, and do not currently have the requisite knowledge of radiation safety (doctors in specialty training).

Metastasis/Negative Oncologic Findings

hospital. The primary tumor was unknown. It was unclear, whether the nodal involvement resulted from lo-coregional lymph node metastasis or hematogenous metastasis to an axillary node. Dermatologists speculated that skin biopsies taken 3 and 7 years earlier (right shoulder, diagnosed as acanthotic variant of seborrheic keratosis; right supraclavicular region, diagnosed as papillomatous compound nevus) may have been misinterpreted as benign and may have represented the primary tumor. Whole-body PET/CT scans had shown no evidence of a primary tumor or additional metastases. The patient later presented for approximately 3-month-interval follow-ups consisting of a clinical examination, laboratory determination of serum S-100β marker level, and ultrasound scanning of the cervical soft tissues, axillae, and groin.

Two years after the initial diagnosis, the patient's serum S-100β level rose from values in the range of 0.07–0.14 μg/L to 0.86 μg/L (< 0.12 μg/L is normal, 0.12 –0.20 μg/L is borderline, and > 0.20 μg/L is abnormal). To exclude growth of the previously unknown primary tumor or

History and Clinical Findings

Two years before his current presentation, a 53-year-old man underwent excision of a right axillary lymph node metastasis from amelanotic melanoma at a different

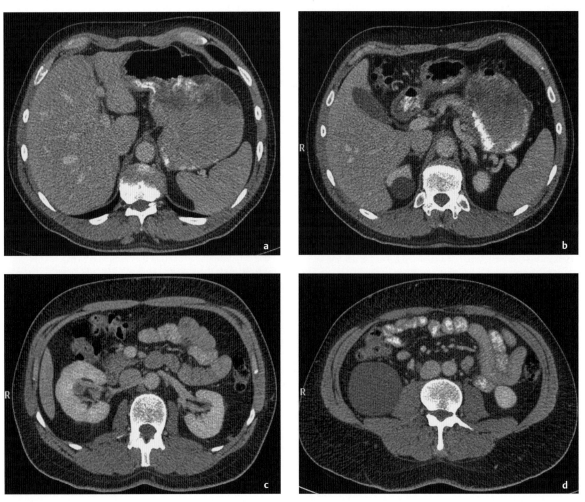

Fig. 4.74 a–h These abdominal CT scans were interpreted as negative for cancer. Dysontogenetic cysts were noted in the right kidney as an incidental finding (**c–f**).

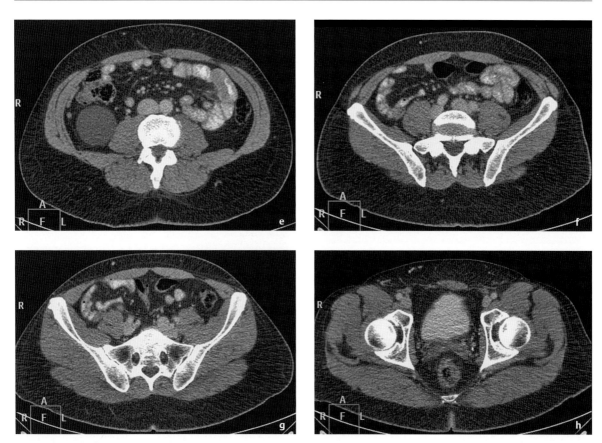

Fig. 4.74 e–h Continued

metastasis, the patient was evaluated by thoracic and abdominal CT (**Fig. 4.74**) and cranial MRI, which yielded normal findings. Given the only slight elevation of the borderline S-100β levels, the patient was scheduled for a clinical and laboratory follow-up at 3 months.

Further Case Summary

When he returned 3 months later, the patient complained of pain in his left thigh. Other clinical findings were normal. The serum S-100β level had risen to 1.34 μg/L. CT scans of the abdomen and thigh showed thickening of the small-bowel wall at the jejunoileal junction, which was not yet associated with bowel obstruction (**Fig. 4.75 a, b**). The differential diagnosis of this finding included the primary tumor and hematogenous metastasis. CT also showed an osteolytic metastasis with a soft-tissue component in the mid-diaphysis of the left femur (**Fig. 4.75 c, d**)/FDG/PET showed foci of increased glucose metabolism at the sites of the two CT-confirmed tumors with no other focal abnormalities. By 8 weeks after the second CT examination, the patient's serum S-100β level had risen to 2.14 μg/L. The small-bowel tumor was resected. Immunohistology identified the lesion as metastatic to amelanotic malignant melanoma. Hence the primary tumor was still unknown. The metastasis in the left femur was excised for histopathology and to reduce the tumor volume. The bone was stabilized by composite internal fixation and treated with postoperative radiotherapy. The serum S-100β level declined postoperatively to a range of 0.37–0.89 μg/L. No additional metastases were found during 1 year of follow-up.

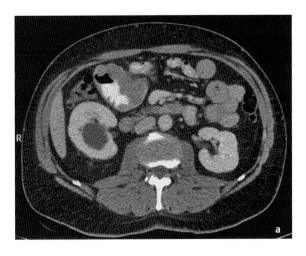

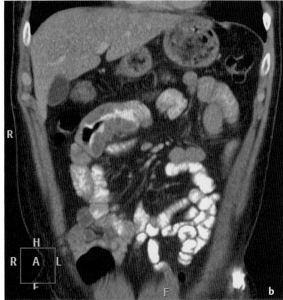

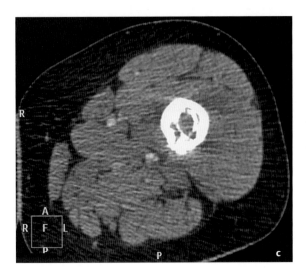

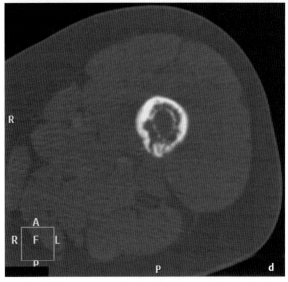

Fig. 4.75 a–d CT follow-up at 3 months.
a Axial data acquisition.
b Coronal reformatted image.

c Magnified image of the left thigh with a soft-tissue window.
d Magnified image of the left thigh with a bone window.

Error Analysis and Strategy for Error Prevention

The eccentric thickening of the small bowel at the jejunoileal junction was already detectable at the first CT follow-up prompted by an elevated serum S-100β and had increased since the previous examination. Its variable location in the right (**Fig. 4.74 e**) and left mid-abdomen (**Fig. 4.75 a, b**) is explained by the mobility of the small bowel within the abdominal cavity, as the bowel loops are tethered to the retroperitoneum only by their mesenteric pedicle. The lesion was missed (see **Fig. 4.76**) because the possibility of enteric tumor involvement was not con-

sidered and it had produced no clinical symptoms. It is rare for a malignant melanoma to arise from small-bowel mucosa. The primary hematogenous metastasis of malignant melanoma occurs in only 30% of affected patients. At the time of primary diagnosis 50% of tumors undergo locoregional lymphogenous metastasis, and 20% produce satellite or in-transit metastases. Based on the analysis of clinical and radiologic studies, we know that the hematogenous metastasis of malignant melanoma occurs most frequently to the lung (18–36% of patients), followed by the liver (14–20%), brain (2–20%), skeleton (4–17%), adrenal glands (1–11%), and gastrointestinal tract (1–8%, two-thirds to small bowel, one-third to colon).

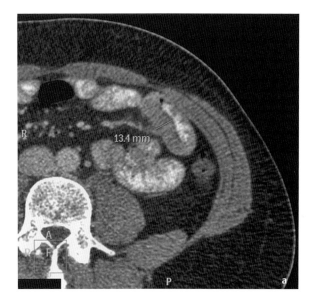

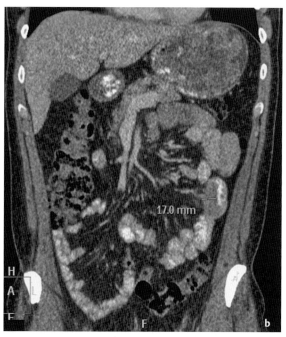

Fig. 4.76 a,b   Eccentric thickening of the small bowel at the jejunoileal junction. This finding was missed in the first two CT examinations (see **Fig. 4.74 e**).

S-100β Tumor Marker

The S-100β protein is expressed by cells of the nervous system, cartilage cells, fat cells, and cells of melanocytic origin. Because it is expressed in the central nervous system, S-100β was long used as a marker protein for malignant melanoma in the serum and CSF. It was first described as a serum marker for melanoma in the mid 1990s. Since then, the determination of serum S-100β levels has proven to be a good indicator of tumor burden, disease progression, and treatment response in patients with metastatic melanoma. Because the serum S-100β level correlates with the tumor mass present in the patient's body, a level above the normal range provides an indicator of tumor growth. The S-100β marker is also useful for evaluating response in patients with hematogenous metastasis. Due to the small tumor mass in patients with primary-stage melanoma, the serum S-100β protein level is not useful for screening, diagnosing primary tumors, or differentiating nevus from melanoma. Because the serum S-100β level correlates with tumor burden, it correlates with total survival in patients with metastatic disease. Serum S-100β does not correlate with total or disease-free survival in tumor-free patients.

References and Further Reading

Ghanem G, Loir B, Morandini R, et al. On the release and half-life of S100β protein in the peripheral blood of melanoma patients. Int J Cancer 2001; 94: 586–590

Guo HB, Stoffel-Wagner B, Bierwirth P, Mezger J, Klingmüller D. Clinical significance of serum S100 in metastatic malignant melanoma. Eur J Cancer 1995; 31: 924–928

Hauschild A, Engel G, Brenner W, et al. Predictive value of serum S100β for monitoring patients with metastatic melanoma during chemotherapy and/or immunotherapy. Br J Dermatol 1999;140: 1065–1071

Hauschild A, et al. S100β protein detection in serum is a significant prognostic factor in metastatic melanoma. Oncology 1999; 56: 338–344

Jury CS, McAllister EJ, MacKie RM. Rising levels of serum S100 protein precede other evidence of disease progression in patients with malignant melanoma. Br J Dermatol 2000; 143: 269–274

Leiter U, Meier F, Schittek B, Garbe C. The natural course of cutaneous melanoma. J Surg Oncol 2004; 86: 172–178

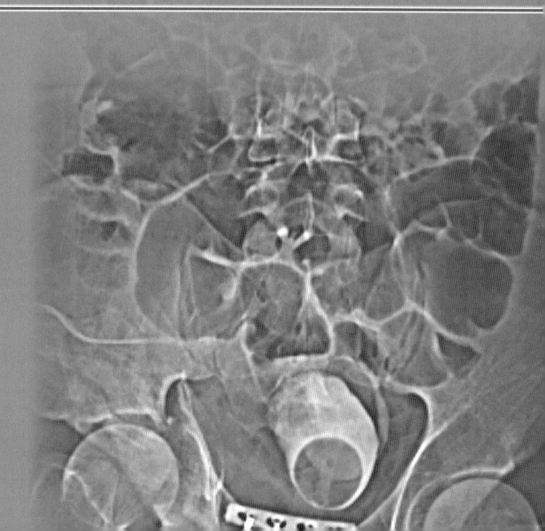

Abdomen
Urogenital Tract

Renal Parenchymal Damage/ Contrast Infusion Error

History and Clinical Findings

A 64-year-old man receiving chemotherapy for malignant lymphoma in an oncology ward complained of noncolicky pain in both flanks. A urologist was called in and ordered an IVP. When he arrived at radiology, the patient had a serum creatinine of 1.8 mg/dL. Intravenous pyelography was performed using standard technique (infusion of 100 mL of a nonionic iodinated contrast agent, iodine concentration 300 mg/dL). An abdominal radiograph taken 15 minutes after IV contrast administration showed contrast medium in the bladder with poor visualization of the upper urinary tract (**Fig. 4.77**).

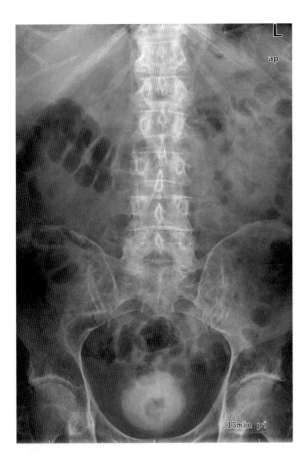

Fig. 4.77 Abdominal radiograph taken 15 minutes after IV contrast administration.

Further Case Summary

When the ward physician was questioned, it was learned that before receiving the IVP the patient had been given 1 liter of IV NaCl solution for volume replacement due to compensated renal failure. The diluting effect of this solution led to poor opacification of the renal pelves and ureters. The IVP was not repeated the next day because of the clinical improvement.

Error Analysis and Strategy for Error Prevention

The IV infusion of NaCl solution before the IVP resulted in poor visualization of the kidneys and ureters. Intravenous saline to promote diuresis is appropriate only after the IV administration of an iodinated contrast agent in patients with compensated renal failure. In effect, the IV infusion of NaCl solution (1000 mL) before the study reduced the iodine concentration of the contrast medium (100 mL) from 300 mg/dL to only 30 mg/dL. The infusion of Ringer solution temporarily lowered the colloidal osmotic pressure in the blood plasma. From the formula

$$P_{eff} = P_C - P_B - \pi$$

where P_{eff} is the effective filtration pressure, P_C is the hydrostatic capillary pressure, P_B is the hydrostatic pressure in the Bowman capsule, and π is the colloidal osmotic pressure, we see that the reduced colloidal osmotic pressure causes a rise in the effective filtration pressure, resulting in an increased volume of filtered primary urine (**Fig. 4.78**). Since the volume and iodine concentration of the administered contrast medium are normalized, the same number of contrast molecules were excreted into Bowman's space as under normal conditions, and therefore the concentration of iodine atoms in the primary urine was lower than it would have been if the patient had not been "prehydrated." This disproportion was not offset by physiologic water and electrolyte shifts during tubular transit due to the reduction of plasma and primary-urine osmolarity by the infusions. Instead, the contrast medium itself functioned as an additional diuretic as the tubular concentration of contrast medium in the descending limb of Henley's loop increased through the physiologic tubular resorption of water, thereby raising the osmolarity of the primary urine and, in an extreme case, preventing any further reabsorption.

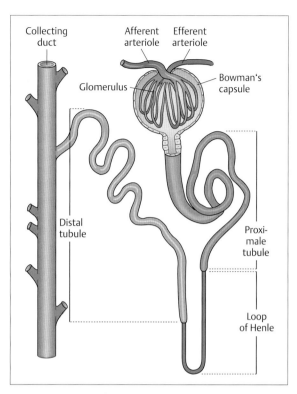

Fig. 4.78 Structure of a nephron. (Source: Schurek H.-J., Neumann K-H. Physiologie der Niere. In: Koch K-M, ed. Klinische Nephrologie. Munich: Urban & Fischer; 2000. Reprinted with permission.)

Another factor was that the IV infusion increased the urine volume. This caused an increase in tubular flow with a more rapid passage of opacified urine into the bladder than if preliminary volume replacement had been withheld.

References and Further Reading

Schurek H-J, Neumann K-H. Physiologie der Niere. In: Koch K-M, ed. Klinische Nephrologie. Munich: Urban & Fischer; 2000

Walsh PC, Retik AB, Vaughan ED, Wein AJ, eds. Campell's Urology. Philadlephia: WB Saunders; 2002

Wein JA, Kavoussi LR, Novick AC, Partin AW, Peters CA, eds. Campell-Walsh Urology. 9th ed. New York: Elsevier; 2007

Urine Formation

The primary urine is formed in the glomeruli of the kidneys. It is an almost protein-free fluid that is filtered from the glomerular capillaries into Bowman's space, which marks the start of the excretory portion of the urinary tract. The glomerular capillary wall has endothelial pores that make it highly permeable to water and low-molecular-weight compounds such as iodinated contrast agents. Only larger molecules are unable to pass through this filtration barrier.

The driving force for glomerular filtration is the hydrostatic capillary pressure (P_C). This pressure is opposed by the hydrostatic pressure in Bowman's space (P_B) and the colloidal osmotic pressure in the capillaries (π), which is determined by the concentration of protein molecules in the blood plasma. Thus, the effective filtration pressure (P_{eff}) is given by the formula

$$P_{eff} = P_C - P_B - \pi.$$

As the blood passes through the glomerular capillaries, the hydrostatic capillary pressure (P_C) falls only slightly due to the low flow resistance, with the result that the transcapillary pressure difference remains almost constant throughout capillary transit. By contrast, the colloidal osmotic pressure (π) increases significantly along the capillary pathway, causing the effective filtration pressure (P_{eff}) to decline toward the end of the capillary. Approximately 180 L/day of primary urine is formed in healthy individuals. As it passes through the tubules, this glomerular filtrate is concentrated to a final urine volume of approximately 1.5 L/day. This is accomplished by the hormonally modulated interaction of various passive transport processes (osmosis, countercurrent concentration mechanism with H_2O exchange between the tubular loop and peritubular capillaries) and active transport mechanisms (Na^+ and Cl^- transfer, etc.).

Four Errors in Examination Technique

History and Clinical Findings

An 82-year-old bed-confined patient was referred for IVP to evaluate the urinary tract on the left side, having undergone a right nephroureterectomy for urothelial carcinoma 4 months earlier. She had undergone a total left hip replacement 17 years earlier. Ultrasound did not show a urinary tract obstruction. Her serum creatinine was 1.9 mg/dL. Intravenous pyelography (**Fig. 4.79**) was performed using standard technique (infusion of 100 mL of a nonionic contrast medium, iodine concentration 300 mg/dL). The IVP report noted dilatation of the left pelvicaliceal system and proximal left ureter, surgical clips projected over the right upper quadrant of the abdomen, osteochondrosis of the lower lumbar spine, osteoarthritis of the right hip, and a total hip replacement on the left side. A cause was not given for ectasia of the left renal pelvis and proximal left ureter because of overlying bowel gas and poor opacification of the ureter.

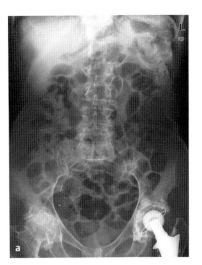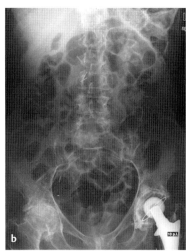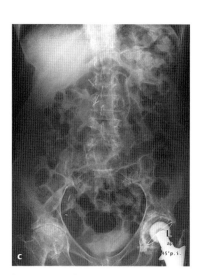

Fig. 4.79 a–c Intravenous pyelography.
a Abdominal radiograph before contrast administration.

b Abdominal radiograph 10 minutes after contrast administration.
c Abdominal radiograph 45 minutes after contrast administration.

Further Case Summary

Comparison with the preoperative IVP and retrograde fluoroscopically guided visualization of the left collecting system by the urologist showed that the patient did not have a left-sided urinary tract obstruction but an ampullary pelvicaliceal system (**Fig. 4.80**). There was no evidence of a new urothelial carcinoma or urolithiasis.

Error Analysis and Strategy for Error Prevention

Intravenous pyelography was not indicated in this case because ultrasound had excluded a urinary tract obstruction and the patient had an elevated serum creatinine. Errors in examination technique related to collimation and the sequence of the abdominal radiographs:

- The radiographs were not collimated, which violates standard practice guidelines for x-ray quality assurance. Collimating the emerging x-rays to the region of interest reduces scattered radiation within the patient's body by restricting the exposed body volume. The rays emanating from the x-ray tube are confined to the region of interest by attaching a collimator to the tube. Collimation is confirmed on the film by noting the collimated edges of the x-ray field.
- Examination of the right hemiabdomen was unnecessary. Besides the history and clinical findings, the surgical clips in the right medial retroperitoneum and at the detachment site of the right ureter indicated that the patient had undergone a right nephroureterectomy.
- Given the massive distention of the small and large bowel and the state of compensated renal failure, the examination should have been discontinued after the abdominal radiograph and before contrast administration. A detailed analysis of the collecting system to detect or exclude a small urothelial carcinoma (irregular urinary tract outlines, signs of incipient urinary stasis) was not possible under these circumstances.
- The abdominal radiograph obtained 10 minutes after contrast infusion was taken too soon. Even in patients with normal renal function, it takes approximately 20 minutes for IV contrast medium to fully opacify the kidney and ureter. In the era before color duplex sonography, a film was often taken 5 minutes after contrast

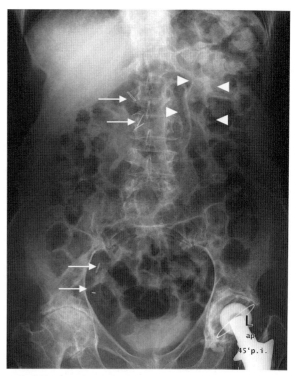

Fig. 4.80 Ampullary left renal pelvis (arrowheads). Surgical clips are projected over the bed of the extirpated right kidney and over the right lesser pelvis (arrows).

infusion to evaluate contrast inflow and the uptake of contrast medium in the renal parenchyma. A discrepancy between the two sides suggested renal artery stenosis and/or unilateral renal parenchymal damage. Today this early view is considered obsolete.

Scattered Radiation

When x-rays encounter atoms, the processes of penetration and absorption are accompanied by the production of scattered radiation. Most of these scattered rays are not directed parallel to the primary beam and therefore do not have a meaningful geometric relationship to structures in the object under study. Superimposition of scattered radiation on the primary x-ray image causes a uniform darkening of the image that reduces contrast and hampers the visualization of fine details. Scattered radiation can be reduced by collimating the x-ray beam (tube, collimator), compressing the abdomen (reducing the object thickness), increasing the object–film distance, and using a scatter-reduction grid. When a collimator is attached to the x-ray tube, it reduces scattered radiation by restricting the x-rays emerging from the tube to the body region under study.

Urinary Tract Obstruction/ Parapelvic Renal Cysts

History and Clinical Findings

A 79-year-old man was referred for abdominal CT with noncolicky flank pain and new grade I hydronephrosis detected on the left side by ultrasound (**Fig. 4.81**). He had a known prior history of parapelvic renal cysts. His urinary status and CBC were normal.

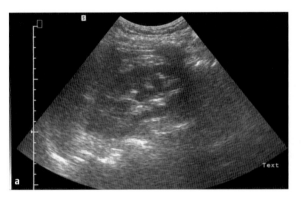
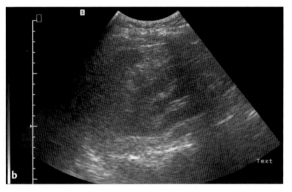

Fig. 4.81 a, b B-mode ultrasound examination of the left kidney. Longitudinal scans at two different angles.

Further Case Summary

CT demonstrated parapelvic cysts in both kidneys (**Fig. 4.82 a–c**). Each kidney was found to have an ampullary pelvis as a normal variant. The cause of the flank pain was not identified. Several days later the patient's complaints improved; to date they have not recurred over a 3-year follow-up period.

Error Analysis and Strategy for Error Prevention

The serous fluid in the parapelvic cysts and the urine in the pelvicaliceal system have the same echogenicity. In this patient the walls separating the adjacent cysts were so thin that they could not be identified sonographically. Ultrasound also failed to demonstrate the stretching of the caliceal necks caused by the mass effect of the parapelvic cysts. As a result, the string of parapelvic cysts (**Fig. 4.82**) created the impression of a dilated pelvicaliceal system. Ultrasound scanning of the kidney in an angled transverse plane would have supplied the correct diagnosis by displaying the normal size of the ureteropelvic junction and proximal ureter. The ureteropelvic junction is the key anatomic feature that can distinguish urinary obstruction from a parapelvic cyst (**Fig. 4.82 b, c**).

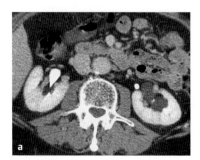 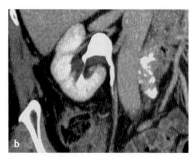 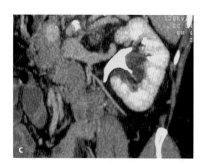

Fig. 4.82 a–c Abdominal CT demonstrates bilateral parapelvic renal cysts.

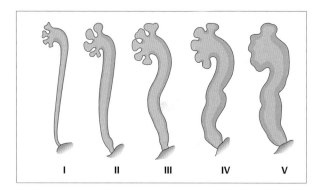

I   II   III   IV   V

Fig. 4.82 d Grades of hydronephrosis (from Bücheler et al, 2006).

References and Further Reading

Bücheler E, Lackner K-J, Thelen M. Einführung in die Radiologie. Diagnostik und Interventionen. 11th ed. Stuttgart: Thieme; 2006

Hepatitis/Pancreatitis/Nephritis/Gastrointestinal Infection

History and Clinical Findings

A 63-year-old woman had experienced nausea and diarrhea for several days. When hospitalized, she had a fever of 40 °C. Her upper abdomen was tender to pressure. The patient stated that she had fallen approximately 5 weeks earlier while in Africa, sustaining a fracture of the left ischium. Her laboratory tests showed elevated inflammatory markers with a CRP of 28 mg/L and WBC of 12 000/µL. The referring internist suspected hepatitis, pancreatitis, or a gastrointestinal infection. He initially reviewed representative abdominal CT scans with the patient and declared that they showed no abnormalities (**Fig. 4.83**).

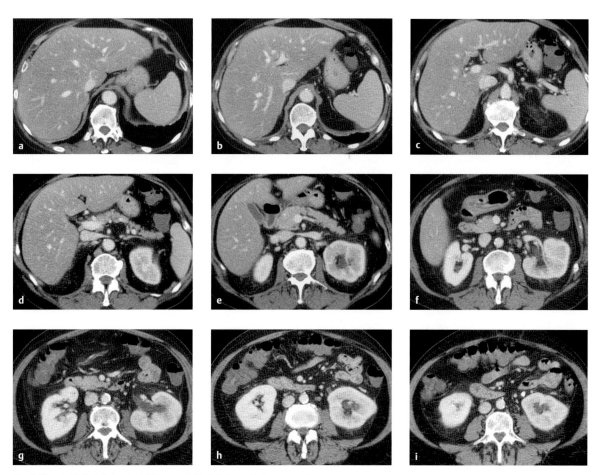

Fig. 4.83 a–i   Spiral abdominal CT scans, initially interpreted as normal.

Further Case Summary

After conferring with radiology, the internist requested a nephrology consult. The nephrologist noted tenderness to percussion in the left renal bed. When all CT images were reviewed again, radiopaque stones were detected in both pelvicaliceal systems and one stone was found in the left ureter (**Figs. 4.83i, 4.84**), leading to grade I hydronephrosis. The parenchyma of the left kidney showed less enhancement in the early and late perfusion phases after IV contrast injection than the right kidney (**Figs. 4.83e–i, 4.84b,c**). The urologists initially performed an ultrasound-guided percutaneous nephrostomy to relieve the obstruction. The nephrostomy yielded urine with a high content of WBCs. The following day, the ureteral stone was disintegrated by extracorporeal shock-wave lithotripsy (ESWL). The stone fragments were excreted with the urine over the next several days. The patient defervesced and was discharged home 1 week later.

Error Analysis and Strategy for Error Prevention

Guided by the clinical impression, the radiologist limited his attention to CT scans acquired in the late perfusion phase after IV contrast administration. While the abnormalities were visible on these images (**Figs. 4.83i, 4.84c**), the increased density of the renal parenchyma and urine in the late phase made the stones more difficult to detect than in the precontrast and early-phase scans, and consequently the findings were missed.

References and Further Reading

Walsh PC, Retik AB, Vaughan ED, Wein AJ, eds. Campell's Urology. Philadelphia: WB Saunders; 2002

Wein JA, Kavoussi LR, Novick AC, Partin AW, Peters CA, eds. Campell-Walsh Urology. 9th ed. New York: Elsevier; 2007

Hydronephrosis/Pyonephrosis

Pyonephrosis (infected hydronephrosis) is defined as a collection of pus in a dilated pelvicaliceal system. It develops in the setting of an obstructive uropathy.

- A complete ureteral obstruction leads to a rise of pressure in the obstructed pelvicaliceal system. The pressure increase is transmitted through the collecting ducts into the renal tubules and Bowman's spaces (increased intranephron pressure). This reduces the pressure gradient between the hydrostatic pressure in the glomerular capillaries and the pressure in Bowman's space (which receives the filtered primary urine) and adjacent tubules. The result of this pressure equalization is an initially short-term fall of the glomerular filtration rate in the affected nephrons.

- A second phase, lasting only a few hours, is marked by an autoregulatory increase in renal blood flow as vasoactive hormones (prostaglandins) dilate the afferent vessels. This leads to an increase in the glomerular filtration rate and a further rise of pressure in the collecting system.

- In a third phase, which lasts weeks to months, activation of the renin–angiotensin system in response to catecholamine secretion leads to decreased renal blood flow and a consequent fall in the glomerular filtration rate with ischemic injury to the tubules.

- In a fourth "steady-state" phase, renal function is irreversibly impaired even if the obstruction is relieved.

Hydronephrosis and pyonephrosis are associated with a risk of urosepsis caused by rapid bacterial proliferation in the obstructed pelvicaliceal system. Even today, this condition has a mortality rate of 70%.

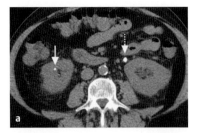 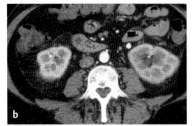 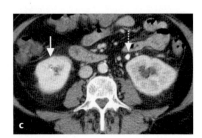

Fig. 4.84a–c CT scans at the level of the calculi in the right pelvicaliceal system (solid arrows) and left ureter (dotted arrows). Comparison of the sides shows decreased enhancement of the cortex (**b, c**) and medullary pyramids (**c**) in the left kidney.

a Before contrast administration.
b Early perfusion phase.
c Late perfusion phase.

Nephroblastoma/ Neuroblastoma/ Ganglioneuroma

History and Clinical Findings

A 7-year-old boy presented with left flank pain. His IVP showed a mass in the upper left quadrant of the abdomen (**Fig. 4.85**). Subsequent CT confirmed a soft-tissue mass with coarse calcifications arising from the upper pole of the left kidney (**Fig. 4.86**). The pelvicaliceal system was indented and displaced downward by the mass. The upper group of calices showed no evidence of infiltration or destruction. A nephroblastoma (Wilms tumor) was diagnosed based on a review of both imaging studies.

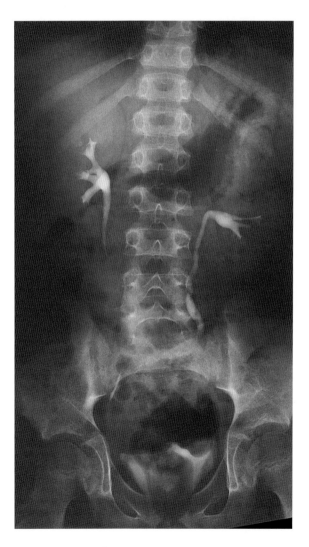

Fig. 4.85 IVP was described as showing inferior displacement of the left pelvicaliceal system and a mass of soft-tissue density at the upper pole of the left kidney.

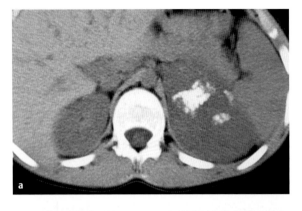

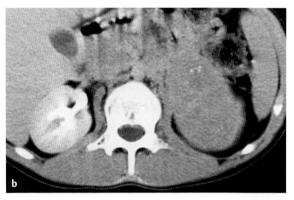

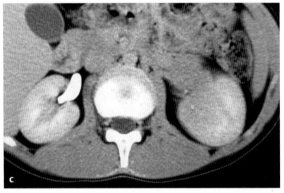

Fig. 4.86 a–d CT demonstrates a mass of soft-tissue density with coarse calcifications (**a**) that is inseparable from the upper pole of the left kidney (**b, c**). It was identified as a nephroblastoma.

a Precontrast scan at the level of the lower pole of the spleen.
b–d Scans after IV contrast administration.

Further Case Summary

A B-mode ultrasound examination showed that the tumor was located outside the kidney and was impressing upon its upper pole (**Fig. 4.87**). MIBG scintigraphy showed increased uptake projected onto the left adrenal gland. Urinalysis revealed catecholamines, homovanillic acid, and neuron-specific enolase (NSE), changing the preoperative diagnosis to neuroblastoma. The tumor was completely removed at operation. Specimen histology established a diagnosis of ganglioneuroma arising from the left adrenal gland.

Error Analysis and Strategy for Error Prevention

The following signs of an extrarenal tumor location were missed on the IVP (**Fig. 4.88**):

- The right kidney, because of its relationship to the liver, normally occupies a level that is approximately one vertebral body lower than the left kidney. In this case the relations were reversed, however: due to pressure from the adrenal tumor, the left kidney occupied a lower position than the right kidney.
- The outlines of the left kidney were definable even at its upper pole.

The slice thickness of the CT scans, at 10 mm, was so great that a single slice encompassed the diagnostically crucial region between the tumor and upper renal pole (**Fig. 4.86 c**). As a result, partial volume effects made it difficult to evaluate the topography of the lesion in the axial plane. The digital image data were not reformatted in coronal or sagittal planes. Calcifications are a nonspecific feature that may occur in both nephroblastomas and neuroblastomas.

References and Further Reading

Georger B, Hero B, Harms D, Grebe J, Scheidhauer K, Berthold F. Metabolic activity and clinical features of primary ganglioneuromas. Cancer 2001; 91: 1905–1913

Lonergan GJ, Schwab CM, Suarez ES, Carlson CL. Neuroblastoma, ganglioneuroblastoma, and ganglioneuroma: radiologic-pathologic correlation. Radiographics 2002; 22: 911–934

Wittmann S, Wunder C, Zirn B, et al. New prognostic markers revealed by evaluation of genes correlated with clinical parameters in Wilms tumors. Genes Chromosomes Cancer 2008; 47: 386–395

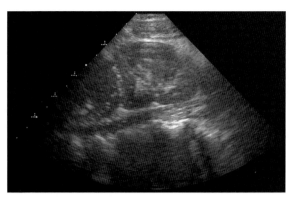

Fig. 4.87   B-mode ultrasound. The suprarenal tumor is not delineated from the kidney in this longitudinal scan.

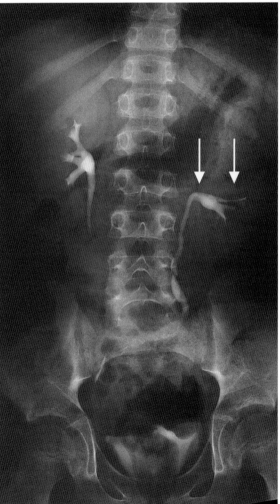

◀ **Fig. 4.88**   IVP shows inferior displacement of the left kidney. The upper pole of the left kidney has been flattened by pressure from the adrenal tumor (arrows). The renal outlines are preserved, however.

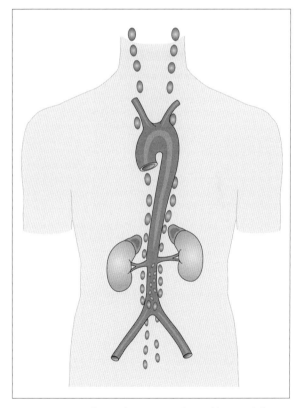

Fig. 4.89   Potential sites of occurrence of neuroblastoma follow the distribution of the sympathetic ganglia.

Nephroblastoma (Wilms Tumor)

Nephroblastoma is the most common renal malignancy in children. It arises from the metanephrogenic blastema, which normally regresses by the 36th week of gestation. Children under 4 years of age are predominantly affected. The tumor reportedly affects approximately 1 in 10 000 children. Besides sporadic unilateral nephroblastomas, 5% of affected children have bilateral Wilms tumors with a familial occurrence. Genetic abnormalities appear to play a causal role, especially mutations in the suppressor gene WT-1 on chromosome 11p13, which suppresses growth factors such as IGF-2.

The clinical manifestations are usually nonspecific. A painless increase in abdominal circumference is often found. Abdominal pain and a palpable upper abdominal mass may also occur. Hematuria is observed in only 5–10% of patients. The recovery rate with appropriate treatment is >90%.

Neuroblastic Tumors: Neuroblastoma, Ganglioneuroblastoma, Ganglioneuroma

Definition. Neuroblastomas, ganglioneuroblastomas, and ganglioneuromas are known collectively as "neuroblastic tumors." They reflect a spectrum of sympathetic neuroectodermal tumors ranging from neuroblastoma (high malignant potential) and ganglioneuroblastoma (intermediate malignant potential) to ganglioneuroma (little or no malignant potential). Neuroblastic tumors develop from sympathicoblasts of the sympathetic trunk, the sympathetic ganglia, the thoracoabdominal sympathetic nerve plexuses, and the ectodermal adrenal medulla. They may remain undifferentiated (neuroblasts) or mature to gangliocytes and Schwann cells. Neuroblastic tumors differ from one another in their degree of cellular and extracellular maturation. Neuroblastomas are composed of immature neuroblasts while ganglioneuroblastomas consist of neuroblasts and gangliocytes, and ganglioneuromas consist entirely of gangliocytes and mature stroma.

Sites of occurrence. Neuroblastic tumors may occur at any sites where sympathetic nervous tissue is located (**Fig. 4.89**). The adrenal medulla (approximately 35% of patients) is most commonly affected, followed by the extra-adrenal retroperitoneum (30–35%), the posterior mediastinum (20%), the neck (1–5%), and the pelvis (1–3%). In 1% of patients with an initial diagnosis of metastatic neuroblastoma, a primary tumor cannot be found. Atypical sites of occurrence are the thymus, lung, kidneys, anterior mediastinum, stomach, and cauda equina.

Epidemiology and prognosis. The incidence of neuroblastoma is 0.8% of the population under 15 years of age. Despite therapeutic advances (surgery, chemotherapy), neuroblastoma is still a malignancy that accounts for 10% of pediatric tumors and 15% of cancer deaths. Poorly differentiated neuroblastomas most commonly occur in small children (average age at diagno-

sis <2 years). Sporadic cases are also diagnosed in newborns and fetuses. Older children present with more mature tumors (average age at diagnosis 7 years). On the other hand, neuroblastomas—even those that have metastasized—may take a relatively benign course. There have been numerous reports of spontaneous regression as well as maturation to more highly differentiated, less aggressive forms. Most spontaneous remissions are believed to result from a genetic apoptosis code that is enabled during the embryonic period and becomes active after birth. The prognosis is influenced by radiologic, histologic, immunocytochemical and genetic information (amplification of the proto-oncogene *Myc-N*).

Clinical manifestations. Neuroblastomas and ganglioneuroblastomas generally present clinically with pain (primary tumor, metastases) and intra-abdominal masses. Other common symptoms are lethargy, poor concentration, weight loss, dyspnea (large intra-abdominal tumor), and peripheral neurologic deficits (invasion of the spinal canal through the intervertebral foramina, nerve compression). While 90–95% of neuroblastomas and ganglioneuroblastomas express vanillylmandelic acid and homovanillic acid, catecholamine expression is usually not symptomatic.

Ganglioneuromas. Ganglioneuromas may arise primarily or may result from the spontaneous or chemotherapy-induced maturation of a neuroblastoma or ganglioneuroblastoma. The peak age incidence is 7 years. Ganglioneuromas most commonly occur in the posterior mediastinum (42%), followed by the extra-adrenal retroperitoneum (38%), adrenal glands (21%), and neck (8%). Most are asymptomatic and are detected incidentally on chest radiographs. Approximately 37% of patients have elevated catecholamine levels in the serum and urine.

Renal Cell Carcinoma/ Oncocytoma

History and Clinical Findings

A 57-year-old man had been receiving medical treatment for Schoenlein–Henoch purpura for several years. A routine ultrasound examination revealed a mass on the left kidney. CT was subsequently performed, and the report confirmed suspicion of a renal cell carcinoma (**Fig. 4.90**). The patient felt well physically; he had no unspecific paraneoplastic symptoms like weight loss, tiredness, or fever. His serum creatinine was 2.62 mg/dL. Differential creatinine clearance was 23% on the left side and 77% on the right side.

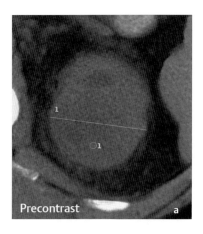
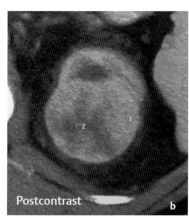

Precontrast a

Postcontrast b

Fig. 4.90 a, b CT scans display a solid, well-circumscribed tumor at the upper pole of the left kidney. The mass shows peripheral enhancement comparable to renal parenchyma after IV contrast injection. It contains a central, stellate hypodensity both before (**a**) and after contrast administration (**b**).

Further Case Summary

The patient underwent a left nephrectomy for suspected renal cell carcinoma. Specimen histology revealed an oncocytoma. Postoperative serum creatinine rose to 6.54 mg/dL, but the patient was not considered to require hemodialysis.

Error Analysis and Strategy for Error Prevention

Renal oncocytoma is an essentially benign tumor composed predominantly of classic oncocytes (round or polygonal cells with a granular, eosinophilic cytoplasm and small round nuclei). There have been occasional reports of malignant transformation and metastasis. Renal oncocytoma is difficult to distinguish radiologically from chromophobic and eosinophilic renal cell carcinoma due to their similar imaging appearances (**Table 4.6**). Hence the diagnosis should always be established histologically (ultrasound- or CT-guided percutaneous biopsy, tumor enucleation, nephrectomy). Oncocytomas less than 4 cm in diameter can be managed by radiologic surveillance (CT, MRI). If the tumor enlarges or changes its configuration,

Table 4.6 CT differentiation of oncocytoma and renal cell carcinoma

Imaging findings	Oncocytoma	Renal cell carcinoma
Sharp margins relative to renal parenchyma	Common	Rare
Intense arterial contrast enhancement	Rare	Common
Central necrosis	Rare	Common
Infiltration of renal vein	Never	Occasional
Lymph node metastasis	Never	Occasional

and in patients with a larger oncocytoma (risk of intratumoral hemorrhage), it is advisable to remove the tumor surgically (enucleation, nephrectomy) or by radiofrequency ablation. The tumor is comparable to renal angiomyolipoma in its differential diagnosis and treatment options (**Fig. 4.91**).

In the present case, a benign renal tumor was not considered in the differential diagnosis due to the high incidence of renal cell carcinoma in urologic surgical popula-

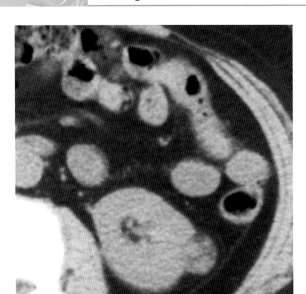

Fig. 4.91 Renal angiomyolipoma in a different patient, misinterpreted as renal cell carcinoma on postoperative CT scans. Intravenous contrast administration was withheld because of an autonomous thyroid adenoma. Tumor elements with attenuation values less than − 70 HU are considered proof of angiomyolipoma. The diagnosis in this case was established by surgical enucleation of the tumor.

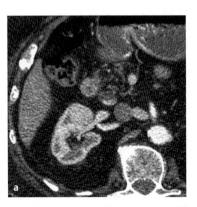
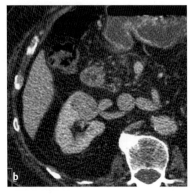
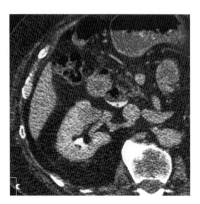

Fig. 4.92 a–c Renal cell carcinoma in a different patient. A protein-rich cyst was initially diagnosed based on a failure to analyze and properly interpret enhancement kinetics. The diagnosis was established by a segmental resection with curative intent.

a Early arterial phase. Tumor density is 116 ± 24 HU.
b Parenchymal phase. Tumor density is 81 ± 28 HU.
c Renal or late phase. Tumor density is 61 ± 23 HU.

tions (relative frequency of oncocytomas is 2–18%). Meanwhile, the extent of parenchymal damage in the contralateral kidney was underestimated despite laboratory findings of compensated renal failure, and so the less-invasive treatment options of ultrasound- or CT-guided percutaneous biopsy followed by imaging surveillance or tumor enucleation were not pursued.

The errors of image interpretation in this patient resulted in a failure to make the correct clinical and surgical decisions.

In some cases even a benign renal mass may present atypical imaging features causing it to be confused with a malignant tumor (**Fig. 4.92**).

References and Further Reading

Amin MB, Crotty TB, Tickoo SK, Farrow GM. Renal oncocytoma: a reappraisal of morphologic features with clinicopathologic findings in 80 cases. Am J Pathol 1997; 21: 1–12

De Carli P, Vidiri A, Lamanna L, Cantiani R. Renal oncocytoma: image diagnostics and therapeutic aspects. J Exp Clin Cancer Res 2000; 19: 287–290

Heidenreich A, Ravery V. Preoperative imaging in renal cell cancer. World J Urol 2004; 22: 307–315

Li GR, Soulie M, Escourrou G, et al. Renal oncocytomas. Report of 13 cases. Ann Urol 1997; 31: 123–130

Perez-Ordonez B, Hamed G, Campbell S, et al. Renal oncocytoma: a clinicopathologic study of 70 cases. Am J Pathol 1997; 21: 871–873

Revascularization of a Solitary Kidney in Acute Renal Failure: Correct Indication? Sound Interventional Technique?

History and Clinical Findings

A 58-year-old woman was hospitalized with suspected terminal renal failure of acute onset. Her history indicated a nonfunctioning atrophic left kidney. Two years earlier, stenosis of the right renal artery had been treated by balloon dilatation and stent implantation by interventional radiology. Serologic renal function had not been followed since then. For the previous 3 weeks, the patient had complained of vomiting and watery diarrhea. When hospitalized, she already had a significant decrease in diuresis and was in a debilitated state. Serum creatinine was 20 mg/dL, blood urea was 255 mg/dL.

Color duplex sonography showed a normal-sized right kidney with normal parenchymal thickness. Waveforms sampled from the segmental arteries showed a flattened upstroke, a low systolic amplitude, a flattened postsystolic downstroke, and an absence of retrograde diastolic flow— all consistent with a significant vascular stenosis.

Given the suspicion of a hemodynamically significant restenosis or occlusion of the right renal artery, it was decided, after consulting with the nephrologist, to proceed with digital subtraction angiography (DSA) while having facilities ready for an interventional procedure. Although the prospects for organ salvage by vascular recanalization appeared slim due to the apparent 2- to 3-week period of diminished blood flow, the attempt was considered to be justified, when the risks were weighed against the definite need for dialysis, if the intervention were withheld.

The diagnostic study confirmed an occlusion of the right renal artery (**Fig. 4.93**). A catheter and hydrophilic wire were advanced through the occlusion. Manual injection of a nonionic, low-osmolarity iodinated contrast medium (iodine content 350 mg/mL) demonstrated an approximately 3-cm long occlusion of the renal artery. A self-expanding stent 4 cm long (6 mm diameter) was advanced into place and used to dilate the occlusion.

The postinterventional image showed a normal luminal size of the renal artery with copious blood flow even in the segmental arteries, the subsegmental arteries, and the interlobular arteries. The rapid tapering from the subsegmental to arcuate arteries was interpreted as a result of the previous ischemic injury to the organ.

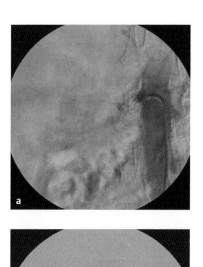
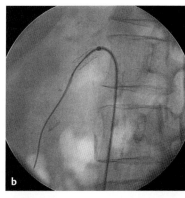
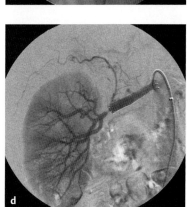

Fig. 4.93 a–d Interventional recanalization of the right renal artery.
a   Occlusion of the renal artery after previous stent-assisted PTA. Status post left nephrectomy.
b, c Recanalization of the right renal artery.
d   Appearance following stent implantation and recanalization. Vasospasms are noted at the distal end of the stent.

Further Case Summary

One hour after the intervention, the patient complained of increasing pain in her right flank. Ultrasound revealed hypoechoic to echo-free zones distributed diffusely throughout the renal parenchyma, which were interpreted as hemorrhagic areas. Renal blood flow was substantially reduced. CT confirmed the impression of a new impairment of renal blood flow and parenchymal tears (**Fig. 4.94**). A large extracapsular hematoma was noted at the upper pole of the kidney. A steady fall in the hemoglobin level was discovered and was considered to warrant nephrectomy. Surgery confirmed the presence of extensive parenchymal lacerations, intraparenchymal hemorrhages, a laceration of the renal capsule at the upper pole, and an extracapsular hematoma in the same region. The operation was uneventful. Following a brief stay in the ICU, the patient was placed in the care of a nephrologist and has undergone regular hemodialysis. The histopathology report described significant, long-standing ischemic damage to the renal parenchyma. There was no evidence of injury to the renal artery or segmental arteries.

Error Analysis and Strategy for Error Prevention

The disseminated intraparenchymal hemorrhages were a result of reperfusion injury to the kidney, which had already sustained ischemic damage (**Table 4.7**). The presumed progressive decline in renal blood flow over a 2- to 3-week period was sufficient to cause disseminated areas of cellular necrosis that had not yet healed by scarring. This must have been particularly damaging to the medullary pyramids, which are sensitive to ischemic injury. The metabolic state of the organ deteriorated in response to the sudden reperfusion. The effects on a cellular level included massive intracellular edema and cell destruction; the macroscopic effects were generalized swelling of the organ and a rise of parenchymal pressure due to the rigidity of the renal capsule. This was the mechanism that caused the parenchymal tears and hemorrhages. Finally, the pressure within the renal capsule was so high that the capsule ruptured at its upper pole, producing an extracapsular hematoma.

The kidney did not rupture as a result of interventional manipulations. This is suggested by the uneventful course of the procedure and the minimal histopathologic findings. The administration of a nonionic, low-osmolarity contrast medium, which was essential for planning the intervention, may have compounded the parenchymal damage. This type of contrast material may cause biphasic hemodynamic changes in a previously damaged kidney—phase 1 consisting of an increase in perfusion and phase 2 of a gradual decrease in perfusion. The material may also

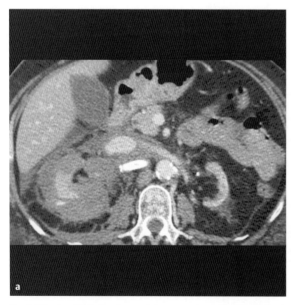

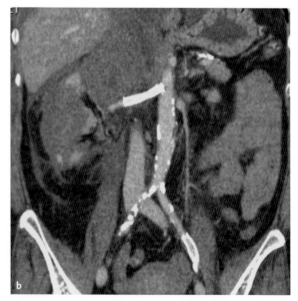

Fig. 4.94 a, b CT during the portal venous phase after IV contrast administration shows perfusion of the newly implanted stent in the right renal artery (**a**) with occlusion of the segmental arteries. The parenchyma of the right kidney is thickened and does not enhance because of parenchymal destruction. An extrarenal hematoma is visible at the upper pole of the right kidney (**b**). Fluid in the right renal hilum, in the perirenal fibrofatty tissue, and in the perihepatic peritoneal compartment has blood-equivalent attenuation values (approximately 20 HU). The patient has a small, nonfunctioning left kidney (**a**). Atherosclerotic wall calcifications are visible in the aorta and iliac arteries. A stent was previously implanted in the left external iliac artery (**b**).

Table 4.7 Pathogenesis of acute renal failure. (Source: Neumayer 1993. With permission from the author)

Vascular disorders

- Decreased renal perfusion pressure
  - Increased tone of the afferent arterioles
  - Decreased tone of the efferent arterioles

- Reduction of glomerular permeability
  - Decrease in ultrafiltration coefficient

- Medullary congestion with corticomedullary blood redistribution and predominantly cortical ischemia

Tubular disorders

- Tubular obstruction
  - Swelling of the tubular epithelium
  - Cellular debris
  - Myoglobin
  - Bilirubin
  - Paraproteins
  - Crystals, etc.

- Tubular leak
  - Tubulorrhexis
  - Tubular necrosis

Cellular disorders

- Decreased mitochondrial respiration

- Intracellular calcium overload

- Excess of free radicals

- Lipid peroxidation

have a direct toxic effect on the renal tubular epithelium. The contrast administration is not considered to have causal significance, however, since a rise of serum creatinine due to contrast nephropathy usually does not occur until 24–48 hours after contrast administration.

It must be considered that the temporal dynamics of the renal artery occlusion were unknown and that, given the complexity of pathophysiologic variables, there is no fixed correlation between (1) the duration and degree of decreased renal blood flow and (2) the extent of preexisting parenchymal damage and the degree of damage that would likely result from reperfusion. For these reasons we feel that, even in retrospect, the attempt to revascularize the kidney was justified. In a similar situation, the stent-assisted revascularization of a renal artery occlusion in a different patient had a more favorable outcome (**Fig. 4.95**). Moreover, a complication of the type experienced here had not been previously described in the literature. The intervention offered the only chance for the patient to avoid compulsory dialysis. An open revascularization procedure would have raised the same pathophysiologic problems and general surgical risks. The risk of a fatal outcome from the intervention and subsequent nephrectomy was extremely low, given adequate surveillance in the ICU. By contrast, hemodialysis means a permanent compromise in quality of life, heightened susceptibility to secondary diseases, and a shortening of life expectancy.

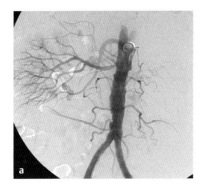 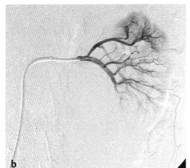 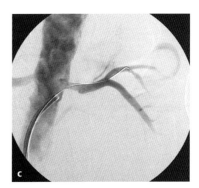

Fig. 4.95 a–c Successful stent PTA of a 3-month-old occlusion of the left renal artery. Six weeks before the intervention, functional renal scintigraphy with differential clearance showed a non-functioning left kidney under baseline conditions and during captopril administration.

a Occlusion of the left renal artery.
b Appearance following catheterization of the occluded left renal artery.
c Appearance following stent-assisted PTA of the left renal artery.

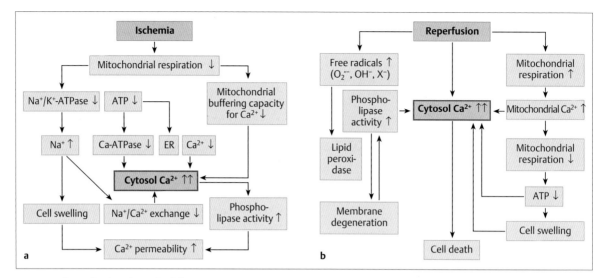

Fig. 4.96 a, b Pathophysiology of cellular damage due to ischemia and reperfusion. (Source: Neumayer 1993. With permission from the author.)

a Ischemia-induced changes in the intracellular calcium ion balance.

b Changes in the intracellular calcium ion concentration, free radical formation, and lipid peroxidation during the reperfusion phase.

Pathophysiology of Renal Ischemia (Fig. 4.96)

Renal Ischemia Stage

Prolonged ischemia leads to the suppression of mitochondrial energy production and a decrease in the ATP content of the cell. This triggers a change from an aerobic to an anaerobic metabolic state and the development of acidosis. As pump mechanisms such as sodium–potassium ATPase and calcium ATPase begin to fail, the intracellular sodium concentration rises, the cell membrane becomes more permeable to Ca^{2+} ions, and intracellular edema develops. As increased amounts of Ca^{2+} ions enter the cell from the extracellular space and are released from intracellular stores, sufficient numbers of these ions can no longer be transported from the cell. The damaged mitochondria can buffer the Ca^{2+} ion excess only to a limited degree. Loss of the mitochondrial buffering capacity leads to phospholipase activation and to the disintegration of cellular membrane structures.

Reperfusion Stage

With the onset of reperfusion, the metabolic situation does not improve. Instead, the reoxygenation induced by vascular recanalization plus a new influx of Ca^{2+} ions and a simultaneous correction of cellular acidosis are the most damaging factors in terms of cellular metabolism. As oxygen enters the system, the xanthine oxidase that forms from xanthine dehydrogenase under the influence of Ca^{2+} ions during the ischemic phase (breakdown of ATP and its incorporation into the uric acid cycle) leads to the formation of inorganic free radicals (O_2-, H_2O_2, OH-). These compounds, together with the lipid peroxidation of phospholipid-containing membrane structures, contribute to the further acceleration of cell destruction.

References and Further Reading

Neumayer H.-H. Akutes Nierenversagen. In: Franz HE, Risler T, eds. Klinische Nephrologie. Handbuch für Klinik und Praxis. Landsberg: Ecomed; 1993

Walsh PC, Retik AB, Vaughan ED, Wein AJ (eds.). Campell's Urology. Philadelphia: WB Saunders; 2002

Wein JA, Kavoussi LR, Novick AC, Partin AW, Peters CA, eds. Campell-Walsh Urology. 9th ed. New York: Elsevier; 2007

Extragonadal Choriocarcinoma/ Residual Scar/Lymph Node Metastasis/ Mature Teratoma

History and Clinical Findings

A 26-year-old man presented with a one-month history of intermittent fever, fatigue, bloating, and nausea. Gastroscopy showed no abnormalities. Ultrasound demonstrated a retroperitoneal mass. CT detected masses in both lungs and the liver as well as enlarged retroperitoneal lymph nodes (**Fig. 4.97 a**). Laboratory tests showed elevation of β-HCG (330000 U/L), LDH (520 U/L) and CRP (110 mg/L). AFP was within normal limits at 2 U/L. Ultrasound-guided biopsy of a retroperitoneal tumor yielded the diagnosis of an extragonadal β-HCG-expressing choriocarcinoma. A "burned out" testicular tumor (i.e., one that was regressive when the metastases were diagnosed) was discussed as a possible source. The tumor was classified as stage III (pulmonary, hepatic, and retroperitoneal lymph node metastases).

During the next 12 months the patient underwent four cycles of high-dose chemotherapy with cisplatin, bleomycin, and etoposide; four cycles of high-dose chemotherapy with paclitaxel and ifosfamide; and an autologous stem-cell transplantation. The pulmonary, hepatic and most of the retroperitoneal lymph node metastases showed excellent response to this regimen (RECIST 1.1 criteria, see p. 161). By contrast, the largest retroperitoneal lymph node metastasis showed very little shrinkage during the first 7 months of chemotherapy and no additional change thereafter. For this reason, a mature teratoma was included in the differential diagnosis along with still-active choriocarcinoma tissue.

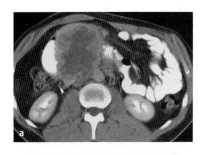
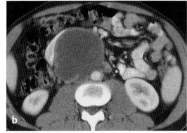
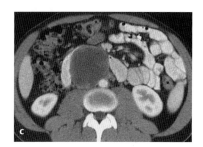
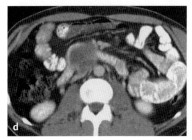
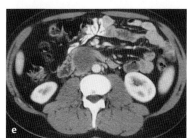

Fig. 4.97 a–e Response to chemotherapy of a retroperitoneal, precaval lymph node metastasis. CT scans during the first 7 months of chemotherapy show a slight degree of tumor shrinkage with an increase in central necrosis (**a–d**). The tumor appears unchanged from months 7 to 12 (**d, e**). The differential diagnosis included active residual tissue of metastatic choriocarcinoma and the development of a mature teratoma.

a CT scan at initial diagnosis.
b Three months after image **a**.
c Five months after image **a**.
d Seven months after image **a**.
e Twelve months after image **a**.

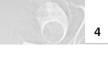

Further Case Summary

Twelve months after the initial diagnosis, the retroperitoneal tumor was resected. Histologic analysis of the surgical specimen revealed nonspecific tissue with a fibrous capsule and no signs of malignancy.

Error Analysis and Strategy for Error Prevention

In the benign/malignant differentiation of a mass, imaging studies must rely on indirect criteria such as size, shape, tumor matrix, density characteristics before and after IV contrast administration, and a possible relationship to the underlying disease. Scar tissue or remission can be diagnosed at follow-up only if the residual process shows no change in size or configuration for several months without chemotherapy. In the case presented here, the absence of change during the last 5 months before the operation should have raised the possibility that the lesion had resolved to form a pseudocyst with scar tissue. Another possibility was active residual tumor tissue in the pseudocyst wall, whose growth had been suppressed by the last chemotherapy cycle. On the other hand, the maturation of a teratoma was unlikely due to the central necrosis, since mature teratomas typically appear on CT as solid masses with an inhomogeneous texture and calcifications.

Because both scar tissue and mature teratomas have a relatively low glucose metabolism, positron emission tomography with [^{18}F]fluorodeoxyglucose (FDG/PET) would not have contributed to the diagnosis. The same applies to the serum β-HCG, which may be normal after high-dose chemotherapy in the case of necrosis, scar tissue, or even a mature teratoma.

References and Further Reading

Kumano M, Miyake H, Hara I, et al. First-line high-dose chemotherapy combined with blood stem cell transplantation for patients with advanced extragonadal germ cell tumors. Int J Urol 2007; 14: 336–338

Petura JL, Lawrentschuk N, Ballok Z, et al. 18F-Fluorodeoxyglucose positron emission tomography in evaluation of germ cell tumor after chemotherapy. Urology 2004; 64: 1202–1207

Rabbani F, Gleave ME, Coppin CM, Murray N, Sullivan LD. Teratoma in primary testis tumor reduces complete response rates in the retroperitoneum after primary chemotherapy. The case for primary retroperitoneal lymph node dissection of stage IIb germ cell tumors with teratomatous elements. Cancer 1996; 78: 430–436

Germ Cell Tumors in Males

Histopathology and growth characteristics. Testicular tumors may be classified as germ cell tumors (95% of testicular neoplasms) or gonadal stromal tumors (Leydig and Sertoli cell tumors, malignant in approximately 10% of cases). The group of germ cell tumors includes seminomas (approximately 40% of germ cell tumors) and, in descending order of malignancy, nonseminomatous embryonal cell carcinomas, choriocarcinomas, and teratomas. Sixty percent of the tumors have a uniform histologic pattern. In forms with a mixed histopathology, embryonal cell carcinoma and teratoma ("teratocarcinomas") are the most frequent combination. Burned-out tumors are testicular neoplasms whose metastases determine the clinical picture while the primary tumor has regressed and appear histologically as a scar embedded in the testicular tissue.

Primary extragonadal germ cell tumors, which originate from germ cells deposited outside the gonads during embryonic development, are rare. They are most commonly located in the mediastinum. While benign germ cell tumors do not show an age or sex predilection, malignant forms predominantly affect young males.

Cystic tumors are usually benign, while solid tumors tend to be malignant. Intratumoral calcifications are common in both benign and malignant forms. If a nonseminomatous germ cell tumor does not fully regress in response to chemotherapy, it is reasonable to assume that it consists of approximately equal parts of residual tumor tissue, scar tissue, and well-differentiated mature teratoma.

Tumor markers. Alpha-fetoprotein (AFP) and the beta chain of human chorionic gonadotropin (β-HCG) provide effective serum markers for nonseminomatous germ cell tumors. Because β-HCG is not normally produced in the placenta, the detection of an elevated serum level in males is pathognomonic for the presence of a tumor with trophoblastic elements. An elevated serum β-HCG is a poor prognostic sign. The half-life of AFP is 4.5 days, while that of β-HCG is 1–2 days. As a result, β-HCG is particularly useful for monitoring treatment response and should be determined before the affected testis is removed. Lactate dehydrogenase (LDH) is a nonspecific tumor marker that is most important for evaluating treatment response and prognosis in patients with advanced seminomas.

Extent of Injuries?

History and Clinical Findings

A 22-year-old woman was involved in a motor vehicle accident on the freeway at night while riding as a passenger. The emergency physician had intubated her, placed a central line, and delivered her to an interdisciplinary emergency unit. On admission the patient was evaluated by spiral CT scanning of the skull, cervical spine, chest, and abdomen. The CT report described a ruptured liver, free intraperitoneal air (suspected bowel rupture), and complex, bilateral anterior and posterior pelvic ring fractures (**Fig. 4.98**). No neurologic or urologic abnormalities were found. On the same night the patient underwent laparotomy by a visceral surgeon, who oversewed the ruptures in the liver and small bowel. Next a trauma surgeon treated the pelvic ring fractures by external skeletal fixation and a pelvic C-clamp.

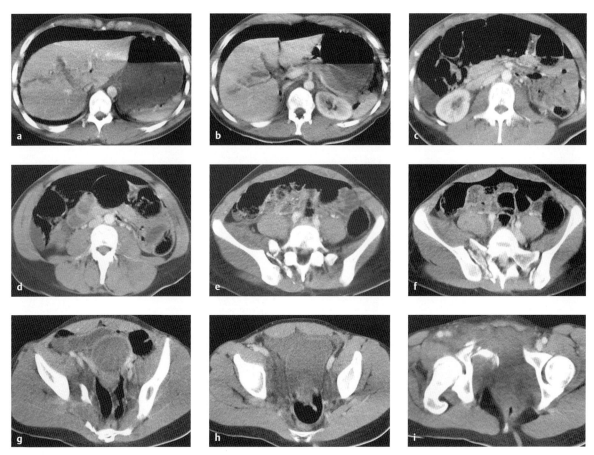

Fig. 4.98 a–i   Abdominal spiral CT scans demonstrate a hepatic rupture (**a, b**) and bilateral anterior (**i**) and posterior pelvic ring fractures (**e–g**). With a soft-tissue window, free intraperitoneal air is not distinguishable from air contained in bowel loops.

Further Case Summary

One week after the accident the patient developed fever accompanied by swelling and local warmth of the right groin and upper right thigh. When CT was repeated, both the scans and a subsequent Lauenstein view (**Fig. 4.99**) showed contrast extravasation arising from the bladder and spreading into the anteromedial soft tissues of the right thigh. CT imaging after retrograde contrast instillation via the urethra confirmed the diagnosis of an initially-missed bladder rupture with avulsion of the urethra (**Fig. 4.100**).

Error Analysis and Strategy for Error Prevention

A retrospective analysis showed that the initial emergency placement of a bladder catheter had been unsuccessful. This fact plus the absence of urinary excretion were initially ignored due to the critical condition of the patient. When another bladder catheter was introduced in the ICU, it yielded a blood-tinged fluid.

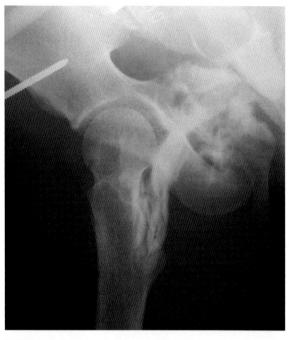

Fig. 4.99   Lauenstein view shows contrast extravasation originating from the bladder. An external fixation pin is projected over the right iliac wing.

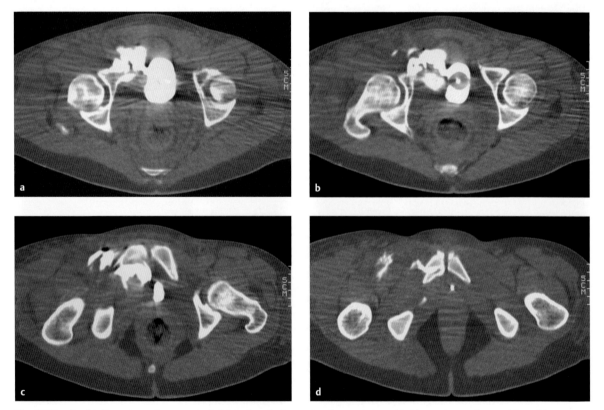

Fig. 4.100 a–d   CT after retrograde contrast administration via the urethra demonstrates a bladder rupture and an avulsion of the urethra.

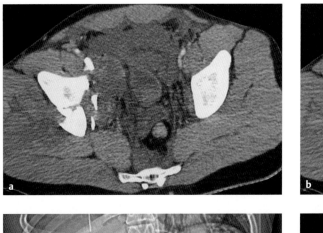

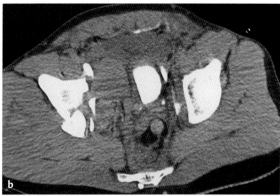

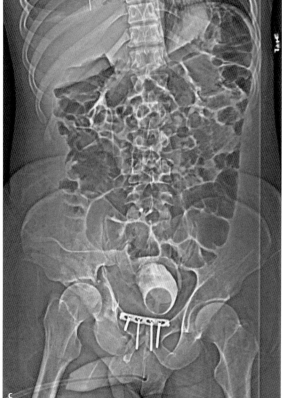

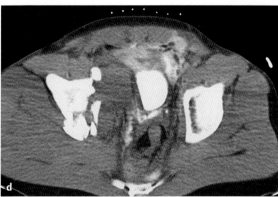

Fig. 4.101 a–d A different multiply injured patient with a right-sided pelvic ring fracture, a hematoma in the lesser pelvis, and avulsion of the urethra from the bladder. Extraluminal contrast medium lateral and anterolateral to the bladder was missed on initial CT scans (**a, b**). A urethral avulsion was suspected when the retrograde bladder catheter did not provide adequate urinary drainage. After surgical stabilization of the fractures, a new bladder catheter was placed via a suprapubic approach under CT guidance. A scout view before the CT-guided aspiration shows the high position of the bladder in the lesser pelvis (**c**). The bladder is filled with opacified urine from the previous IV contrast injection. The scout images confirmed that a significant amount of urine mixed with contrast medium had tracked into the soft tissues of the pelvic floor (**d**).

a Diagnostic examination before IV contrast administration.
b Diagnostic examination after IV contrast administration.
c Scout view prior to CT-guided bladder aspiration.
d Planning the CT-guided bladder aspiration.

When the initial CT examination was interpreted, it was not considered that comminuted fractures of the anterior pelvic ring can cause injuries to the urinary bladder and urethra (**Fig. 4.98 i**). The fluid collection along the right anterolateral aspect of the bladder (**Fig. 4.98 h, i**) should have been interpreted as a urinoma. Its CT density (approximately 80 HU) corresponded to a mixture of blood and urine and was lower than that of the iliac hematoma (**Fig. 4.98**). The fluid anterolateral to the bladder could not be interpreted as ascites because it was extraperitoneal.

As the case of a different multiply injured patient illustrates, a high position of the bladder in the lesser pelvis provides further evidence of a urethral avulsion (**Fig. 4.101**). The bladder moves upward because it has been released from its anatomical attachment to the pelvic floor.

References and Further Reading

Greenspan A. Orthopedic Imaging: A Practical Approach. 4th ed. Philadelphia: Lippincott Williams & Wilkins; 2005

Siegmeth A, Müllner T, Kukla C, Vècsei V. Begleitverletzungen beim schweren Beckentrauma. Unfallchirurg 2000; 103: 572–581

Injuries That May Accompany Pelvic Ring Fractures

The prognosis of severe pelvic injuries is significantly worsened by the presence of associated injuries. Concomitant injuries to the urogenital organs, vessels, nerves, and parenchymal abdominal organs are the most common. Siegmeth et al. (2000) reported on 39 of 126 (31%) consecutive patients with pelvic ring fractures who had associated peripelvic injuries. Sixteen of the 39 patients (41%) had a type B fracture and 23 patients (59%) had a type C fracture. The most common associated injuries involved the liver, spleen, kidney, and pancreas (59%), followed by urogenital injuries (47%). Peripheral nerve injuries were present in 26% of the 39 patients, and vascular injuries were present in 15%. Mesenteric ruptures, vascular trauma, and degloving injuries were also observed. Extrapelvic injuries predominantly involved the chest (56%) and head (33%). Twenty-eight of the 39 patients survived. Seven patients died during the acute phase, and four patients died from multisystem organ failure while in intensive care.

5

Spinal Column

Normal Findings/ Bony Injury

History and Clinical Findings

A 23-year-old man sustained a serious head injury in a motor vehicle accident. Radiographs taken on admission (**Fig. 5.1**) were considered to exclude bony injuries of the cervical spine.

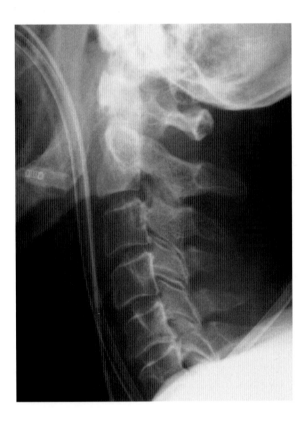

Fig. 5.1   Radiographic examination of the cervical spine in the intubated patient did not reveal any bony injuries.

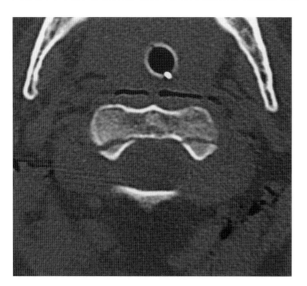

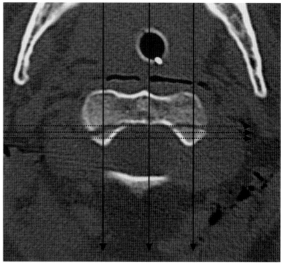

Fig. 5.2 Axial CT of the upper cervical spine on the same day shows an essentially nondisplaced fracture running through the base of the dens in the coronal plane.

Fig. 5.3 Axial CT of the upper cervical spine. The fracture was not detected on radiographs because the beam passed through roughly equal portions of the cortex, cancellous bone, and fracture line in both the frontal projection (solid arrows) and lateral projection (dotted arrows). Consequently, the absorption differences were inadequate to permit visual detection of the fracture.

Further Case Summary

Given the severity of the cranial injuries, it was decided to include the upper cervical spine in a subsequent CT examination of the skull (**Fig. 5.2**). The scans revealed a fracture line running through the base of C2 in the coronal plane.

Error Analysis and Strategy for Error Prevention

Even when the CT findings were known, the dens fracture could not be identified on the cervical radiographs. This is due to the characteristics of the fracture (thin fracture line, coronal orientation, nondisplaced fragments) and the limitations of projection radiographs (**Fig. 5.3**). Radiographs are two-dimensional images that reflect the summation of x-ray absorption that occurs in a series of tissues having different densities. The fracture cannot be detected in the frontal projection because the x-rays pass equally through all portions of the vertebral body—the cortex, cancellous bone, and fracture. This summation effect does not yield a perceptible density or absorption difference between the fracture and vertebral body. The fracture was undetectable in the lateral projection for the same reason. The fracture line was thin, the fragments were minimally displaced, and the coronal orientation of the fracture resulted in insufficient image contrast for detection.

Because injuries of the upper cervical spine are not clinically apparent in up to 50% of serious-accident victims and are often missed on admission, cranial CT in all patients with serious head injuries should include scanning of the upper cervical spine. Disability resulting from a missed cervical fracture (e.g., cord impingement and paralysis caused by moving the patient before stabilizing the fracture) could have significant medicolegal consequences.

References and Further Reading

Berne JD, Velmahos GC, El-Tawil Q, et al. Value of complete cervical helical computed tomographic scanning in identifying cervical spine injury in the unevaluable blunt trauma patient with multiple injuries: a prospective study. J Trauma 1999; 47: 896–902

Davids JW, Phreaner DL, Hoyt DB, Mackersie RC. The etiology of missed cervical spine injuries. J Trauma 1993; 34: 342–345

Deliganis AV, Baxter AB, Hanson JA, et al. Radiologic spectrum of craniocervical distraction injuries. Radiographics 2000; 20: 237–250

Jelly LME, Evans DR, Easty MJ, Coats TJ, Chan O. Radiography versus spiral CT in the evaluation of cervicothoracic junction injuries in polytrauma patients who have undergone intubation. Radiographics 2000; 20: 251–259

Dislocation/ Pseudodislocation

History and Clinical Findings

A 6-year-old boy fell approximately 2 meters to the ground from a window. Afterward he complained of posterior neck pain. No other clinical abnormalities were found. Radiographs of the cervical spine in two planes showed an anterior offset of C2 relative to C3. The patient was hospitalized in the pediatric unit with a suspected ligamentous injury and dislocation at the C2–C3 level. The pediatrician requested a CT examination of the cervical spine. Because plain films taken elsewhere did not accompany the patient, the radiographic examination was repeated in pediatric radiology (**Fig. 5.4**). When the radiographs confirmed anterior displacement of the C2 vertebral body relative to C3 (approximately 2 mm on the film), CT scans were obtained of the craniovertebral junction and upper cervical spine, confirming the x-ray findings (**Fig. 5.5**).

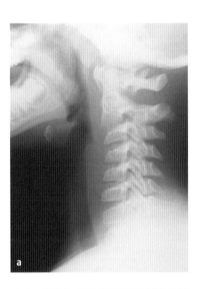

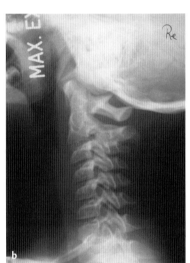

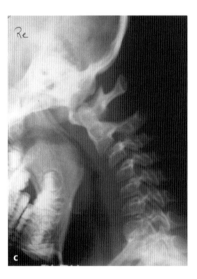

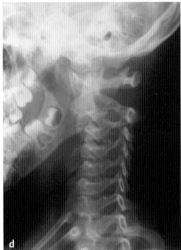

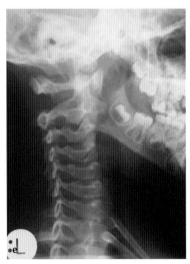

Fig. 5.4a–e Radiographic examination shows a slight anterior offset of C2 relative to C3 in the neutral position (**a**). The vertebra occupies a normal position when the head is tilted back (**b**). Tilting the head forward increases the relative offset of C2 (**c**). There is no evidence of bony injuries.
a Lateral view in the neutral position.
b Lateral view in retroflexion.
c Lateral view in anteflexion.
d Oblique view of the right intervertebral foramina.
e Oblique view of the left intervertebral foramina.

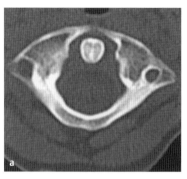
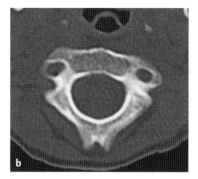
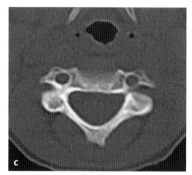

Fig. 5.5 a–c Noncontrast CT scans of the cervical spine show no evidence of bony injuries.

a Axial scan at the level of C1 and the dens of C2.
b Axial scan at the C2 level.
c Axial scan at the C3 level.

Further Case Summary

A pseudodislocation at the C2–C3 level was diagnosed from the radiographs (**Fig. 5.4**) based on a normal position of the posterior cervical line (**Fig. 5.6**). There was no evidence of bony injuries or ligament instability (**Fig. 5.7**). When a neck brace was applied, the complaints improved within a few days and the patient was able to return to school.

Error Analysis and Strategy for Error Prevention

When an anterior offset of the posterior border of C2 relative to the posterior border of C3 is found in the neutral position in children and adolescents, it may represent a physiologic pseudodislocation or a pathologic dislocation associated with a C2 fracture (hangman's fracture = fracture through the pedicles of the C2 vertebra). A pseudodislocation is a relatively common condition resulting from the natural compliance of pediatric ligaments. Differentiation from a true dislocation is based on the alignment of the anterior surfaces of the C1 through C3 spinous processes in the lateral radiographic view (posterior cervical line). With a pseudodislocation, the anterior surface of

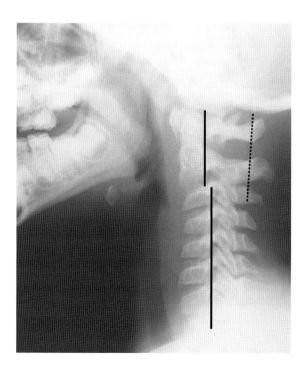

Fig. 5.6 Pseudodislocation at the C2–C3 level is evidenced by a discontinuity in the posterior vertebral body line (solid line) and a normal position of the posterior cervical line (dotted line).

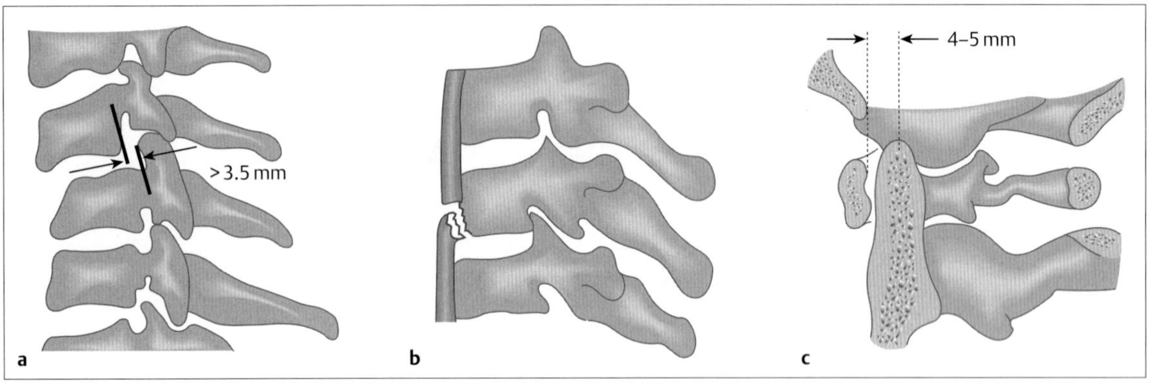

Fig. 5.7 a–c   Signs of instability in the upper cervical spine following trauma in adults (after Bücheler et al. 2006).

a Posterior borders of the vertebral bodies displaced by more than 3.5 mm.
b Anterior corner fracture of the vertebral body end plate.
c Increased distance between the anterior surface of the dens and the posterior border of the anterior arch of the atlas.

the C2 spinous process may deviate up to 2 mm from a line tangent to the anterior surfaces of the C1 and C3 spinous processes. If the deviation is greater than 2 mm, a true dislocation should be diagnosed (**Fig. 5.6**).

From a radiation safety standpoint, it would have been preferable to obtain the cervical spine radiographs taken elsewhere and merely supplement them with functional and oblique views. Based on the guidelines of the American College of Radiology, sagittal and coronal reformatted CT images and/or MRI are indicated in children and adolescents with a suspected bony and/or ligamentous injury of the cervical spine (history, clinical examination, radiographs). The information from both imaging modalities is frequently combined to evaluate the skeleton (CT) and the soft tissues (MRI).

References and Further Reading

American College of Radiology ACR Appropriateness Criteria. Suspected Spine Trauma. http://www.acr.org/Secondary-MainMenuCategories/quality_safety/app_criteria/pdf/ExpertPanelonNeurologicImaging/HeadTraumaDoc5.aspx (accessed November 10, 2010)

Bücheler E, Lackner K-J, Thelen M. Einführung in die Radiologie. Diagnostik und Interventionen. Stuttgart: Thieme; 2006

Greenspan A. Orthopedic Imaging: A Practical Approach. 4th ed. Philadelphia: Lippincott Williams & Wilkins; 2005

Swischuk LE. Anterior displacement of C2 in children: physiologic or pathologic. Radiology 1977; 122: 759–763

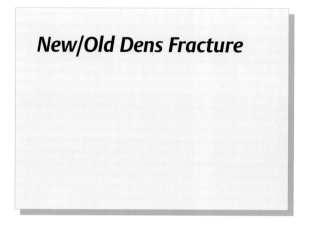

New/Old Dens Fracture

History and Clinical Findings

A 16-year-old boy was injured in a motorcycle accident while wearing a helmet, sustaining head trauma with a subdural hematoma in the right occipital area. He complained of decreased vision in the right eye. When the patient was hospitalized, CT scans of the skull and upper cervical spine were taken because clinically occult fractures of that region are common in traffic accident victims (present in approximately 20% of fatal traffic accidents) and are missed in one-half of accident survivors unless a routine CT examination is performed. In the present case an oblique, nondisplaced fracture of the dens extending from the level of the anterior atlas arch to the base of the dens was diagnosed from the CT images (**Fig. 5.8**). The written report stated that the anterior cortex was disrupted and the fracture margins were not sclerotic.

Two days later the cervical spine was evaluated by MRI. These images were described as showing a physiologic growth plate between the dens and body of the axis (**Fig. 5.9**). Additionally, the fracture line in the dens was described as subtle because of the absence of visible bone-marrow edema. There was still no evidence of displacement. A hematoma was not visible. On the basis of these findings, the most likely diagnosis was felt to be a congenital normal variant or an old fracture that had undergone fibrous union. The findings were considered atypical of a recent fracture, and further evaluation by functional MRI was recommended.

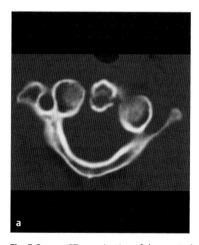
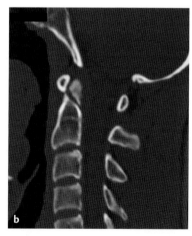
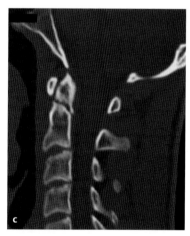

Fig. 5.8 a–c CT examination of the cervical spine. The report described a fresh oblique fracture through the apex of the dens.

a Axial scan at the level of the dens.
b Sagittal reformatted image in the midline.
c Sagittal reformatted image 4 mm to the left of **b**.

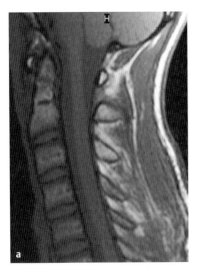
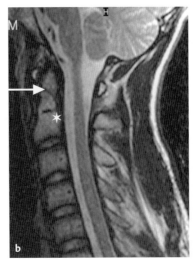
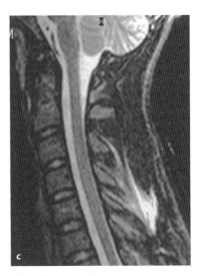

Fig. 5.9 a–c MRI of the cervical spine. A physiologic growth plate was described between the dens and body of the axis (asterisk) along with a subtle fracture line (arrow). There is no evidence of displacement, bone bruising, or hematoma formation. Differential diagnosis: congenital normal variant or the fibrous consolidation of an old fracture. Edema or hemorrhagic areas are visible in the nuchal soft tissues (**b, c**).

a T1-weighted image without fat suppression.
b T2-weighted image without fat suppression.
c T2-weighted fat-suppressed image (STIR sequence).

Further Case Summary

The patient was treated conservatively with a cervical collar. MRI follow-up 6 weeks later showed a more conspicuous fracture line (**Fig. 5.10**). Even on the basis of MRI criteria, disruption of the cortex was apparent. Posterior displacement of the dens, bone-marrow edema, and hematoma formation at the fracture site had developed since the previous examination. CT scans 2 weeks later confirmed the increasing dehiscence of the fracture site and the posterior deviation of the longitudinal axis of the dens

(**Fig. 5.11**). No signs of incipient bony consolidation were visible 8 weeks after the injury. The lesion was therefore classified as an Anderson–D'Alonzo type II fracture of the dens, subcategory B in the Eysel–Rosen classification, that was progressing to nonunion (**Figs. 5.12, 5.13**). Two months after the injury, the fracture was stabilized by minimally invasive internal fixation with screws and a single titanium compression plate. The surgery was uneventful. One day later the patient was feeling well and was released from the hospital.

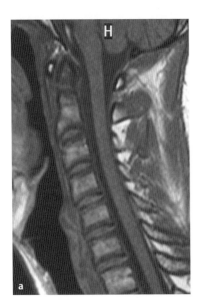
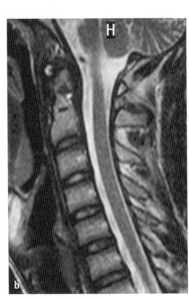

Fig. 5.10 a, b MRI follow-up 6 weeks after the first examination shows slight displacement of the dens apex, gapping of the fracture line, and a new bone bruise close to the fracture site (hypointense in **a**, hyperintense in **b**).
a T1-weighted image.
b T2-weighted image.

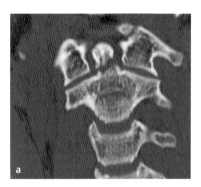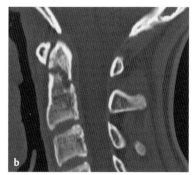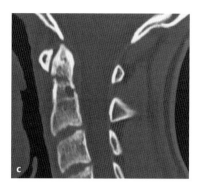

Fig. 5.11 a–c CT of the cervical spine 8 weeks after the first examination shows increasing dehiscence of the fracture site and slight posterior angulation of the apical fragment.

a Coronal reformatted image.
b Sagittal reformatted image in the median plane.
c Sagittal reformatted image 4 mm to the left of **b**.

Error Analysis and Strategy for Error Prevention

The initial CT diagnosis was correct. Misinterpretation of the first MRI was based on the absence of visible bone-marrow edema and soft-tissue hematoma on the initial images. The attending radiologist believed incorrectly that both signs would have been present during the first few days after the injury if a new fracture had occurred. There are no hard and fast empirical rules on the time required for bone-marrow edema to develop. Fracture healing is divided into stages of inflammation and granulation-tissue formation, new bone formation, and remodeling of the injured bone. The time course of bone healing is subject to large interindividual variations relating to many factors such as the patient's age, the static loads on the affected region, the degree of fracture immobilization, reapproximation of the fracture surfaces, and the patient's nutritional status and hormonal status. Lack of fracture immobilization and an incongruent reduction of the fragments will interfere with healing and promote bone resorption and secondary callus formation, which may culminate in a nonunion.

The treatment of an Anderson–D'Alonzo type II fracture of the dens is a controversial issue. Conservative treatment is justified for a primarily nondisplaced fracture (halo fixation or stiff-neck collar for at least 8 weeks). Surgical stabilization is indicated for a posteriorly displaced fracture to prevent a nonunion. In surgical cases, the type II fracture is the classic indication for anterior lag-screw fixation using one or two bone screws.

References and Further Reading

Anderson LD, D'Alonzo RT. Fractures of the odontoid process of the axis. J Bone Joint Surg Am 1974; 56: 1663–1674

Deliganis AV, Baxter AB, Hanson JA, et al. Radiologic spectrum of craniocervical distraction injuries. Radiographics 2000; 20: 237–250

Eysel P, Roosen K. Ventral or dorsal spondylodesis in dens basal fracture – a new classification for choice of surgical approach. Zentralbl Neurochir 1993; 54: 159–164

Imhof H, Fuchsjäger M. Traumatic injuries: imaging of spinal injuries. Eur Radiol 2002; 12: 1262–1272

Ulrich C, Bühren V. Verletzungen der Halswirbelsäule. Orthopädie und Unfallchirurgie up2date 2006; 1: 415–441

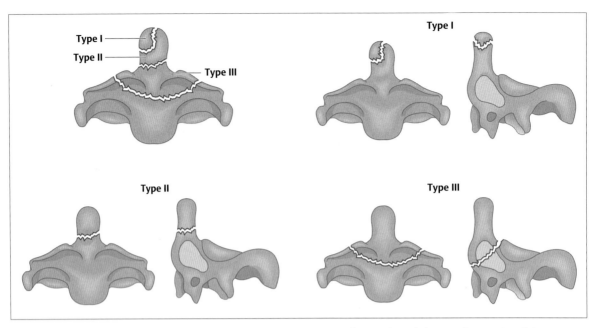

Fig. 5.12   Anderson and D'Alonzo classification of dens fractures.
Type I: oblique fracture of the dens apex and bony avulsion of the alar ligaments.
Type II: extra-articular fracture through the apophysis of the dens.

Type III: fracture through the cancellous portion of the axis body.
Dens fractures may be caused by a combination of vertical compression and horizontal shear. Type III lesions most commonly result from a hyperextension mechanism. Type II lesions are typically caused by a shear force acting from the anterolateral direction.

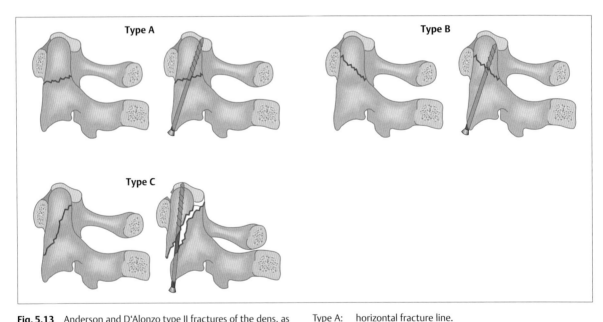

Fig. 5.13   Anderson and D'Alonzo type II fractures of the dens, as subclassified by Eysel and Rosen. Lag screw placement for internal fixation is also shown.

Type A: horizontal fracture line.
Type B: anterosuperior to posteroinferior fracture line.
Type C: posteroinferior to anterosuperior fracture line.

Normal Findings/ Bony Injury

History and Clinical Findings

A 47-year-old man presented in orthopedics with severe upper thoracic back pain after a fall. Spinal radiographs were taken and were interpreted as normal (**Fig. 5.14**).

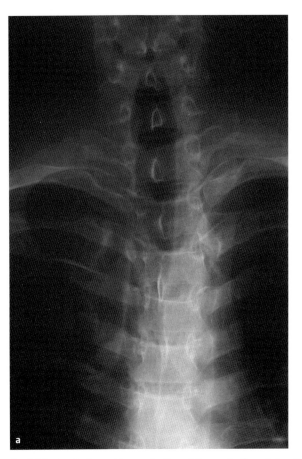
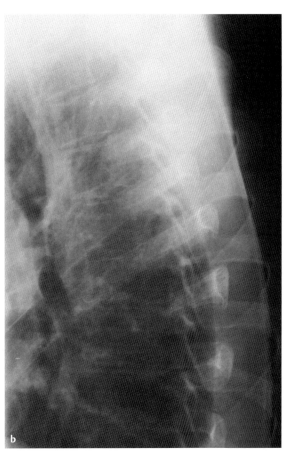

Fig. 5.14 a, b Radiographic examination of the cervicothoracic junction. The films were interpreted as normal.

Further Case Summary

The patient returned 3 days later in severe distress from continued back pain. On physical examination, the T4 vertebral body was tender to percussion. Subsequent MRI showed a bandlike zone of low T1-weighted and high T2-weighted signal intensity in the bone marrow of the T4 vertebral body (**Fig. 5.15**). The finding was interpreted as traumatic bone-marrow edema. During the next few weeks, the patient's complaints improved in response to conservative immobilization.

Error Analysis and Strategy for Error Prevention

Two relevant findings had been missed on the frontal radiograph: slight left convex scoliosis at the T3–T4 level and the slightly decreased height of the T4 vertebral body on the left side (**Fig. 5.16**). A review of the lateral radiograph confirmed the absence of visible abnormalities. MRI is superior to radiographs for detecting postcontusional bone marrow changes owing to its excellent soft-tissue contrast (**Fig. 5.17**).

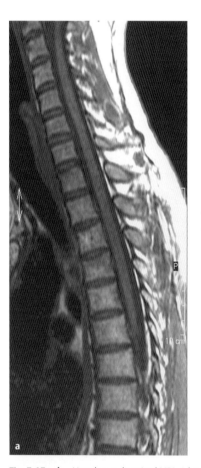
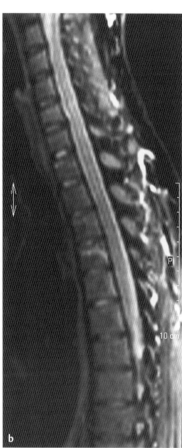

Fig. 5.15 a, b Unenhanced sagittal MRI. A bandlike zone of bone-marrow edema in T4 appears hypointense on the T1-weighted image and hyperintense on the T2-weighted image.
a T1-weighted image.
b T2-weighted image.

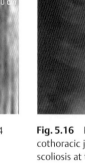

Fig. 5.16 Frontal radiograph of the cervicothoracic junction. Slight left convex scoliosis at the T3–T4 level and slightly diminished height of the left lateral border of the T4 vertebral body had been missed on initial interpretation. 1 = T1 vertebra, 4 = T4 vertebra.

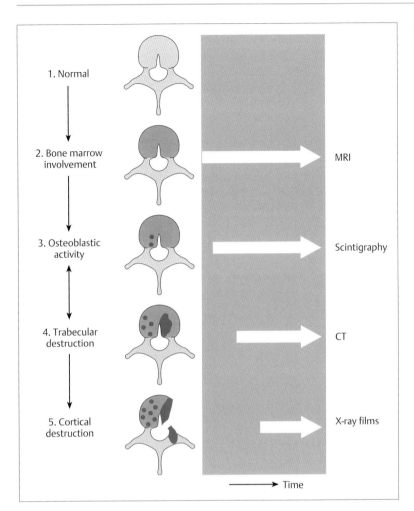

Fig. 5.17 Sensitivity of various imaging modalities in the detection of bone-marrow and skeletal changes.

1. Normal

2. Bone marrow involvement

3. Osteoblastic activity

4. Trabecular destruction

5. Cortical destruction

MRI

Scintigraphy

CT

X-ray films

Time

Bone Bruise

A bone bruise is characterized on MRI by low signal intensity of the bone marrow on T1-weighted images and high signal intensity on T2-weighted images in patients with a trauma history. Comparative histopathologic studies have shown that a bone bruise represents a combination of bone-marrow edema and small intraosseous hemorrhages that may result from fractures of cancellous trabeculae. Bone bruises may be caused by direct, violent trauma or by repetitive or chronic unphysiologic loading of the bone. On average, a bone bruise will appear 12 hours after the injury (no less than 1 hour and no more than 30 hours post trauma). Often it is the only morphologic imaging sign that an injury has occurred and should prompt a detailed search for associated injuries. In patients who have not sustained a trauma, the alteration of bone marrow signal intensity may be a result of bone-marrow edema secondary to inflammation, neoplasia, or avascular necrosis.

References and Further Reading

Blanenbaker DG, De Smet AA, Vanderby R, et al. MRI of acute bone bruises: timing of the appearance in a swine model. AJR 2008; 190: W1–W7

Oda H, Igarashi M, Sase H, Sase T, Yamamoto S. Bone bruise in magnetic resonance imaging strongly correlates with the production of joint effusion and knee osteoarthritis. J Orthop Sci 2008; 13: 7–15

Thiryayi WA, Thiryayi SA, Freemont AJ. Histopathological perspective on bone-marrow edema, reactive bone change and haemorrhage. Eur J Radiol 2008; 67: 62–67

Underdiagnosis/ Appropriate Work-up

History and Clinical Findings

A 61-year-old woman fell down stairs. She loss consciousness briefly after the fall but did not experience prolonged impairment of consciousness. She complained of gross hematuria during the initial hours after the accident. Clinical examination revealed no abnormalities. No neurologic deficits were found, and there was no tenderness to percussion of the skull or spinal column. The hematuria was investigated by abdominal B-mode ultrasound, which was negative although scanning conditions were unfavorable due to overlying bowel gas (**Fig. 5.18**). CT was recommended in the event that gross hematuria persisted.

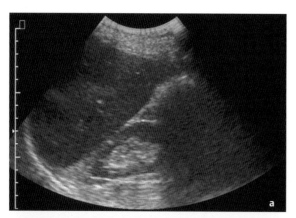

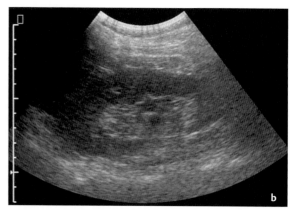

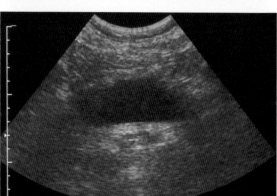

Fig. 5.18 a–c Abdominal ultrasound scans were described as normal, although interpretation was hampered by overlying bowel gas.
a Longitudinal scan through the right kidney.
b Longitudinal scan through the left kidney.
c Transverse scan through the bladder.

Further Case Summary

Ten days later the patient developed a conus medullaris syndrome marked by bladder dysfunction and sensory disturbances in the genital region. MRI of the lower thoracic spine and lumbar spine revealed a vertebral fracture involving the posterior margin of the T12 vertebral body and the pedicles (**Fig. 5.19**). A detached bone fragment was encroaching on the spinal canal, narrowing its AP diameter by approximately 50%. CT scans of the thoracolumbar junction were obtained for preoperative planning. The scans showed a multipart fracture of the T12 vertebral body with involvement of the posterior margin and the intraspinal displacement of a loose bone fragment (**Fig. 5.20**). The adjacent T11–T12 and T12–L1 intervertebral disks showed vacuum signs resulting from the distraction injury. The injury was classified as a Magerl type B unstable osteoligamentous fracture (**Table 5.1, Fig. 5.21**). A lumbosacral transitional vertebra with the partial sacralization of L5 on the left side was noted as an incidental finding.

Table 5.1   Magerl classification of spinal injuries (after Magerl et al. 1994)

Type	Description of injury
A	Vertebral body compression
B	Anterior and posterior element injuries with distraction
C	Anterior and posterior element injuries with rotation

Error Analysis and Strategy for Error Prevention

The initial diagnostic work-up was inadequate. The severity of the trauma was underestimated during clinical examination.

- The brief period of unconsciousness after the fall indicated craniocerebral trauma. Based on the interdisciplinary guidelines of the American College of Radiology and the German Society for Neurosurgery, CT examination of the skull and upper cervical spine without IV contrast administration would have been appropriate due to the initial loss of consciousness.

- The transient gross hematuria suggested significant trauma to the retroperitoneum including the kidneys and ureters. Ultrasound was not suitable for the detection or exclusion of urinary tract injuries due to limited visualization of the retroperitoneum. Abdominal CT scans after IV contrast administration, including coverage of the lower thoracic spine, would have been a better option.

- From 15% to 20% of all serious head and abdominal injuries are associated with injuries to the craniovertebral junction and spinal column. From 70% to 80% of all spinal injuries affect the thoracic and lumbar spine, with more than 50% involving the thoracolumbar junction. The vulnerability of this region is explained by the natural transition from thoracic kyphosis to lumbar lordosis and the fact that the thoracic spine is stabilized by the thoracic cage. An analysis of 775 spine-injured patients from the trauma registry of the German

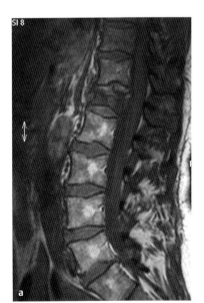 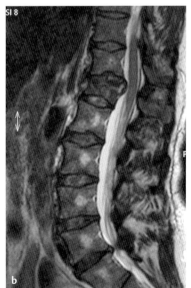 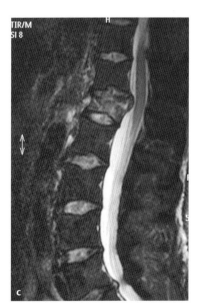

Fig. 5.19 a–c   MR images of the lower thoracic spine and lumbar spine demonstrate a fracture of T12 involving the posterior vertebral margin, both pedicles, and the posterior column. The height of the T12 vertebral body is diminished anteriorly. Lordosis is increased. The bony spinal canal is narrowed by a posteriorly displaced bone fragment.

a   T1-weighted image.
b   T2-weighted image.
c   STIR sequence.

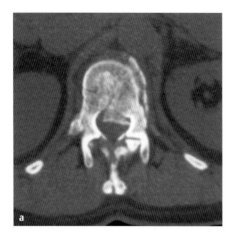 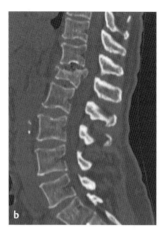

Fig. 5.20 a, b   CT scans of the thoracolumbar junction and lumbar spine for preoperative planning show distraction of the T11 and T12 spinous processes and posttraumatic gas collections in the T11–T12 and T12–L1 intervertebral disks. The fracture was classified as unstable due to involvement of the posterior vertebral body margin, pedicles, and posterior column.

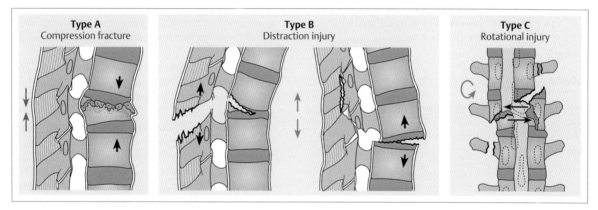

| Type A | Type B | Type C |
| Compression fracture | Distraction injury | Rotational injury |

Fig. 5.21   Magerl classification of thoracolumbar vertebral fractures (after Gonschorek and Bühren 2006).

Society for Trauma Surgery indicated that motor vehicle accidents (49%) and falls from a height (20%) were the most common mechanisms of injury. Fractures of the cervical spine (34%), thoracic spine (40%), and lumbar spine (31%) occurred with approximately equal frequencies. In nearly half of the spine-injured patients reviewed, the emergency physician found no evidence of injury to the spinal column. For this reason, a radiographic examination of the axial skeleton should have been performed to exclude a fracture despite the absence of spinal tenderness to percussion.

Craniocerebral Trauma

Craniocerebral trauma is a head injury characterized by functional alteration and/or damage to the brain. An injury not associated with brain damage or dysfunction is called a head contusion. Typical subjective complaints following craniocerebral trauma are headache, impairment of consciousness, nausea, dizziness, diplopia, and hearing loss. Objective signs of injury include soft-tissue swelling, bleeding, gashes and lacerations, and cranial deformation. Neurologic injury may be manifested by amnesia, decreased alertness, disorientation, vomiting, paralysis, speech and coordination difficulties, cranial

nerve deficits, seizures, and autonomic dysfunction. Impairment of consciousness indicates a severe alteration of brain function. A distinction is drawn between impaired consciousness (decreased alertness; diminished orientation to person, place, and time; the patient is able to open the eyes) and loss of consciousness (loss of mental perception of surroundings and self).

Cranial CT is an essential diagnostic study in head-injured patients who present with coma, impaired consciousness, amnesia, other neurologic deficits, vomiting, a seizure, and/or clinical or radiographic signs of a skull fracture.

Classification of Spinal Fractures

A classification should permit the identification of any injury based on a simple clinical and radiological algorithm. It should also supply reproducible information on the severity of the injury and provide guidance for treatment planning and clinical studies. The definition of stability in spinal injuries is complex and remains a controversial issue.

Clinical stability categories. An injury may be classified clinically as "stable" (no further position change should occur at rest or with exercise), "slightly unstable" (should heal without significant deformity or neurologic deficits), or "highly unstable" (significant deformity and neurologic deficits would occur with functional therapy).

Two-column and three-column models. In 1977 Whitesides introduced a two-column model of the spine: an anterior column consisting of the vertebral bodies and intervertebral disks, and a posterior column consisting of the vertebral arches, vertebral processes, and ligaments. The anterior column is subjected mainly to compression, the posterior column to tension. In 1983 Denis added a third, middle column consisting of the posterior wall of the vertebral bodies, the posterior portion of the annulus fibrosus, and the posterior longitudinal ligament.

ASIF classification. The classification introduced by the Association for the Study of Internal Fixation (ASIF) is most commonly used in Europe for the classification of spinal injuries (Magerl 1994, **Table 5.1**). It is based on the two-column model of Whitesides and ranks injuries from category A through C according to increasing degree of instability. Isolated fractures of the transverse and spinous processes are disregarded. Type A fractures involve the vertebral body, or anterior column, which generally is injured by a compression mechanism. Type B and C injuries involve both columns. Type B is characterized by a flexion–distraction mechanism, and type C by rotational instability. Each of the three types is further classified into subgroups 1–3 based on increasing degree of severity. Injuries involving the posterior margin of the vertebral body and posterior column (corresponding to columns 2 and 3 in the Denis model) as well as distraction and rotational injuries are assumed to be unstable.

Treatment. Approximately 80% of spinal injuries are treated conservatively. Type A1 and A2 fractures are generally referred for early conservative functional therapy (physical therapy plus analgesics). Surgical treatment is indicated in patients with angular and rotational deformities, narrowing of the bony spinal canal (usually by a posteriorly displaced vertebral body fragment), or instability. The goals of surgical treatment are to correct the deformity, decompress the spinal canal, and restore stability.

References and Further Reading

American College of Radiology. Appropriateness Criteria. Neurologic Imaging. Head Trauma. http://www.acr.org/SecondaryMainMenuCategories/quality_safety/app_criteria/pdf/ExpertPanelonNeurologicImaging/HeadTraumaDoc5.aspx (accessed November 10, 2010)

Deutsche Gesellschaft für Neurochirurgie. Leitlinie "Schädel-Hirn-Trauma im Erwachsenenalter." In: AWMF online (Arbeitsgemeinschaft der Wissenschaftlichen Medizinischen Fachgesellschaften). http://www.uni-duesseldorf.de/WWW/AWMF/ll/ (accessed November 10, 2010)

Gonschorek O, Bühren V. Verletzungen der thorakolumbalen Wirbelsäule. Orthopädie und Unfallchirurgie up2date 2006; 1: 195–222

Magerl F, Aebi M, Gertzbein SD, Harms J. Nazarian S. A comprehensive classification of thoracic and lumbar injuries. Eur Spine J 1994; 3: 184–201

Schinkel C, Frangen TM, Kmetic A, et al. AG Polytrauma der DGU. Wirbelsäulenverletzungen bei Mehrfachfrakturen. Eine Analyse des DGU-Traumaregisters. Unfallchirurg 2007; 100: 946–952

Assessing the Risk of Spinal Instability: CT, Radiographs, or Both?

History and Clinical Findings

A 79-year-old man had undergone previous surgical removal of an adenocarcinoma of the left parotid gland with an ipsilateral neck dissection. CT examination of the facial skeleton and neck was done postoperatively for restaging and mainly showed multiple osteolytic bone metastases (**Fig. 5.22**). Degenerative spinal changes were also noted as incidental findings. Based on the CT findings, the patient was referred the next day for radiographic examination to check for possible instability of the cervical spine (**Fig. 5.23**).

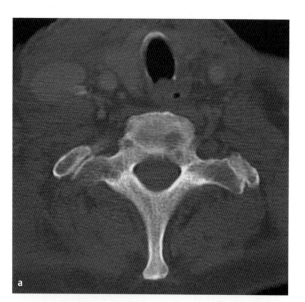

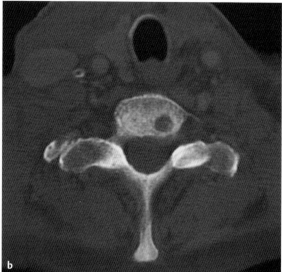

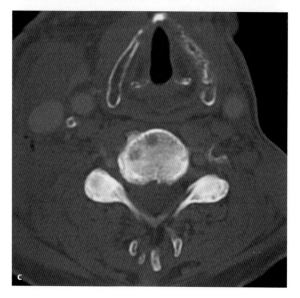

Fig. 5.22a–c   Axial CT scans of the neck.

Further Case Summary

The radiographic examination revealed kyphosis of the midcervical spine (possibly of the postural type) and osteochondrosis in the C6–C7 segment. Osteolytic lesions were not detected. A review of the CT and radiographic findings excluded any immediate risk of instability.

Error Analysis and Strategy for Error Prevention

The plain radiographs had not been ordered by a physician with expertise in radiation safety and were not indicated for the following reasons:

- Because plain films yield a summation image, they are inherently inferior to sectional CT images for detecting small osteolytic foci. As a rule, an absorption difference between healthy cancellous bone and cancellous bone permeated by one or more osteolytic lesions can be detected on plain films only when approximately 30% of the bone matrix has been destroyed (see **Fig. 5.17**).
- CT had already excluded a risk of instability. Sufficient bone stock was still present to withstand pressure loads from the head and neck, and there were no destructive changes in the posterior vertebral body margins or pedicles that involved the cortical bone. The ligaments that stabilize the spine against rotation and shear were intact.

References and Further Reading

Council Directive 96/29/EURATOM of 13 May 1996 laying down basic safety standards for the protection of the health of workers and the general public against the danger arising from ionizing radiation. http://ec.europa.eu/energy/nuclear/radioprotection/doc/legislation/9629_en.pdf (accessed January 10, 2011)

Council Directive 97/43/EURATOM of 30 June 1997 on health protection in individuals against the dangers of ionizing radiation in relation to medical exposure, and repealing Directive 84/466 Euratom. http://ec.europa.eu/energy/nuclear/radioprotection/doc/legislation/9743_en.pdf (accessed January 10, 2011)

Ecker RD, Endo T, Wetjen NM, Kraus WE. Diagnosis and treatment of vertebral column metastases. Mayo Clin Proc 2005; 80: 1177–1186

Fourney DR, Gokaslan ZL. Spinal instability and deformity due to neoplastic conditions. Neurosurg Focus 2003; 15: 14

Greenspan A. Orthopedic Imaging: A Practical Approach. 4th ed. Philadelphia: Lippincott Williams & Wilkins; 2005

Pathria M. Imaging of spine instability. Semin Musculoskelet Radiol 2005; 9: 88–99

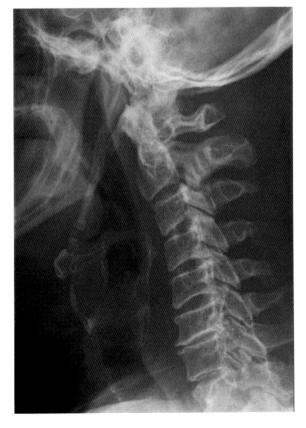

Fig. 5.23 Lateral radiograph of the cervical spine.

Plain Radiography/ MRI to Exclude Skeletal Metastasis

History and Clinical Findings

A 63-year-old symptomatic woman underwent bone scintigraphy for restaging of breast cancer (**Fig. 5.24**). The bone scans showed increased uptake in the right shoulder, in the spinal column (lateral portions of the midcervical spine, L4–L5 vertebral bodies), and in the left hip. The increased uptake in the lower lumbar spine had been unchanged for 1½ years. Although all scintigraphic findings were interpreted as degenerative, radiographic examination (**Figs. 5.25a, 5.26a**) and MRI of the lumbar spine and pelvis (**Figs. 5.25b, 5.26b**) were scheduled on the same day.

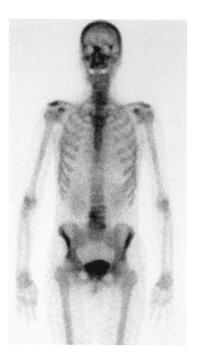

Fig. 5.24 Radionuclide bone scan in the supine position.

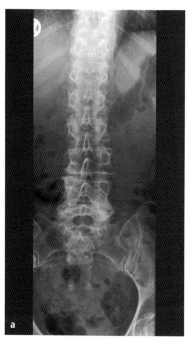

Fig. 5.25a, b Examination of the lumbar spine.

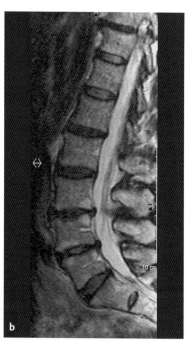

a Radiographic examination.
b MRI.

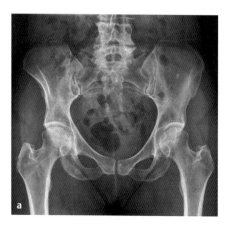

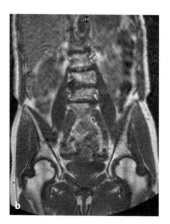

Fig. 5.26a, b Examination of the pelvis.
a Radiographic examination.
b MRI.

Further Case Summary

The radiographic and MRI examinations revealed osteochondrosis of the lumbar spine with intervertebral disk protrusions and incipient osteoarthritis of the hip as correlating with the areas of increased uptake on the radionuclide scans. There was no evidence of metastasis—a diagnosis that was confirmed by an additional 3 years of follow-up.

Error Analysis and Strategy for Error Prevention

Scheduling MRI and radiography of the same body region on the same day constituted an excessive work-up. The lumbar examinations were not indicated because the scintigraphic finding had remained unchanged for 18 months, confirming a benign cause. MRI would have been better than radiography for excluding metastasis in the left hip owing to its greater sensitivity (**Table 5.2**).

Table 5.2   Diagnostic strategies for detecting skeletal metastases

Clinical findings	Diagnostic procedure	Goal
Curative indication		
Asymptomatic patient	Bone scintigraphy	Search for foci of increased uptake anywhere in the skeleton (DD: metastases, degenerative changes, posttraumatic changes, etc.)
■ Apparently benign scintigraphic focus	Plain radiography	Topographic correlation of the scintigraphic finding with a benign skeletal finding (osteochondrosis, old fracture, spondylarthrosis, etc.)
■ Indeterminate scintigraphic focus	MRI	Characterization of scintigraphic foci in cases with therapeutic implications
	CT-guided percutaneous or open biopsy	Histologic confirmation in cases with therapeutic implications
Symptomatic patient	MRI	Investigation of local finding
	CT-guided percutaneous or open biopsy	Histologic confirmation in cases with therapeutic implications
Palliative indication		
Symptomatic patient	Plain radiography	Assess instability risk
	MRI	Investigate local finding only if there will be therapeutic implications

Skeletal Metastases

Skeletal metastases are by far the most common neoplastic skeletal disease in adults. They are particularly common with breast cancer (47–85% of deaths), lung cancer (32%), prostate cancer (54–85%), and renal cell carcinoma (33–40%). More than 90% of skeletal metastases involve the spinal column and pelvis owing to the rich vascularity of the hematopoietic red bone marrow. Metastasis occurs by the hematogenous route through the haversian canals into the bone marrow, spreading later to involve the cancellous trabeculae and cortical bone. The most frequent initial complaint is back pain, which is caused by neoplastic infiltration of the richly innervated periosteum via the haversian canals and cortical bone.

Imaging modalities. MRI is the most sensitive imaging modality for detecting changes in the medullary cavity because of its excellent soft-tissue contrast (see **Fig. 5.17**). Bone scintigraphy is the second most sensitive procedure, demonstrating the compensatory increase in bone metabolism due to cortical invasion based on a focal increase in the uptake of radiolabeled technetium-99m methyldiphosphonate (^{99m}Tc-MDP). Experience has shown that the erosion of cancellous trabeculae in itself is not sufficient for a scintigraphic diagnosis of metastasis. Osteolytic metastases are not visible on plain radiographs until 30–50% of the bone matrix has already been destroyed. CT detects cortical bone erosion earlier than plain films but cannot demonstrate changes within the medullary cavity. Unless the findings are very prominent, all of these imaging studies are nonspecific, and histologic confirmation by CT-guided percutaneous or open biopsy should be sought in an appropriate clinical context (suspicion of a solitary initial metastasis, therapeutic implications).

References and Further Reading

Altehoefer C, Ghanem N, Hogerle S, Moser E, Langer M. Comparative detectability of bone metastases and impact on therapy of magnetic resonance imaging and bone scintigraphy in patients with breast cancer. Eur J Radiol 2001; 40: 16–23

Ecker RD, Endo T, Wetjen NM, Kraus WE. Diagnosis and treatment of vertebral column metastases. Mayo Clin Proc 2005; 80: 1177–1186

Even-Sapir E. Imaging of malignant bone involvement by morphologic, scintigraphic, and hybrid modalities. J Nucl Med 2005; 46: 1356–1367

Soderlund V. Radiological diagnosis of skeletal metastases. Eur Radiol 1996; 6: 587–595

Toaka T, Mayr NA, Lee HJ, et al. Factors influencing visualization of vertebral metastases on MR imaging versus bone scintigraphy. AJR 2001; 176: 1525–1530

6

Musculoskeletal System

Bony Injury?

History and Clinical Findings

A 31-year-old man had fallen 4 weeks earlier during a soccer match. He had attempted to break his fall with his hands. Afterward he complained of pain on the radial side of his right wrist and painful limitation of motion, especially on extension. He reported that his hand had been swollen for several days after the fall. Radiographs of the right wrist were interpreted as normal (**Fig. 6.1**).

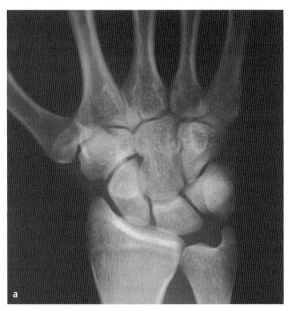
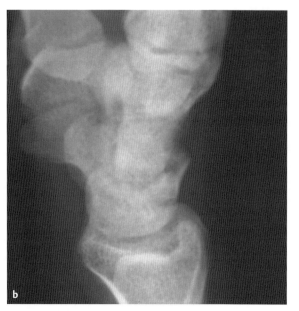

Fig. 6.1 a, b   Radiographic examination of the right wrist after trauma. The radiographs were interpreted as normal.

Further Case Summary

The attending trauma surgeon was sure that the patient had sustained a scaphoid fracture due to the typical clinical findings (tenderness over the snuffbox, pain on axial compression of the thumb). This prompted him to request spot radiographs of the scaphoid in two different oblique projections. The spot films revealed a Herbert type B2 scaphoid fracture (unstable, nondisplaced fracture through the middle third of the scaphoid, **Figs. 6.2, 6.3**).

Error Analysis and Strategy for Error Prevention

As in the present case, up to 70% of scaphoid fractures are missed on standard radiographic projections in two planes because the capsule and ligaments tend to reduce the fragments to an anatomical position. When clinical findings are suspicious for a scaphoid fracture, the wrist should first be radiographed in two planes to provide an overview of the radius, ulna, and carpal bones. With the hand in a neutral position, these survey views may not demonstrate the fine line of a fresh, nondisplaced fracture due to the minimal absorption differences and superimposed shadows, even when the injury is known (**Fig. 6.1**). Given the doubly oblique orientation of the scaphoid bone, spot views in pronation and supination are often better for positioning the scaphoid parallel to the imaging plane. The purpose of these oblique projections is to correct for the palmar angulation of the scaphoid and image the bone perpendicular to its long axis (the four views in **Fig. 6.1** and **Fig. 6.2** are called the "scaphoid quartet"). If the survey and spot films do not reveal a scaphoid fracture in clinically suspicious cases, the prognostic and therapeutic implications of this injury warrant investigation by CT or MRI to prevent the fracture from going on to necrosis or nonunion.

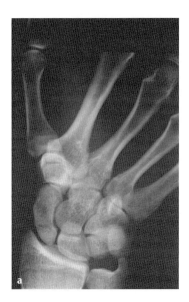 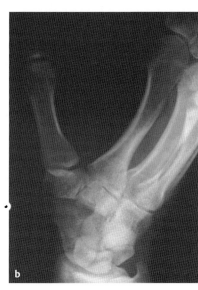

Fig. 6.2 a, b Spot radiographs of the scaphoid bone in the dorsovolar projection demonstrate a nondisplaced, horizontal fracture through the middle third of the scaphoid (Herbert type B2).

a View with the wrist pronated approximately 15°.

b View with the wrist supinated approximately 15°.

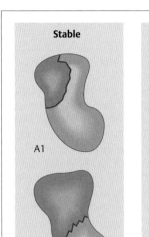
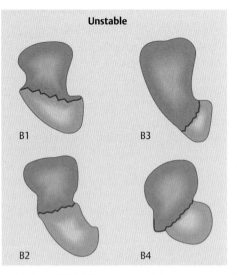
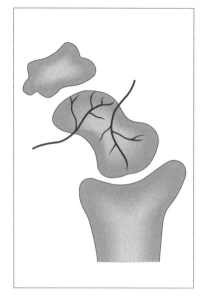

Fig. 6.3 Herbert classification of acute and subacute scaphoid fractures (after Treitl et al. 2002). A1 = fracture of the scaphoid tubercle, A2 = incomplete fracture of the middle third, B1 = distal oblique fracture, B2 = complete fracture of the middle third, B3 = fracture of the proximal pole, B4 = transscaphoid perilunar fracture with carpal dislocation.

Fig. 6.4 Arterial blood supply of the scaphoid in the lateral view (after Treitl et al. 2002).

Scaphoid Fractures

Approximately 60% of wrist fractures involve the scaphoid bone. The ratio of scaphoid to radial fractures is approximately 1:10. Males between 15 and 40 years of age are predominantly affected. Most scaphoid fractures are caused by a fall onto the hyperextended hand. This mechanism drives the scaphoid bone up against the posterior margin of the radius, which acts as a fulcrum. While the proximal scaphoid is fixed to the radius by the radioscaphocapitate ligament, the force vector acts directly on the distal pole of the scaphoid. Even with a complete scaphoid fracture, the fragments are often undisplaced because the extrinsic capsule and ligaments hold them in an approximately normal position. The middle third of the scaphoid is most commonly affected. Scaphoid fractures are often associated with other fractures and tendon/ligament injuries. The exact location of the fracture has prognostic importance because the distal and middle portions of the scaphoid have a better blood supply than the proximal pole (**Fig. 6.4**). As a result, proximal scaphoid fractures are more likely to go on to nonunion than fractures at other sites.

Stability and treatment. The imaging goal in patients with an acute (< 2 weeks post injury) or subacute scaphoid fracture (2–6 weeks post injury) is to distinguish a stable fracture, which can be managed conservatively, from an unstable fracture, which requires surgical treatment.

Stable: Fractures of the scaphoid tubercle, incomplete fractures, and nondisplaced transverse fractures of the middle third.

Unstable: Distal oblique fractures, displaced transverse fractures of the middle third, all proximal third fractures, and transscaphoid perilunar fracture-dislocations.

References and Further Reading

Greenspan A. Orthopedic Imaging: A Practical Approach. 4th ed. Philadelphia: Lippincott Williams & Wilkins; 2005

Treitl M, Stäbler A, Reiser M. Bildgebende Diagnostik der Handwurzel. Radiologie up2date 2002; 1: 93–120

Postoperative Follow-up after Internal Fixation/ Refracture/ Laterality Error

History and Clinical Findings

A 92-year-old woman suffering from osteoporosis was taken to the emergency room with a fracture of the distal left femur. Initial radiographs showed an extra-articular fracture of the distal femoral diaphysis (**Fig. 6.5**). A preoperative lateral view was omitted because of the poor clinical condition of the patient. At operation, the fracture was stabilized with an intramedullary nail under image intensifier control. Postoperative radiographs of the left femur taken in the ICU not only showed the surgically stabilized distal femoral fracture (**Fig. 6.6c, d**) but also revealed a new, posteriorly displaced fracture of the proximal femur, which was visible in the lateral projection in the second round of radiographs (**Fig. 6.6b**).

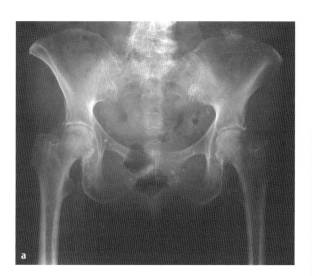

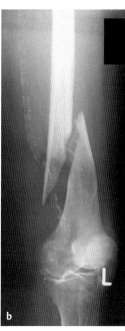

Fig. 6.5a, b Preoperative radiographs showed an extra-articular fracture of the distal left femur with shortening, lateral displacement, and rotational displacement of the distal femur.

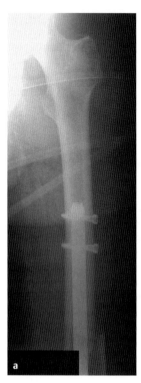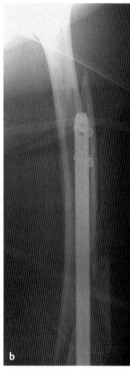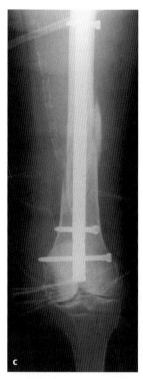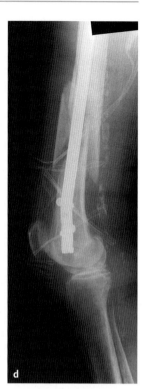

Fig. 6.6 a–d Postoperative radiographs taken in the ICU. The radiographs are presented in chronological order.

Further Case Summary

The image intensifier used at operation confirmed that the original fracture was confined to the distal femoral diaphysis. The postoperative lateral radiograph revealed a new fracture of the proximal femur (**Fig. 6.6 b**).

This fracture, then, occurred while the patient was being positioned for the second round of radiographs. Afterward the patient confirmed that she had felt a sudden pain during the examination. Positioning was difficult due to patient immobility. The intramedullary nail had acted as a lever and pressed sharply against the posterior femoral cortex, which had already been weakened due to osteoporosis. The second fracture was successfully treated by internal fixation on the following day (**Fig. 6.7**).

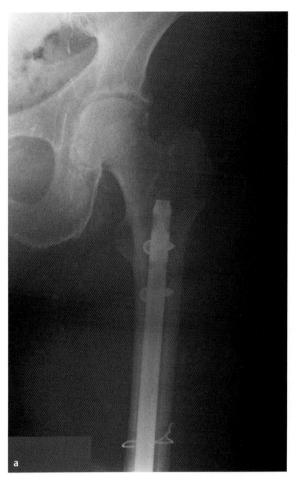 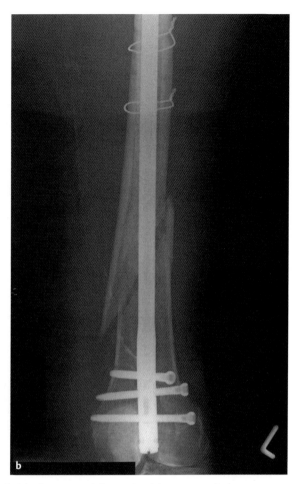

Fig. 6.7 a, b Radiographic examination of the left femur after removal of the first intramedullary nail and the insertion of a longer intramedullary nail with cross screws. The new nail extends the full length of the femoral diaphysis.

Error Analysis and Strategy for Error Prevention

The following errors were made during the postoperative radiographic examination (**Fig. 6.6**):

- Both technologists who performed the radiographic examination on the bed-confined 92-year-old patient had underestimated the fragility of the osteoporotic bone. During positioning of the cassette, the distal femur had been elevated from a relatively fixed position of the hip. During this maneuver the intramedullary nail pressed hard against the posterior femoral cortex, causing the proximal blowout fracture that was visible on postoperative films. This type of error could easily provide grounds for subsequent litigation.

- The mA·s product was set too high for the proximal femoral radiographs (**Fig. 6.6 a, b**). Because of this, the proximal thigh was imaged in the "shoulder" part of the gradation curve rather than its linear portion, and regional differences in the radiation dose delivered to the film were not converted into gray-scale differences in a linear fashion. This resulted in a dark, low-contrast appearance of the fracture zone.

In a different patient 89 years of age, postoperative radiographs were taken to assess the fixation of a left femoral neck fracture with a dynamic hip screw. Initial radiographs of the right hip showed no abnormalities (**Fig. 6.8 a, b**). When the technologist was questioned, it was learned that she had x-rayed the right hip instead of the left hip, where the surgery had actually been performed. Subsequent radiographs of the left hip showed an unstable femoral neck fracture that had been stabilized with a dynamic hip screw. The films showed impaction, shortening, axial rotation, and medial angulation of the femoral diaphysis (**Fig. 6.8 c, d**). As a result of these findings, the femoral head and neck were resected and a total hip replacement was performed. A detailed review of the case showed that the radiology technician had not asked the patient which side required imaging and had failed to note the absence of a surgical scar. There was no valid indication for imaging the right hip, and this type of error would furnish definite grounds for a malpractice claim.

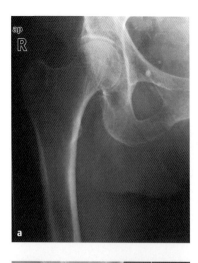

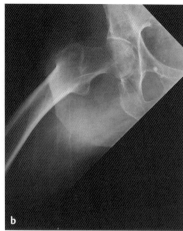

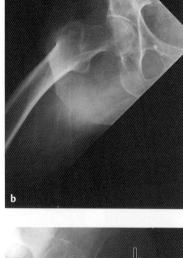

Fig. 6.8 a–d   Radiographs in an 89-year-old woman referred for evaluation of a femoral neck fracture stabilized with a dynamic hip screw.
a, b   Initial radiographic examination of the right hip. A side marker was not placed in **b**.
c, d   Second radiographic examination.

References and Further Reading

American College of Radiology (ACR). ACR Practice Guideline for Diagnostic Reference Levels in Medical X-ray Imaging. http://www.acr.org/SecondaryMainMenuCategories/quality_safety/RadSafety/RadiationSafety/guideline-diagnostic-reference.aspx (accessed November 10, 2010)

Amis ES, Butler PF, Applegate KE, et al. American College of Radiology White Paper on Radiation Dose in Medicine. J Am Coll Radiol 2007; 4: 272–284. http://www.acr.org/SecondaryMainMenuCategories/quality_safety/white_paper_dose.aspx (accessed November 10, 2010)

Council Directive 96/29/EURATOM of 13 May 1996 laying down basic safety standards for the protection of the health of workers and the general public against the danger arising from ionizing radiation. http:// ec.europa.eu/energy/nuclear/radioprotection/doc/legislation/9629_en.pdf (accessed January 10, 2011)

Council Directive 97/43/EURATOM of 30 June 1997 on health protection in individuals against the dangers of ionizing radiation in relation to medical exposure, and repealing Directive 84/466/Euratom. http:// ec.europa.eu/energy/nuclear/radioprotection/doc/legislation/9743_en.pdf (accessed January 10, 2011)

Sonnek C, Bauer B. Die neue Röntgenverordnung. Verordnung über den Schutz vor Schäden durch Röntgenstrahlen (Röntgenverordnung RöV) vom 8. Januar 1987 (BGBl. I S 114), zuletzt geändert durch Verordnung vom 18. Juni 2002 (BGBl. I S 1869). Berlin: H. Hoffmann; 2002

Degenerative Changes/ Osteolytic Lesions

History and Clinical Findings

A 67-year-old man was referred from radiotherapy for pelvic radiographs because of pain in the right hip (**Fig. 6.9**). He had a history of metastatic adenocarcinoma from an unknown primary tumor (CUP) with lesions in the liver, lungs, mediastinal lymph nodes, and ribs. The radiology report described degenerative changes in the lower lumbar spine. Osteolytic and osteoplastic changes were excluded, although the lower portion of the sacrum could not be evaluated due to superimposed iodinated contrast medium in the bladder following a previous examination with IV contrast administration.

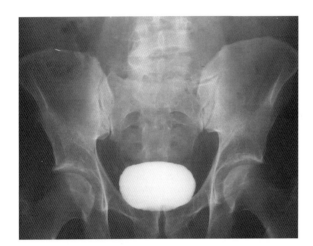

Fig. 6.9   Radiographic examination of the pelvis, interpreted as normal.

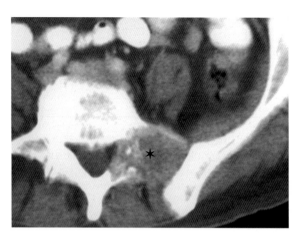

Fig. 6.10   Abdominal CT shows destruction of the left pedicle and left transverse process of L5 with an extraosseous soft-tissue component (asterisk).

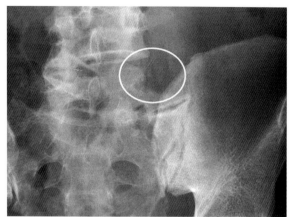

Fig. 6.11   Pelvic radiograph. Magnified view of the osteolytic area (circled).

Further Case Summary

An abdominal CT examination performed earlier in the day showed an osteolytic metastasis in the left pedicle and left transverse process of the L5 vertebra (**Fig. 6.10**). In retrospect, this finding was also visible on the pelvic radiograph (**Fig. 6.11**). A lumbosacral transitional vertebra with degenerative changes was noted on the left side as an incidental finding. Chemoradiation was prescribed for the disseminated metastases. A small-cell lung cancer was later identified histologically as the primary tumor.

Error Analysis and Strategy for Error Prevention

Radiographic examination of the pelvis was not indicated in this patient because the pelvic skeleton had already been evaluated earlier that day by CT, which is superior to plain films. The clinical request for pelvic radiographs contained no information on the CT examination, although scrutiny of the patient's chart and questioning of the patient would have drawn attention to the duplicated examination. When the radiographs were interpreted, the opacified bladder urine should have indicated the previous CT examination and called the radiographic findings into question.

Destruction of the left pedicle and left transverse process of L5 was presumably missed because the original clinical problem was right hip pain.

References and Further Reading

American College of Radiology (ACR). ACR Practice Guideline for Diagnostic Reference Levels in Medical X-ray Imaging. http://www.acr.org/SecondaryMainMenuCategories/quality_safety/RadSafety/RadiationSafety/guideline-diagnostic-reference.aspx (accessed November 10, 2010)

Amis ES, Butler PF, Applegate KE, et al. American College of Radiology White Paper on Radiation Dose in Medicine. J Am Coll Radiol 2007; 4: 272–284.http://www.acr.org/SecondaryMainMenuCategories/quality_safety/white_paper_dose.aspx (accessed November 10, 2010)

Council Directive 97/43/EURATOM of 30 June 1997 on health protection in individuals against the dangers of ionizing radiation in relation to medical exposure, and repealing Directive 84/466/Euratom. http://ec.europa.eu/energy/nuclear/radioprotection/doc/legislation/9743_en.pdf (accessed January 10, 2011)

Sonnek C, Bauer B. Die neue Röntgenverordnung. Verordnung über den Schutz vor Schäden durch Röntgenstrahlen (Röntgenverordnung RöV) vom 8. Januar 1987 (BGBl. I S 114), zuletzt geändert durch Verordnung vom 18. Juni 2002 (BGBl. I S 1869). Berlin: H. Hoffmann; 2002

Skeletal Metastases: CT/Plain Radiographs

History and Clinical Findings

A 63-year-old man had undergone a radical prostatectomy for prostate cancer 10 years earlier. At follow-up he was found to have a serum PSA > 10 µg/mL, which continued to rise in subsequent follow-ups. CT showed multiple sclerotic lesions in the axial skeleton as evidence of osteoplastic bone metastases (**Fig. 6.12**). Six days later the patient was referred by urology for radiographic evaluation of the axial skeleton to verify the CT findings (**Fig. 6.13**).

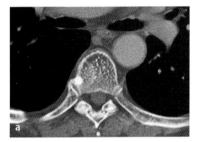 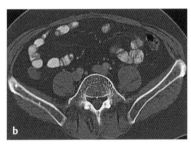 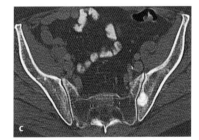

Fig. 6.12 a–c   CT. The report described multiple osteoplastic masses consistent with metastases.

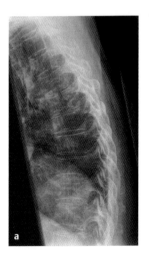 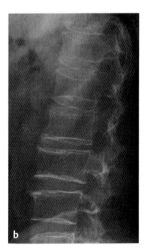 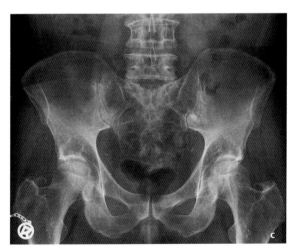

Fig. 6.13 a–c   Representative selection of radiographs. Diagnosis: osteosclerotic metastasis in the left ilium and surgical clips in the lesser pelvis following a prostatectomy.

Further Case Summary

The osteoplastic metastasis in the left ilium close to the sacroiliac joint was visible on the pelvic radiograph (**Fig. 6.13**). Osteoporosis and spondylosis deformans were noted in the mid and lower lumbar spine as incidental findings.

Error Analysis and Strategy for Error Prevention

The radiographic examinations were not indicated for the following reasons:

- The diagnosis of skeletal metastasis was established by the serum PSA level and abnormal CT findings. Any measurable PSA concentration following a radical prostatectomy indicates the continued presence of neoplastic prostatic tissue, which may signify a local recurrence or lymphogenous or skeletal metastasis. A synoptic review of the CT, clinical, and laboratory findings should have identified the rounded sclerotic lesions in the cancellous and cortical bone as skeletal metastases (**Table 6.1**).
- All questions relevant to further management (number and volume of the metastases) were answered by the CT examination. Osteoplastic metastases do not jeopardize the stability of the bones.

Table 6.1   Differential diagnosis of multiple rounded osteoplastic skeletal lesions

Benign
Islands of cortical bone
Osteopoikilosis
Tuberous sclerosis
Malignant
Metastases (especially from prostate and breast cancer)
Malignant lymphoma
Osteosarcoma

- The spatial and contrast resolution of radiographs is inherently inferior to the spatial and contrast resolution of CT slices due to the projection nature of x-ray films. This explains why the smaller metastases detected by CT (**Fig. 6.12**) were not visible on the radiographs (**Fig. 6.13**).

The radiographs could have been avoided by applying careful selection criteria in urology and radiology. Any unnecessary imaging leads to needless costs and may provide legal grounds for bodily injury claims. The incidence of unnecessary radiographs varies greatly from one facility to the next and is in the range of 10–40% (see p. 217).

Prostate Cancer

Prostate-Specific Antigen (PSA)
The most important serum marker for prostate cancer is PSA, a glycoprotein produced in the glandular epithelial cells of the prostate. The normal serum level of PSA is less than 4.0 μg/mL. The level may be slightly elevated in benign prostatic hyperplasia and acute prostatitis. The serum concentration of PSA correlates closely with the mass of PSA-expressing cells. When the levels exceed 10 μg/mL, it should be assumed that prostate cancer is present until proven otherwise. The progression of serum PSA values is just as important as the absolute PSA level. Up to 15% of all prostate cancers do not express PSA. Any measurable PSA concentration after a radical prostatectomy is abnormal and suggests a local tumor recurrence or metastasis.

Serum PSA
- Low: 0–2.5 μg/mL
- Mildly elevated: 2.6–10.0 μg/mL
- Moderately elevated: 10.1–19.9 μg/mL
- Markedly elevated: ≥ 20 μg/mL

Skeletal Metastasis of Prostate Cancer
Metastases from prostate cancer affect the bone in approximately 90% of cases. Approximately 80% of these metastases are osteoplastic, 4% are osteolytic, and 16% are mixed. Metastases involve the obturator and pelvic lymph nodes in 60% of cases, the lung in 40%, and the liver in 25%.

References and Further Reading

American College of Radiology (ACR). ACR Appropriateness Criteria™. Metastatic bone disease. http://www.acr.org/SecondaryMainMenuCategories/quality_safety/app_criteria/pdf/ExpertPanelonMusculoskeletalImaging/MetastaticBoneDiseaseDoc14.aspx (accessed January 13, 2011)

Greenspan A. Orthopedic Imaging: A Practical Approach. 4th ed. Philadelphia: Lippincott Williams & Wilkins; 2005

Krug B, Wolters U, Stützer H, Lackner K. Inadequacies of repeated radiological examinations in a university hospital. Acta Radiol 2001; 42: 612–61

Krug B, Boettge M, Coburger S, et al. Qualitätskontrolle der ambulanten bildgebenden Diagnostik in Nordrhein-Westfalen, Teil I. RöFo 2003a; 175: 46–57

Krug B, Boettge M, Reineke T, et al. Qualitätskontrolle der ambulanten bildgebenden Diagnostik in Nordrhein-Westfalen, Teil II. RöFo 2003b; 175: 346–360

Walsh PC, Retik AB, Vaughan ED, Wein AJ, eds. Campell's Urology. Philadelphia: WB Saunders; 2002

Wein JA, Kavoussi LR, Novick AC, Partin AW, Peters CA, eds. Campell-Walsh Urology. 9th ed. New York: Elsevier; 2007

Flawed Examination Technique?

History and Clinical Findings

A 69-year-old man with a hemangioendothelial sarcoma in the left pelvis complained of increasing pain in the left hip region. He was referred for pelvic radiography to evaluate bone stability (**Fig. 6.14**). The radiographic report described a pathologic fracture of the left acetabulum associated with osteolytic and osteoplastic bone changes.

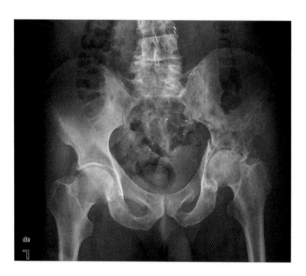

Fig. 6.14   Pelvic radiograph shows a pathologic fracture of the left acetabulum and mixed osteolytic–osteoplastic changes in the left iliac wing in a patient with a known hemangioendothelial sarcoma.

Further Case Summary

Another pelvic radiograph was taken 4 weeks later for restaging prior to chemotherapy (**Fig. 6.15**). When the two images were compared, it was noticed that the "L ap" marker had been placed on the wrong side of the previous radiograph.

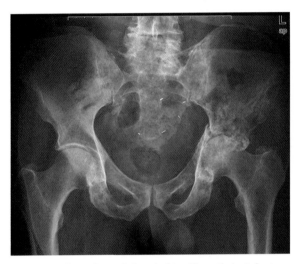

Fig. 6.15 Pelvic radiograph 4 weeks later. The pathologic fracture of the left acetabulum shows increasing marginal sclerosis. New osteolytic lesions in the right ischium and intertrochanteric zone of the left femur were interpreted as hematogenous metastases.

Error Analysis and Strategy for Error Prevention

The RT and attending radiologist had failed to notice the misplaced side marker on the initial pelvic radiograph. The examination had been performed with a digital flat-panel detector system in which side labeling is done automatically when the imaging program is selected. The RT remembered that she had turned the patient 180° due to spatial constraints, positioning the patient's head at the foot of the digital Bucky table. Afterward the image was electronically flipped on the longitudinal body axis, causing the side label to be misplaced. This error went unnoticed until the subsequent restaging radiograph was read.

For accuracy of interpretation and to avoid medicolegal consequences, it is essential that the x-ray film or digital image data set have anatomically correct side labeling.

References and Further Reading

American College of Radiology (ACR). ACR Practice Guideline for Communication of Diagnostic Imaging Findings. http://www.acr.org/SecondaryMainMenuCategories/quality_safety/guidelines/dx/comm_diag_rad.aspx (accessed November 10, 2010)

American College of Radiology (ACR). ACR Practice Guideline for Diagnostic Reference Levels in Medical X-ray Imaging. http://www.acr.org/SecondaryMainMenuCategories/quality_safety/RadSafety/RadiationSafety/guideline-diagnostic-reference.aspx (accessed November 10, 2010)

Amis ES, Butler PF, Applegate KE, et al. American College of Radiology White Paper on Radiation Dose in Medicine. J Am Coll Radiol 2007; 4: 272–284. http://www.acr.org/SecondaryMainMenuCategories/quality_safety/white_paper_dose.aspx (accessed November 10, 2010)

Appropriate Work-up/ Overdiagnosis/ Misdiagnosis

History and Clinical Findings

A 67-year-old woman complained of new pain in the right inguinal region during exertion. Her body weight was 94 kg. She had a history of chronic back pain relating to degenerative spinal changes. She had undergone previous breast-conserving surgery for a ductal carcinoma in situ (DCIS) of the left breast (tumor diameter 0.8 cm).

She had undergone a number of imaging studies at various institutions to investigate her complaints, including radiographs of the lumbar spine, pelvis and right hip (**Fig. 6.16**) and MRI of the lumbar spine 3 months later when her complaints persisted. These studies were oncologically negative. Mammograms were described as showing fibrocystic changes. Pelvic CT scans taken 3 weeks after MRI showed an osteolytic area in the right acetabulum with associated cortical destruction, con-

sidered suspicious for metastasis (**Fig. 6.17**). Bone scintigraphy showed no abnormalities except for focal increased uptake in the same area. Nine days later, CT excluded osteolytic lesions in the femur. CT of the neck and chest was performed 5 days later, and the written report described laryngeal swelling of unknown cause associated with partial destruction of the hyoid bone and a 3-cm mass in the upper lobe of the left lung requiring further investigation. Radiographs of the right hip 3 weeks later confirmed an osteolytic area in the anterior column of the acetabulum (**Fig. 6.18**). Abdominal MRI the following day showed enlargement of the osteolytic soft-tissue mass relative to 4-week-old pelvic CT along with two new satellite lesions in the cancellous bone of the right acetabulum. Since metastatic breast cancer was considered unlikely due to the history of DCIS, positron emission tomography with [¹⁸F]fluorodeoxyglucose (FDG/PET) was performed 7 days later to search for a primary tumor. This study showed abnormally increased glucose metabolism in the apical left lung at the site of the mass detected by CT (**Fig. 6.19 a, b**). A focal increase in glucose metabolism was also found in the anterior column of the right acetabulum. A CT-guided bone biopsy performed the same day yielded a histopathologic impression of Paget disease. This diagnosis was considered unlikely, given the progression of clinical findings. Radiotherapy was prescribed because of the risk of a pathologic fracture. Pelvic CT scans taken to plan the radiotherapy field supplied no new diagnostic information. Ten days after the PET examination, the chest was again evaluated by CT without IV contrast because the initial thoracic CT scans were not available. The new scans confirmed a solid mass in the apical segment of the left

Fig. 6.16 Radiograph of the right hip, interpreted as normal.

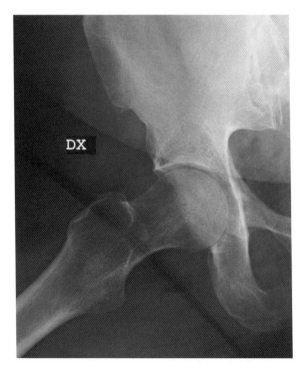

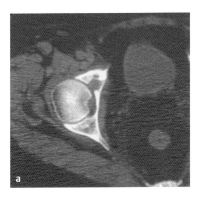
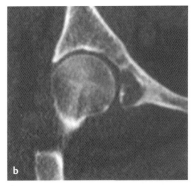

Fig. 6.17 a, b   CT of the pelvis (without IV contrast) demonstrates an osteolytic area in the anterior column of the acetabulum.

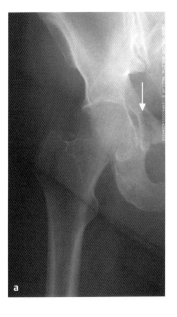

Fig. 6.18 a, b   Radiographs of the right hip 20 weeks after the first radiographic examination (see **Fig. 6.16**) show initial evidence of an osteolytic lesion in the anterior column of the acetabulum (arrows).

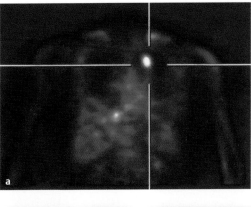
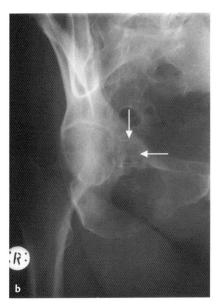
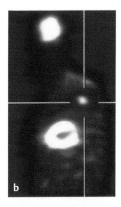
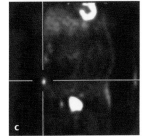
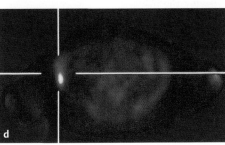

Fig. 6.19 a–d   Whole-body FDG/PET examination. Foci of increased glucose metabolism are detected in the left hilar region or the left lung bordering the hilum (**a, b**) and in the right hip (**c, d**). The high activity in the brain (**b**) and myocardium is due to the high physiologic glucose metabolism in these organs. The activity in the bladder results from the urinary excretion of FDG (**c**).

a Coronal reconstruction of the chest and upper abdomen.
b Sagittal reconstruction of the chest and upper abdomen.
c Coronal reconstruction of the abdomen and pelvis.
d Axial reconstruction of the abdomen and pelvis.

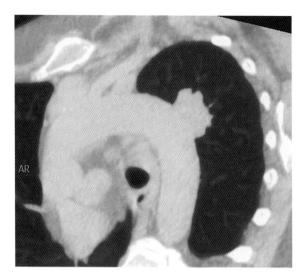

AR

Fig. 6.20 Noncontrast thoracic CT reformatted in an angled coronal plane. The soft-tissue mass in the upper lobe of the left lung is in broad contact with the aorta and has indistinct margins. The report stated that the mass was suspicious for peripheral bronchial carcinoma. Two lymph nodes approximately 7 mm in diameter are visible in the middle mediastinum.

upper lobe in contact with the mediastinal pleura along with multiple mediastinal lymph nodes up to 7 mm in diameter (**Fig. 6.20**). This finding raised an initial suspicion of lung cancer.

Further Case Summary

The mass in the apical segment of the left upper lobe, which bordered directly on the posterior aspect of the aortic arch, was investigated by CT-guided biopsy (**Fig. 6.21a**). This procedure revealed a small, clinically asymptomatic, peritumoral hemorrhage within the lung along with a small posterior pneumothorax, which was absorbed within 24 h (**Fig. 6.21b**). Initially the only histopathologic findings were scar tissue and elastosis. The discrepancy between the radiologic and histopathologic findings was discussed with the pathologist. A new histopathologic work-up of the biopsy cores revealed a well- to moderately-differentiated adenocarcinoma consistent with a primary adenocarcinoma of the lung.

Error Analysis and Strategy for Error Prevention

At least some of the repeated examinations resulted from a lack of awareness of previous imaging studies and the absence of the images themselves. In reviewing the indications, it is helpful to distinguish between diagnostic investigation of the pain symptoms and the search for a primary tumor:

- Based on established guidelines for the etiologic investigation of pain in the right inguinal region, the initial imaging study of choice is pelvic radiography. When radiographs were negative, the next step should have been to proceed with MRI (better than radiographs for defining bone marrow structures and periosseous soft

tissues). Pelvic CT was indicated only for evaluating stability, planning CT-guided bone biopsy, and planning the radiotherapy field.

- Guidelines also state that tests for locating a primary tumor should be limited to mammography, CT of the neck and chest, abdominal MRI (alternative: CT of the abdomen, neck, and chest in one sitting), and bone scintigraphy. Whole-body PET scanning was unnecessary in the present case. It is a very cost-intensive procedure that entails significant radiation exposure (5–8 mSv) and added no new diagnostic information since the left pulmonary mass was already known.

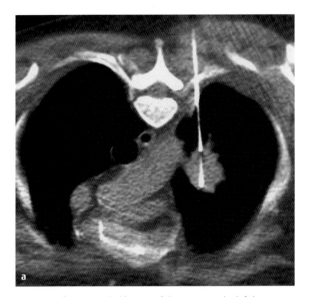

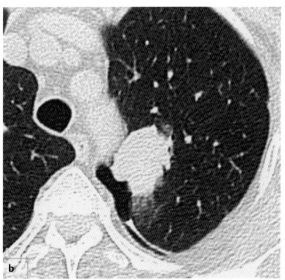

Fig. 6.21 a, b CT-guided biopsy of the tumor in the left lung.
a Axial scan documents the position of the core biopsy needle in the tumor.

b Postinterventional CT shows minimal bleeding sites along the needle tract in proximity to the tumor. A 3- to 4-mm wide pneumothorax is visible posteriorly.

Metabolic Imaging: Positron Emission Tomography (PET)

Principle. PET imaging has been an object of research for more than 25 years. The most commonly used radiotracer is [^{18}F]fluorodeoxyglucose (FDG). Tracers such as [^{11}C]acetate, ^{18}F-choline, and ^{18}F-ethylcholine are being tested for the imaging of prostate cancer. PET displays focal changes in tissue metabolism. Following the IV administration of FDG, the radioactive glucose is disseminated in the bloodstream and enters the intercellular space along an osmotic gradient. From there it is transported into the cells by specific energy-dependent carriers and is incorporated into ATP metabolism. The background activity of the radioactive FDG present in the vascular and intercellular space must be taken into account during qualitative and quantitative evaluation of the scans. Under routine clinical conditions, errors can be minimized by correlating the initial administered activity with the measured locoregional activities. More accurate data (for scientific studies) require a normalizing process based on repeated determinations of the glucose concentration in the blood. False-negative results (saturation of glucose receptors by nonradioactive glucose) are avoided by fasting the patient for several hours before the examination. The locoregional intensity of glucose uptake is found semiquantitatively by determining the standard uptake value (SUV = local activity in tissue [mCi/g]/injected dose [mCi per kg body weight]) 30 or 60 minutes after injection of the activity. The comparability of results is improved by using the same acquisition parameters in follow-ups (fasting, interval to FDG injection, imaging protocol). The glucose concentration in the blood is taken into account by applying the formula

$$SUV_{corrected} = SUV_{uncorrected} \times plasma\ glucose/100.$$

Diagnostic capabilities. A tumor diameter > 10 mm is considered to be the lower limit of detectability by PET due to the dependence of measurable activity on tumor volume, even in metabolically active tumors. Spatial resolution is limited by the edge length of the sensors in the detector. The minimum pixel edge length in clinical whole-body scanners is 3.6 mm. Routine pixel edge lengths in other modalities are 0.3–0.7 mm for CT and 0.6–1.3 mm for MRI. Unlike the one-dimensional gray-scale used to depict focal lesions in CT and MRI, focal increases in metabolic activity are color-encoded in PET, making them easier to recognize during image interpretation. Studies utilizing the criteria of evidence-based medicine have not shown that PET is more sensitive than CT or MRI.

Limitations. One limitation of FDG/PET is that focal changes in glucose metabolism are nonspecific and contribute little to making a specific diagnosis. Smaller lesions in particular may raise problems of differential diagnosis or may be below the detection threshold of PET imaging. PET has the following methodologic limitations:

- Only small malignant tumors with very high glucose metabolism are detectable by FDG/PET due to its relatively low spatial resolution.
- A number of tumors do not have increased glucose metabolism, making them inherently "PET-negative."
- Increased glucose metabolism is a nonspecific finding (differential diagnosis: inflammatory diseases, reparative processes, etc.).
- There are a host of potential pitfalls in PET imaging (contractions of neck muscles and intestinal muscle, radioactive urine in the urinary tract, etc.).

Ductal Carcinoma In Situ (DCIS)

DCIS is the collective term for a heterogeneous group of carcinomas that vary considerably in their histopathology, clinical manifestations, and prognosis. By definition, the malignant cells in DCIS are located exclusively within the ductal structures of the breast. The basement membrane is intact. DCIS lesions undergo contiguous or noncontiguous spread within the ductal system. This explains the frequent multifocality and multicentricity of the disease (see p. 131). When DCIS is characterized by a high proportion of atypical nuclei (Van Nuys score of 2 or 3, see p. 148) and a large tumor volume, progression to invasive ductal carcinoma will occur in up to 50% of cases (criteria: penetration of the basement membrane, invasion of the periductal interstitium). National and international senology guidelines place rigorous quality standards on the histopathologic analysis of biopsied and resected tissues. Nevertheless, it is still possible for pathologists to miss invasive ductal carcinoma within a DCIS in small numbers of cases. DCIS has a reported recurrence rate of 2–3% per year after breast-conserving surgery, corresponding to 10–15% in 5 years and 20–30% in 10 years. Adjuvant radiotherapy or mastectomy is recommended for cases with a higher Van Nuys score, larger tumor volume, and smaller clearance margins. Based on the interdisciplinary S3 guidelines for the diagnosis, treatment and follow-up of breast cancer (Kreinberg et al. 2008), radiotherapy is indicated in all cases where the tumor has not been resected with adequate margins. Radiotherapy may be withheld in cases with a tumor size < 2 cm, a low Van Nuys score, and at least 10 mm clearance between the tumor and resection margins in the surgical specimen. The median 5-year survival rate is 97–100%.

References and Further Reading

American College of Radiology. Practice Guideline for the Management of Ductal Carcinoma In-Situ of the Breast. http://www.acr.org/SecondaryMainMenuCategories/quality_safety/app_criteria/pdf/ExpertPanelonMusculoskeletalImaging.aspx (accessed November 10, 2010)

American College of Radiology. Metastatic Bone Disease. http://www.acr.org/SecondaryMainMenuCategories/quality_safety/app_criteria/pdf/ExpertPanelonMusculoskeletalImaging.aspx (accessed November 10, 2010)

American College of Radiology. Chronic Hip Pain. http://www.acr.org/SecondaryMainMenuCategories/quality_safety/app_criteria/pdf/ExpertPanelonMusculoskeletalImaging.aspx (accessed November 10, 2010)

Buell U, Wieres F J, Schneider W, Reinartz P. 18FDG-PET in 733 consecutive patients with or without side-by-side CT evaluation. Nuklearmedizin 2004; 43: 210–216

Kreienberg R, Kopp I, Lorenz W, et al. Interdisciplinary S 3 guidelines for the diagnosis, treatment and follow-up care of breast cancer. First updated version 2008. http://www.uni-duesseldorf.de/WWW/AWMF/ll/ (accessed November 10, 2010)

Krug B, Dietlein M, Groth W, et al. Fluor-18-fluorodeoxyglucose-positron-emission-tomography (FDG-PET) in malignant melanoma: diagnostic comparison with conventional imaging methods. Acta Radiol 2000; 41, 446–452

Wong W-H, Uribe J, Li H, et al. Principles and instrumentation of positron emission tomography. In: Kim EE, Jackson EF, eds. Molecular Imaging in Oncology. Berlin: Springer; 1999: 71–79

Overdiagnosis/ Misdiagnosis

History and Clinical Findings

A 36-year-old man had been diagnosed 6 months earlier with a high-grade stage IVb lymphoblastic lymphoma. The disease had presented clinically with night sweats and pain in the sacroiliac joints and left knee. MRI elsewhere had shown diffuse bone marrow lesions in the lower limbs. Computed tomography in the initial work-up had detected cervical and retroperitoneal lymphadenopathy accompanied by osteolytic lesions with soft-tissue components in the bodies of the T5 and L4 vertebrae. The histologic diagnosis was established by a transpedicular excisional biopsy from the L3 vertebral body. FDG/PET showed areas of increased uptake distributed throughout the skeleton as evidence of diffuse bone marrow involvement. Combination chemotherapy was instituted according to the protocol of the GERMAN Multicenter Study Group on Adult Acute Lymphoblastic Leukemia (GMALL-Study Group).

A CVC passed through the left internal jugular vein one month after the start of chemotherapy had led to thrombosis of the left brachiocephalic vein (**Fig. 6.22**). At that point the CVC was removed, a vascular access port was implanted via the veins of the right shoulder girdle, and anticoagulant therapy (phenprocoumon) was initiated. Interim CT staging after three chemotherapy cycles documented resolution of the retroperitoneal lymphadenopathy and vertebral soft-tissue masses. Residual thrombus was still present in the left brachiocephalic vein. Whole-body PET/CT scans without iodinated IV contrast were also obtained using low-dose technique and yielded negative oncologic findings (**Fig. 6.23**). After six chemotherapy cycles the patient was restaged by wholebody PET/CT using the same technical factors as before (**Fig. 6.24a, b**). The imaging volume again extended from the skull base to the proximal thighs. The scans continued to show a physiologic radionuclide distribution with no apparent tumor-related increase in FDG uptake. Because the scans did not cover all of the calvaria and lower limbs, hemato-oncology requested scans of the excluded areas due to their possible therapeutic implications. The additional scans were taken two weeks later (**Fig. 6.24c, d**) and confirmed the negative PET findings.

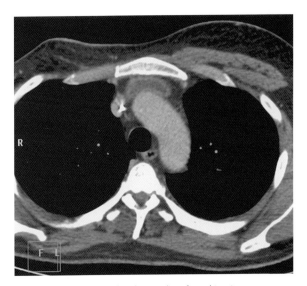

Fig. 6.22 Thoracic CT after four cycles of combination chemotherapy shows a filling defect in the left brachiocephalic vein spreading to the superior vena cava, consistent with recent thrombosis.

Fig. 6.23 Whole-body PET/CT examination after six cycles of ▶ combination chemotherapy. The study employed low-dose technique for emission correction and was done without IV iodinated CT contrast medium.

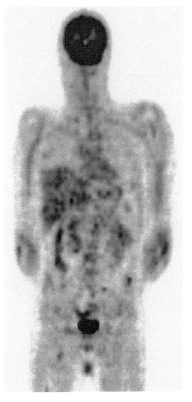

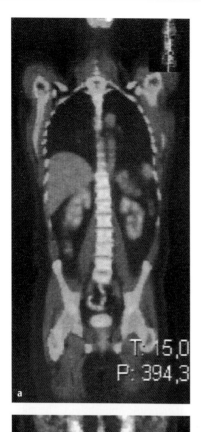

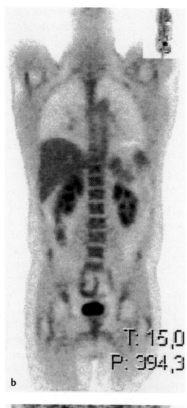

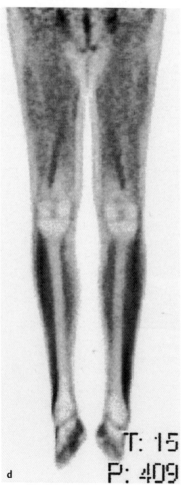

Fig. 6.24 a–d Whole-body PET/CT scans after six cycles of combination chemotherapy show no abnormalities and no changes relative to **Fig. 6.23**. The lower limb scans (**c, d**) were taken 2 weeks after the scans covering the usual acquisition volume (**a, b**) because an initial examination elsewhere had shown areas of increased uptake in that region as well.

a, c PET/CT fusion images.

b, d PET sectional images.

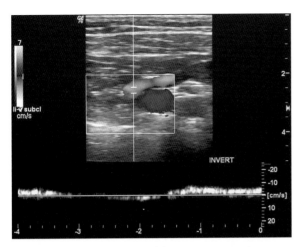

Fig. 6.25 Color duplex ultrasound demonstrates normal morphology of the left subclavian vein and normal modulation of venous blood flow by respiratory intrathoracic pressure variations.

Between the two whole-body PET/CT studies, the patient was referred for color duplex ultrasound (CDU) evaluation of the shoulder-girdle veins to detect or exclude residual thrombosis and thus determine whether to continue or discontinue anticoagulant therapy. Clinical findings were normal. The veins of the neck and shoulder girdle appeared normal at ultrasound (**Fig. 6.25**). The left brachiocephalic vein and superior vena cava could not be visualized, however, and additional sectional imaging studies were recommended as a precaution. Four days later the attending hemato-oncologist referred the patient for thoracic CT angiography. Because the clinical problem related to the cervicothoracic junction, the radiology resident decided to limit CT angiograms to the neck. No abnormalities were found (**Fig. 6.26**).

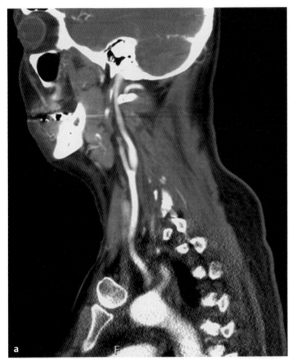

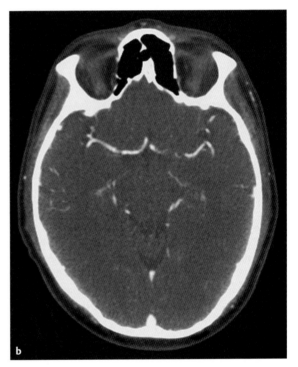

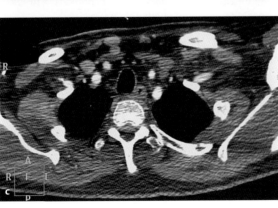

Fig. 6.26 a–c CT angiography was performed for exclusion of residual thrombus in the superior vena cava.

Further Case Summary

The supervising physician noted that the CT study had focused on the arteries from the level of the aortic arch to the skull base and that the large mediastinal veins had not been evaluated (**Fig. 6.26**). When the latter vessels were found to have a normal luminal size, it was unlikely that they were involved by fresh thrombosis, which would have enlarged the vein diameter. The veins may have contained old residual thrombi, however, which would not have expanded the vein lumen but would have required the continuation of anticoagulant therapy. Residual thrombi were subsequently excluded by MRI of the shoulder-girdle veins without IV contrast administration (**Fig. 6.27**).

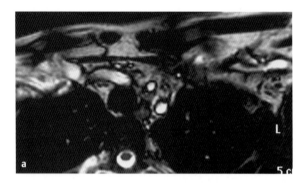

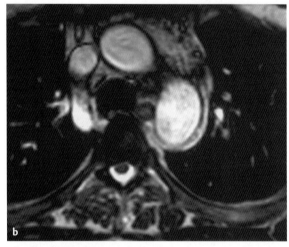

Fig. 6.27 a, b   MRI of the shoulder-girdle veins without IV contrast administration showing a normal morphologic situation. T1-weighted balanced turbo field echo (TFE) sequence.

a Brachiocephalic vessels.
b Superior vena cava at the level of the azygos vein termination.

Error Analysis and Strategy for Error Prevention

The following errors were made in selecting the patient for CT angiography and planning the examinations:

- European atomic energy laws state that preference should always be given to tests that involve either no radiation exposure or the lowest possible level of exposure. Because color duplex ultrasound and MRI do not expose the patient to radiation, either the color duplex scans should have been repeated by an experienced examiner, or the patient should have been referred directly for MRI. This would have had the further advantage of avoiding IV contrast administration.
- Guided by the clinical problem, the radiology resident told the technologist to limit CT angiography to the vessels of the neck. This focused attention on the wrong body region and the wrong vascular system.

- Due to a lack of awareness of previous findings, the scan volume of the first "whole-body" PET/CT study was limited to body regions that are typically covered in this type of examination. This violated European atomic energy laws by making it necessary to repeat the examination to address clinical questions that were relevant to treatment.
- A true whole-body PET/CT study using a higher, diagnostic radiation dose and IV contrast administration for simultaneous evaluation of the shoulder-girdle veins and oncologic soft-tissue status was apparently withheld because oncologic CT findings had been negative after four chemotherapy cycles.

Radiation Safety Directives Issued by the Council of the European Union

Directive 96/29/EURATOM issued by the Council of the European Union on May 13, 1996 (EURATOM Basic Standards), and Directive 97/43/EURATOM issued by the Council on June 30, 1997 (EURATOM Patient Safety Directive), established basic safety standards for protecting workers and the general public from the dangers of ionizing radiation and x-rays. It was mandated that each of these Directives become national law by July 1, 2001, and July 1, 2002, respectively. All member states of the European Union now have a legal framework consisting of laws and their derivative ordinances, guidelines, directives, and standards which translate legal directives issued by the European Union into national law. The Directives of the Council of the European Union define the boundary conditions for the national laws that are adopted by the individual member states. A central theme of the EURATOM Patient Safety Directive addressed in article 3 ("Justification") is the concept of the "justified indication," which entered into the provisions of the Radiation Protection Ordinance (StrSV) and X-Ray Ordinance (RöV) in Germany. (The concept of "justified indication" is described more fully on p. 217).

Image Fusion with Hybrid Systems

CT and MRI supply morphologic information while PET, usually performed with the tracer ^{18}F-FDG, supplies functional information (see "Metabolic imaging: positron emission tomography," p. 289). All three of these modalities are highly sensitive in the detection of abnormalities. Difficulties relate to their specificity. PET scans can be electronically superimposed upon CT scans or MR images to define regions of increased metabolic activity and map their relationship to morphologic features. The alternative technique of electronically fusing separately acquired image data sets is advantageous in that it reduces costs, broadens multimodal options, and does not involve additional radiation exposure.

CT, which requires x-ray exposure, uses radiographic tissue density to produce images while MRI utilizes the T1 and T2 relaxation times, hydrogen content (ϱ), and chemical shifts of tissues. These tissue-specific parameters can be modified by the intravenous (IV) administration of contrast agents to supply information on the perfusion and permeability of blood vessels in pathologic tissues. CT and MRI are classified as morphologic modalities owing to their superior spatial resolution. PET, which has low spatial resolution, is considered a functional modality because it can selectively map metabolic processes following the administration of suitable radioactive tracers.

CT, MRI, and PET, which were developed and introduced clinically at approximately the same time, trace their origins to nuclear physics research in the early 1900s, and since then have undergone varying rates of technological development. Major equipment manufacturers claim that they stopped producing PET-only scanners because the technology had reached an end point that was technically and medically unsatisfactory. This gave impetus to the alternative solution of utilizing the synergistic effects of individual, established imaging technologies. The first prototype of an integrated PET/CT system was introduced in 1998. The goal of the fusion technology was to shorten the examination time by using the CT data set for attenuation correction and to offset the inherent disadvantage of low spatial resolution by superimposing the PET images over CT scans. The technology of the CT and PET components conforms to that of the separate scanners. Hybrid technology does not produce any new diagnostic image parameters. The further development of integrated PET/CT scanners basically followed that of CT technology, lagging behind it by approximately one developmental step. The first integrated PET/MRI and PET/SPECT (single-photon emission computed tomography) systems are already on the market.

As a rule, modern CT and MRI scanners can reliably detect tumors greater than 0.5 cm in diameter (standard minimum edge length of the acquisition matrix: 0.3 mm for CT, 0.6 mm for MRI). With lesions more than 10 mm in diameter, both technologies can contribute to benign/malignant differentiation by evaluating the tumor matrix (density, calcification, necrosis, signal characteristics before and after IV contrast administration), tumor margins, and neighboring structures. Often a conclusive diagnosis can be made within the context of the history, clinical presentation, and associated findings.

Because the signals measured in PET are dependent on tumor volume, even a hypermetabolic tumor generally must be 10 mm or more in diameter before it can be detected on PET scans. Spatial resolution is limited by the edge length of the sensors in the detector. Industry reports a maximum spatial resolution of 3.6 mm for clinical whole-body scanners. Because PET scans display areas of increased or decreased tracer uptake, focal abnormalities are sometimes depicted more clearly and are perceived more easily than on CT and MR images, despite the variety of image information that those modalities provide. While there have been repeated claims of increased sensitivity and the early prediction of treatment response and long-term survival, studies applying the criteria of evidence-based medicine do not support these claims. For biochemical reasons, a combined PET/CT study is rewarding only for tumors that concentrate the tracer compound (usually FDG) that is used. Tumors that do not have increased glucose metabolism are not detected (see p. 289). Data in the literature show that integrated PET/CT scanning would have been indicated in 5–10% of the PET-only examinations that have been performed to date.

Integrated scanners have some inherent disadvantages. One is that a low-dose spiral CT scan lasting up to 20 seconds is followed by an emission scan lasting 25–60 minutes and in some cases by a postcontrast spiral CT scan lasting up to 20 seconds. Even in integrated scanners, patient movements due to respiration, cardiovascular pulsations, and ureteral and intestinal peristalsis must be electronically corrected. Thus, the goal of localizing tiny zones of increased metabolic activity to a specific anatomical structure cannot always be achieved even with hybrid technology. Because the acquisition of CT image data in a PET/CT examination takes approximately 20 *seconds*, while the PET acquisition takes at least 30 *minutes*, we are dealing with the economically unsound combination of fast and slow imaging modalities, neither of which has been improved relative to standard technology. Integrated scanners also raise problems of equipment utilization, since most patients have already been evaluated by one of the two modalities. Another economic drawback of hybrid systems is that one of the two components is standing idle at any given time during the examination.

Artifacts result from the fact that iodinated and barium-containing CT contrast media do not attenuate photons at 511 keV (PET) to the same degree as photons at 110–130 keV (CT). This may result in the incorrect rendering of PET data sets. One possible solution is to acquire CT data sets without IV contrast medium or with dilute contrast medium (< 200 HU), but this significantly limits the diagnostic yield of the CT portion of the hybrid study.

The effective dose from an integrated PET/CT study is in the range 15–26 mSv. Plain spiral CT for attenuation correction accounts for approximately 2 mSv. The PET study delivers approximately 7 mSv, and diagnostic CT delivers approximately 5–16 mSv. Effective exposures of up to 26 mSv have been determined for standard PET/CT protocols carried out at four German universities. While special software can reduce these values slightly by automatically regulating the CT exposure dose, PET/CT still exposes patients to higher radiation levels than any other diagnostic procedure. The radiation exposure from PET/CT is 2–4 times higher than the average exposure from a diagnostic cardiac catheterization. The following technical scenarios are distinguished in PET/CT examinations:

– *CT for attenuation correction only.* Low-dose CT is used as a component of the PET examination (better transmission source). In this scenario, only a very limited amount of diagnostic information can be gleaned from the CT data set (e.g., larger osteolytic lesions or lung tumors). There is no need for patient selection or interpretation by a radiologist.

– *Diagnostic utilization of the CT component.* Separate "justified indications" are established for PET and CT in accordance with article 80 of the German Radiation Protection Ordinance and article 23 of the X-Ray Ordinance. Combined PET/CT is appropriate only if a fully justified indication exists for both PET and CT, or if relevant additional diagnostic information cannot be adequately obtained by any other means. The justified indication is determined by physicians with up-to-date credentials in CT and PET imaging. The findings should be interpreted on an interdisciplinary basis by a proficient radiologist and nuclear medicine physician or by physicians trained in both specialties.

– *Radiotherapy planning.* The role of integrated PET/CT in radiotherapy planning has yet to be established by studies that include a cost–benefit analysis. It is essential that the PET and CT scans be acquired in the same body position as the image-guided radiotherapy planning, regardless of whether a hybrid system or separate PET and CT scanners are used.

References and Further Reading

Antoch G, Saoudi N, Kuehl H, et al. Accuracy of whole-body dual-modality fluorine-18–2-fluoro-2-deoxy-D-glucose positron emission tomography and computed tomography (FDG-PET/CT) for tumor staging in solid tumors: Comparison with CT and PET. J Clin Oncol 2004; 22: 4357–4368

Brix G, Beyer T. PET/CT Dose-escalated image fusion? Nuklearmedizin 2005; 44: 51–57

Brix G, Lechel U, Glatting G, Ziegler S I, et al. Radiation exposure of patients undergoing whole-body dual-modality ^{18}F-FDG PET/CT examinations. J Nucl Med 2005; 46: 608–613

Council of the European Union. Council Directive 96/29/EURATOM of 13 May 1996 laying down basic safety standards for the protection of health of workers and the general public against the danger arising from ionizing radiation. http://ec.europa.eu/energy/nuclear/radioprotection/doc/legislation/9629_en.pdf (accessed November 10, 2010)

Council of the European Union. Council Directive 97/43/EURATOM of 30 June 1997 on health protection of individuals against the danger of ionizing radiation in relation to medical exposure, and repealing Directive 84/466/Euratom. http://ec.europa.eu/energy/nuclear/radioprotection/doc/legislation/9743_en.pdf (accessed November 10, 2010)

Goerres GW, Burger C, Schwitter MR, Heidelberg T-NH, Seifert B, von Schulthess GK. Respiration induced attenuation artifacts at PET/CT: Technical considerations. Radiology 2003; 226: 906–910

Juweid ME. Utility of positron emission tomography (PET) scanning in managing patients with Hodgkin lymphoma. Hematology 2006; 1: 259–265

Juweid ME, Cheson BD. Positron emission tomography and assessment of cancer therapy. N Engl J Med 2006; 354: 496–507

Strahlenschutzkommission Online. Strahlenschutz bei der Anwendung der Positronen-Emissions-Tomographie/Computer-Tomographie (PET/CT). Stellungnahme der Strahlenschutzkommission. http://www.ssk.de/werke/2005/kurzinfo/ssk0513.htm vessels (accessed January 13, 2011)

von Schulthess GK, Steinert HC, Hany TF. Integrated PET/CT: current applications and future directions. Radiology 2006; 238: 405–422

Septic Thrombosis/ Pyomyositis/Malaria

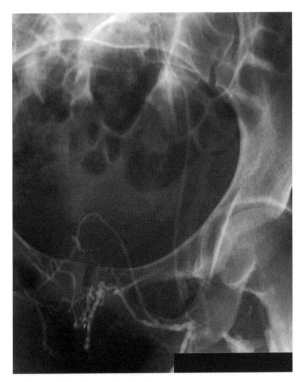

Fig. 6.28 Venogram of the left groin region and left pelvis. Occlusions of the femoral vein and iliac vein are collateralized via the long saphenous vein and pelvic wall veins. The sparse collateralization suggests the recent onset of the thrombosis.

History and Clinical Findings

A 25-year-old African woman came to the emergency room with a 4-day history of fever to 39 °C, night sweats, and chills and a 3-day history of swelling of the left leg and painful limitation of motion in the left hip and left knee. One month earlier she had vacationed in Uganda for 3 weeks without taking malaria prophylaxis. Her family doctor suspected malaria and treated her with doxycycline and tramadol for 3 days before she was hospitalized. Clinical examination revealed redness, local warmth, tenderness, and induration of the skin and subcutaneous tissue of the left groin and left thigh. Laboratory HIV and parasitology tests were negative. CRP was 369 mg/L, WBC 13 800/μL, ESR 99 mm/h, D-dimers 3.1 mg/L, and protein S was 25 % (normal range is 65–140 %).

Color duplex sonography and subsequent venography of the left pelvic and lower extremity veins revealed fresh thrombosis of the deep femoral and pelvic veins extending from the level of the popliteal vein to the iliac vein, with incipient collateralization and lymph node enlargement in the left groin (**Fig. 6.28**). These findings, taken with the fever history and laboratory inflammatory markers, raised suspicion of septic thrombosis. Because the upper end of the thrombosis could not be defined by ultrasound and venography, abdominal CT was performed the same day (**Fig. 6.29**). CT showed that the thrombosis extended into the lower part of the inferior vena cava. The report also described left inguinal soft-tissue edema and a soft-tissue mass that was in contact with the left iliac wing and involved the iliac and psoas major muscles. The differential diagnosis included an inflammatory process, malignant lymphoma, and a tumor. Unenhanced MRI also demonstrated the thrombosis and showed that the edema of the left psoas muscle, left pelvic-wall and thigh muscles, and left inguinal soft tissues was regressive in relation to CT scans taken the previous day (**Fig. 6.30**).

Radiographs of the chest, lumbar spine and pelvis, transcutaneous echocardiography, and abdominal ultrasound showed no abnormalities.

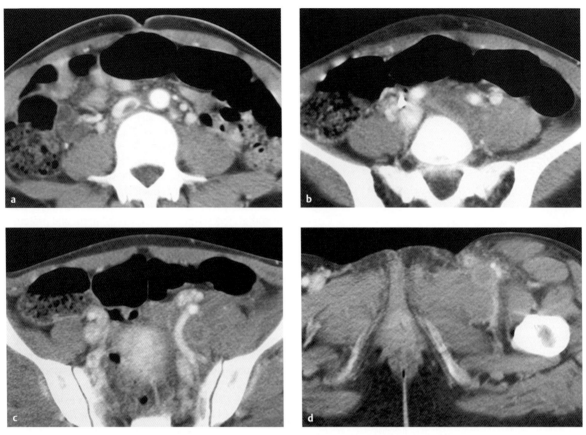

Fig. 6.29 a–d Abdominal CT. The report described acute thrombosis extending from the femoral vein to the inferior vena cava, a soft-tissue mass encompassing the left iliopsoas muscle and left thigh muscles, and left inguinal edema.

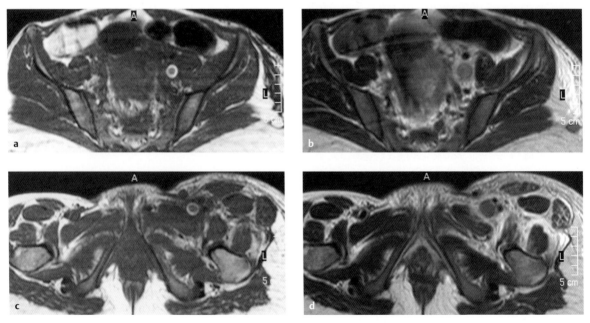

Fig. 6.30 a–d Abdominal MRI. The report described edema of the left pelvic wall muscles, the distal portions of the psoas muscle, and the proximal thigh muscles with involvement of the left inguinal subcutaneous fat, most likely due to an inflammatory cause.

a T1-weighted image at the level of the external iliac vein.
b T2-weighted image at the level of the external iliac vein.
c T1-weighted image at the level of the common femoral vein.
d T2-weighted image at the level of the common femoral vein.

Further Case Summary

On account of suspicion of septic venous thrombosis, systemic thrombolytic therapy and surgery were withheld in favor of full heparinization and 10 days of bed rest. Body temperature and leukocytosis normalized in response to antibiotic therapy with clindamycin and ciprofloxacin. CRP remained elevated at 330 mg/L, however. Multiple blood cultures were sterile, probably because they had been taken after the primary care physician had started antibiotics. Repeated blood smears excluded a malarial infection. Because of clinical suspicion of tropical polymyositis caused by the opportunistic pathogen *Staphylococcus aureus*, the patient was treated empirically with IV cefazolin. With this therapy the CRP fell steadily to a normal level over a 15-day period. When questioned in more detail, the patient recalled having an infected mosquito bite during her stay in Uganda, and this was identified as the cause of the pyomyositis. The development of venous thrombosis was attributed to the interaction of several factors:

- The edema caused by local inflammation led to compression and irritation of the pelvic and femoral veins.
- Prolonged sitting during the return flight from Uganda caused venous pooling in the lower leg due to vessel angulation and loss of the muscle pump.
- A protein S deficiency, possibly hereditary, promoted the development of thrombosis.

Three weeks after she was hospitalized, the patient was free of infection and was discharged with a recommendation for 6 months' anticoagulant therapy.

Error Analysis and Strategy for Error Prevention

Tropical polymyositis is extremely rare on a worldwide scale and occurs only sporadically in Central Europe, so the initial misinterpretation of clinical, sonographic, and venographic findings as septic thrombosis is understandable. The CT and MR findings were descriptive in nature and did not include substantial differential diagnostic considerations. The localization of the changes to various muscles of the pelvis and thigh made malignant lymphoma unlikely and excluded a carcinoma or other tumor (**Fig. 6.31**). MRI should have included a T1-weighted sequence after IV contrast for the reliable detection of inflammatory hyperemia and incipient abscess formation.

The diagnosis was apparent from the color duplex and abdominal CT findings. Abdominal MRI including data acquisition after IV contrast administration would have been an alternative to CT given the clinical presentation and known thrombosis, but there was no need to perform both modalities within a 24-hour period since they were likely to supply redundant information. Venography, radiography of the lumbar spine and pelvis, and abdominal ultrasound were not indicated because they were less powerful techniques than the color duplex scans, CT, and MRI that had already been scheduled or completed.

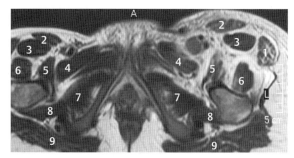

Fig. 6.31 T2-weighted MRI shows increased signal intensity of the left tensor fasciae latae (1), sartorius (2), pectineus (4), iliopsoas (5), and vastus lateralis (6) relative to the opposite side. 3 = Rectus femoris, 7 = obturator externus, 8 = quadratus femoris, 9 = gluteus maximus.

Pyomyositis (Tropical and Nontropical)

Pyogenic myositis (pyomyositis) is a severe inflammatory disease of skeletal muscle that is most prevalent in tropical countries and typically affects children or adolescents following a penetrating injury. Without appropriate treatment, it may lead to sepsis and death. By far the most common causative organism is *Staphylococcus aureus*, followed by *Escherichia coli* and *Klebsiella species*. Once antibiotic therapy has been initiated, however, often it is not possible to identify a causative organism. HIV infections, IV drug abuse, malnutrition, diabetes mellitus, and chronic renal failure are predisposing factors. Patients present clinically with muscle pain, swelling, local warmth and redness, painful limitation of motion, fever, and laboratory signs of inflammation. The quadriceps, gluteus, and psoas muscles are commonly affected. Multiple muscle groups are affected in approximately 40% of patients. Due to its rarity and atypical clinical symptoms, the disease is often mistaken for thrombophlebitis, osteomyelitis, septic arthritis, hematoma, lymphedema, or neoplasia.

Imaging is of key importance in the detection and localization of inflammatory muscle changes and determining their extent. Treatment requires the prompt initiation of aggressive antibiotic therapy and, if necessary, percutaneous or open abscess drainage.

References and Further Reading

Christin L, Sarosi GA. Pyomyositis in North America: case reports and review. Clin Infect Dis 1992; 15: 668–677

Jou IM, Chiu NT, Yang CY, et al. Pyomyositis—with special reference to the comparison between extra- and intrapelvic abscess. Southeast Asian J Trop Med Public Health 1998; 29: 835–840

Martinelli I, Mannucci PM, de Stefano V, et al. Different risks of thrombosis in four coagulation defects associated with inherited thrombophilia: a study of 150 families. Blood 1998; 92: 2353–2358

Patel SR, Olenginski TP, Perruquet JL, Harrington TM. Pyomyositis: clinical features and predisposing conditions. J Rheumatol 1997; 24: 1734–1738

Theodorou SJ, Theodorou DJ, Resnick D. MR imaging findings of pyogenic bacterial myositis (pyomyositis) in patients with local muscle trauma: illustrative cases. Emerg Radiol 2007; 14: 89–96

Adverse Reaction to Contrast Medium?

History and Clinical Findings

A 70-year-old man had undergone a transurethral resection of the prostate (TUR P) for prostate cancer 1 year earlier. The lesion was staged postoperatively as pT1 G1 N0 M0. Due to a rise in the serum level of prostate-specific antigen (PSA), the patient was scheduled for a prostatectomy. Preoperative staging included abdominal CT scans. When questioned before the examination, the patient reported having a prior allergic reaction (itching and skin rash) to IV contrast administration. For this reason, 1 amp clemastine, 1 amp ranitidine, and 250 mg methylprednisolone were administered intravenously 30 minutes before the contrast injection. The CT examination was uneventful and showed no abnormalities other than an old parenchymal defect in the right kidney (**Fig. 6.32**).

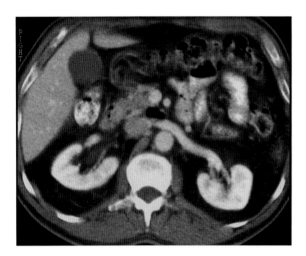

Fig. 6.32 Abdominal CT after IV contrast administration shows no abnormalities besides a parenchymal defect in the right kidney consistent with an old postischemic or postinflammatory scar.

Further Case Summary

Two days after the CT examination, the patient developed a headache, fever, and itchy, weeping skin rash on his back that quickly spread to cover the torso. Detailed questioning revealed that the original contrast reaction had been associated with protracted, weeping skin eruptions. Dermatologic allergy testing (prick test, intradermal test, skin biopsy) established the diagnosis of a delayed contrast reaction. The skin changes cleared with 1 week of IV corticosteroid therapy.

Error Analysis and Strategy for Error Prevention

The rate of adverse reactions to nonionic, water-soluble iodinated contrast media is low. Late reactions occurring days to weeks after IV contrast injection may include renal dysfunction (especially in patients with preexisting renal parenchymal disease), the induction of hyperthyroidism (in patients with thyroid autonomy), and hypersensitivity reactions. Due to the potentially long interval between IV contrast injection and overt complications, late reactions in many patients are not attributed to the contrast agent and are not reported to radiology.

In the case presented above, a detailed allergy history had not been taken prior to the examination. If the severity of the initial contrast reaction had been known, abdominal CT could have been withheld in favor of MRI to avoid the IV administration of an iodinated agent. Premedication with corticosteroids and antihistamines is effective only in preventing early adverse reactions.

References and Further Reading

Kanny G, Pichler W, Morisset M, et al. T cell-mediated reactions to iodinated contrast media: evaluation by skin and lymphocyte activation test. J Allergy Clin Immunol 2005; 115: 179–185

Katayama H, Yamaguchi K, Kozuka T, Takashima T, Seez P, Matsuura K. Adverse reactions to ionic and nonionic contrast media. A report of the Japanese committee on the safety of contrast media. Radiology 1990; 175: 621–628

Kvedariene V, Martins P, Rouanet L, Demoly P. Diagnosis of iodinated contrast media hypersensitivity: results of a 6-year period. Clin Exp Allergy 2006; 36: 1072–1077

Rutten A, Prokop M. Contrast agents in X-ray computed tomography and its application in oncology. Anticancer Agents Med Chem 2007; 7: 307–316

Webb JAW, Stacul F, Thomsen HS, et al. Late adverse reactions to intravascular iodinated contrast media. Eur Radiol 2003; 13: 181–184

Wolf GL, Arenson RL, Cross AP. A prospective trial of ionic vs. nonionic contrast agents in routine clinical practice: comparison of adverse effects. AJR 1989; 152: 939–944

Late Adverse Reactions to Contrast Media

Water-soluble iodinated contrast media are used in a number of radiographic and CT examinations to heighten the contrast of anatomic structures, increase the sensitivity of lesion detection, and improve lesion discrimination.

Nonionic contrast media. Nonionic contrast media have become widely used in the past 15 years. No qualitatively new agents have been developed during that time, and the bulk of pharmacologic and clinical research has focused on improving the tolerance of contrast media and (since the advent of multidetector CT technology) optimizing the contrast injection protocols for nonionic media that are already in clinical use.

From published reports, nonionic contrast media have a 0.7–3.1% rate of clinically mild hypersensitivity reactions and a 0.02–0.04% rate of severe hypersensitivity reactions. The mortality rate is approximately 1 in 100 000 contrast injections.

Early and late reactions. "Early" reactions are those that occur during the first hour after IV contrast administration. "Late" reactions occur from 1 hour to 1 week after the injection. Approximately 75% of all hypersensitivity reactions occur within 5 minutes after contrast administration, and 90% occur within 15 minutes. Late reactions account for approximately 10% of observed contrast reactions. The pathogenic mechanism of late contrast reactions is not yet fully understood. Predominantly

T-cell-mediated reactions are believed to have causal importance, but IgE-mediated allergic effects are also being considered.

Clinical manifestations and diagnosis. Most delayed clinical reactions to contrast media consist of systemic symptoms (headache, nausea, vomiting, fever) and cutaneous manifestations (itching, urticaria, maculopapular eruptions, angioedema, erythema multiforme, cutaneous vasculitis, Stevens–Johnson syndrome, toxic epidermal necrolysis). Patients at highest risk are those with a prior history of contrast allergy or interleukin II therapy. The diagnosis is established by provocation testing (patch test, in which the contrast agent is applied to a pad that is taped to the skin; prick test, in which the agent is pricked into the skin surface with a needle; intradermal test (IDT), in which various concentrations of the agent are injected into the skin; a red, raised area indicates a positive reaction) and by cutaneous biopsy (perivascular infiltrates rich in lymphocytes and eosinophils).

Treatment. Most late reactions are self-limiting and will resolve spontaneously in a matter of weeks. Treatment is symptomatic, like the treatment for other drug-induced skin conditions. Prophylaxis consists of withholding intravenous contrast or, if necessary, premedicating for several days with oral corticosteroids.

Proper Risk Disclosure? Correct Examination Technique?

History and Clinical Findings

A 56-year-old woman had undergone a laparoscopic cholecystectomy. Three weeks later she was referred to the visceral surgery department with severe postoperative upper abdominal pain and fever to 39°C. She was hospitalized and a diagnostic CT examination was performed, at which time an abscess would be drained if necessary under CT guidance. The patient was duly informed about the risks of diagnostic CT (quote from the patient's chart: "hypersensitivity reactions such as nausea, vomiting, erythema, urticaria, bronchospasm, laryngospasm, seizures, anaphylactic shock, death, impaired renal function, organ failure, impaired thyroid function") and the risks of CT-guided drainage ("injury to nerves and vessels, bleeding, infection, organ injury, emergency surgery, intensive care, no guarantee of success, pneumothorax and drainage").

The CT examination was performed according to standard technique. An intravenous line was placed before the examination. Correct intraluminal placement of the line was tested by a trial injection of 20 mL saline. A scout image was taken, and then 100 mL of an iodinated low-osmolarity contrast medium was injected through the line with an injection pump at a perfusion rate of 3 mL/s. Spiral scan coverage was from the diaphragm to the pelvic floor, with data acquisition timed to the portal venous phase. After scanning was completed, it was found that most of the contrast medium had been infused into the soft tissues of the forearm. A heparin dressing was applied, and the ward was notified.

Next an intravenous line was placed in the contralateral arm, and abdominal CT scanning was repeated. A fluid collection with a density of approximately 20 HU and air inclusions was found originating from the bed of the extirpated gallbladder. Because a superinfected hematoma or bilioma was suspected, CT-guided drainage was performed using standard technique. Postinterventional CT confirmed that the drain had been placed in the abnormal fluid collection. The drain yielded a purulent fluid.

Further Case Summary

Over the next few days the patient developed extensive ulcerations in the skin and subcutaneous tissue of the left forearm (**Fig. 6.33**). The lesions healed with scarring in response to appropriate wound care. The abscess that followed the endoscopic cholecystectomy resolved without sequelae in response to CT-guided drainage.

Error Analysis and Strategy for Error Prevention

The abdominal CT examination in this patient was complicated by the extravascular high-pressure injection of 100 mL of a water-soluble, low-osmolarity positive radiographic contrast medium into the forearm.

This complication has a reported incidence of 0.2–0.6% in the literature. Most cases involve the extravasation of small amounts of contrast medium, which are typically absorbed within 24 h. Risk factors include obesity and small or previously damaged veins. A large extravasation is most likely to occur in patients who do not complain of pain during the contrast infusion. From published reports, the frequency of contrast extravasation is independent of the selected flow rate. The extravasation of nonionic contrast medium, as in the present case, is generally less cytotoxic and better tolerated than the extravasation of a high-osmolarity or ionic contrast medium. Severe skin ulcerations and necrosis occasionally occur, as in the present case (**Figs. 6.33, 6.34**).

In this case the patient had not been informed about the possibility of contrast extravasation or its effects. Since current laws require that patients be informed about all risks with an incidence > 1%, and the incidence of contrast extravasation is no greater than 0.6% according to published reports, this disclosure was not strictly necessary. But given the absolute frequency of contrast extravasations, we would recommend that patients be informed accordingly.

In the case shown in **Fig. 6.34**, skin necrosis resulted from contrast extravasation during a CT examination for planning the transapical replacement of a stenotic aortic valve. The peripheral IV line had been placed on the back of the left hand and tested before contrast administration by the trial injection of 20 mL NaCl. Contrast injection by high-pressure pump was not initiated until a normal test had been confirmed. The moment the extravasation was noticed, the contrast injection was discontinued. As a result, only 50 mL of contrast medium had been injected rather than the proposed 100 mL.

Another patient was a 75-year-old woman with cirrhosis of the liver secondary to chronic hepatitis C. While the patient was undergoing the CT-guided radiofrequency ablation of an hepatocellular carcinoma, third-degree skin burns occurred beneath the neutral electrodes on the thighs (**Fig. 6.35**). During the intervention a percutaneous applicator electrode had been passed into the tumor tissue in the liver, and several large neutral electrodes had been placed on the surface of the thighs. Next an AC generator was activated to produce a flow of current between the electrodes. This caused an oscillation of ions within the electric field, heating the tissue through friction and destroying the tumor tissue by thermal necrosis. Generally this effect increases in proportion to the applied energy. Electrodes with a smaller surface area generate a denser pattern of field lines than electrodes with a larger surface area. Applicator electrodes are designed to produce the highest energy density and greatest heating effect in the area immediately surrounding the electrode. As distance from the applicator electrode increases, the energy density is no longer sufficient to cause tissue damage. The skin burns in this patient had the following causes:

- The neutral electrodes were not in full contact with the skin, and so the current flow was not evenly distributed over the skin area where the electrodes were applied. The current peaks that developed in the contract areas led to disproportionate local heating of the skin.

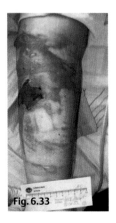

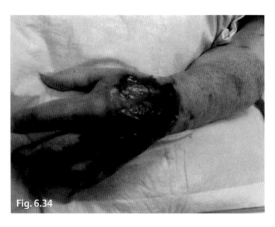

Fig. 6.33 Photographic documentation of skin and subcutaneous tissue necrosis on the left forearm caused by contrast extravasation.

Fig. 6.34 Necrosis of the skin and subcutaneous tissue on the dorsum of the hand in a different patient, also caused by contrast extravasation.

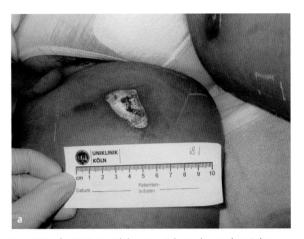

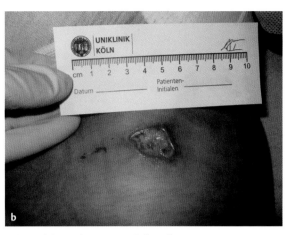

Fig. 6.35 a, b   Patient with hepatic cirrhosis due to chronic hepatitis C. During the CT-guided radiofrequency ablation of a hepatocellular carcinoma of the liver, the patient suffered third-degree skin burns beneath neutral electrodes placed on the thighs. The burns were very slow to heal.

a Wound size and appearance 2 days after radiofrequency ablation.
b The same wound 3 months later.

■ Thermoablation of the tumor tissue required a high generator output (200 watts) and an unusually prolonged application of electric current (40 minutes).

Skin burns occur in up to 2% of all radiofrequency ablations. They can be prevented by performing radiofrequency ablation sequentially with high current levels using multiple large-area neutral electrodes that are securely applied to the skin in order to keep heating and exposure times at levels that will not harm the underlying skin. If the heating effect is excessive, the heat cannot be dissipated by normal heat-exchange processes in the body (radiation, blood flow). Heating above 45 °C causes the breakdown of cellular proteins, resulting in temporary or permanent functional deficits. Localized heating from 45 °C to 50 °C can cause skin damage within minutes, and even higher temperatures can damage the skin within seconds (51 °C to 70 °C) or a fraction of a second (>70 °C). Third-degree skin burns (involving the epidermis, dermis, and subcutaneous tissue) take much longer to heal than first-degree burns (epidermis) and second-degree burns (epidermis and dermis) because they destroy the cutaneous appendages in the dermis and epidermis (hair follicles, sweat glands) that play an essential role in skin repair. As a result, granulation tissue formation in third-degree burns can occur only from the edges of the wound.

References and Further Reading

Bellin M-F. Contrast medium extravasation injury: guidelines for prevention and management. Eur Radiol 2002; 12: 2807–2812

Goette A, Reek S, Klein HU, Geller JC. Case report: severe skin burn at the site of the indifferent electrode after radiofrequency catheter ablation of typical atrial flutter. J Intervent Cardiac Electrophysiol 2001; 5: 337–340

Jacobs JE, Bimbaum BA, Langlotz CP. Contrast media reactions and extravasation: correlation to intravenous injection rates. Radiology 1998; 209: 411–416

7

Vascular Sy

Vascular System

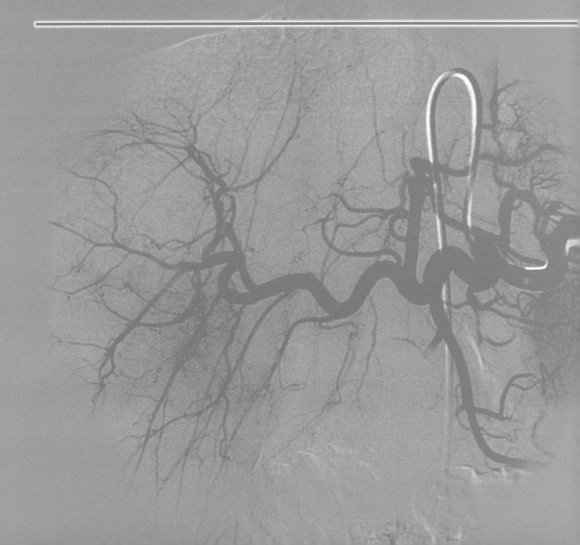

Vasospasm/ Thromboembolism/ Contrast Reaction

History and Clinical Findings

A 36-year-old woman presented at the Neurology Clinic complaining of dizziness that had begun 8 days earlier following a chiropractic manipulation of her cervical spine. Three days earlier she had been hospitalized with a hypertensive episode and had been diagnosed clinically with a suspected vertebral artery dissection. Neurologic examination revealed minimal anisocoria (left < right), mild bradydysdiadochokinesia, slight unsteadiness in stance and gait testing, and hypoesthesia of the radial left fingers and left forearm. Duplex ultrasound and MRI excluded a vascular dissection. MRI showed rounded hyperintensities several millimeters in size distributed in the white matter of both hemispheres and extending to the subcortical level. Microangiopathic changes were considered to be the most likely cause (**Fig. 7.1**). Because the patient had a long known history of asymptomatic Crohn disease, the differential diagnosis also included vasculitis. Laboratory serum and liquor inflammatory markers were not significantly elevated. MR angiography showed long segmental narrowing of the right vertebral artery, predominantly affecting Berguer segments 3 and 4, as a normal variant. The patient was hospitalized. Four days later she was referred to radiology for diagnostic angiography of the cerebral vessels. The clinical question was: High index of suspicion for cerebral vasculitis in Crohn disease, angiography before corticosteroid therapy, vasculitic changes? Informed consent on the day before angiography included disclosure of the following potential complications: allergy, shock, death, bleeding, emergency surgery, vascular injury, vascular dissection, paraplegia, thrombosis, embolism, stroke, and possible need for long-term care. When questioned, the patient denied having any allergies.

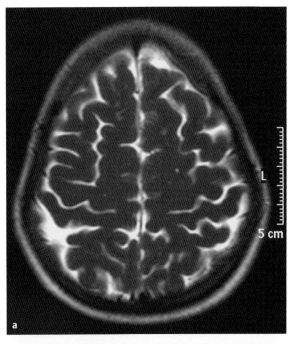

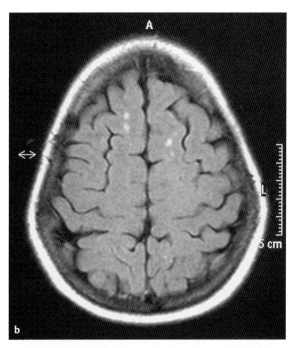

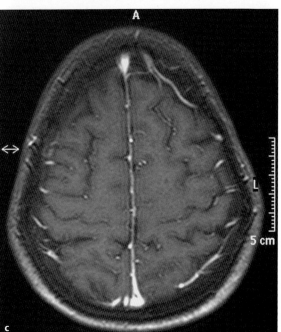

Fig. 7.1 a–d MRI on the day of hospital admission. Rounded, bilateral white-matter lesions up to approximately 5 mm in size have low T1-weighted signal intensity and high signal intensity on T2-weighted and FLAIR images (**a, b**), and do not enhance after contrast administration (**c**). They were considered most likely to have a postischemic or vasculitic cause. Decreased calibers in the right vertebral artery are a normal variant and are most apparent in segments 3 and 4 (**d**).

a T2-weighted image without contrast medium.
b Flair-weighted image without contrast medium.
c T1-weighted image after IV contrast administration.
d MR angiographic sequence.

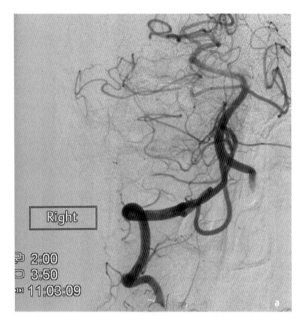

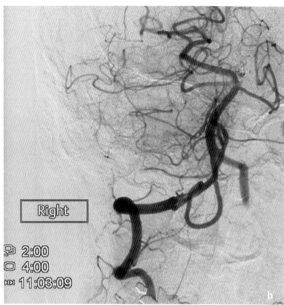

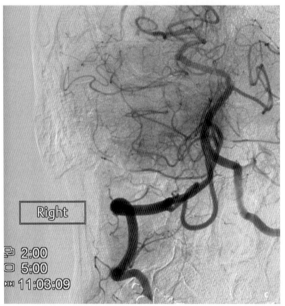

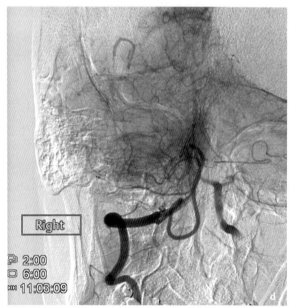

Fig. 7.2 a–e Chronologically first angiographic series in the sagittal projection, taken at 11:03. Representative preexisting segmental images in the early arterial phase (**a**), late arterial phase (**b**), early venous phase (**c**), and late venous phase (**d**). The series confirms hypoplasia of the right vertebral artery and a contrast stasis in the right vertebral artery..

a Chronologically first image documented in the series.
b Chronologically second image documented in the series.
c Chronologically third image documented in the series.
d Chronologically fourth image documented in the series.

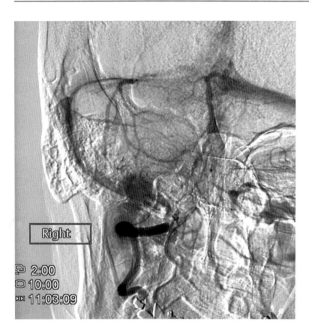

Fig. 7.2 e Chronologically fifth image documented in the series.

The angiographic study was performed by a fourth-year radiology resident who had 8 months' clinical experience in performing diagnostic angiography. He was assisted by a third-year radiology resident. A supervising physician and the department head were standing by in case unexpected problems arose. Despite oral premedication with 1 mg lorazepam, the patient appeared anxious before and during the examination. A Teflon guidewire was placed in the right femoral artery using Seldinger technique. A 5 French (1.67 mm) sheath was introduced over the guidewire, and then a 5 French catheter with a vertebral artery configuration (Cordis) was advanced into the suprarenal aorta. In that position the hydrophilically coated guidewire with a soft, curved tip was inserted (Terumo Europe NV). The vertebral artery catheter was introduced over the Terumo guidewire and advanced into the ascending aorta under fluoroscopic guidance. Next the guidewire was withdrawn into the catheter. Still under fluoroscopic guidance, the catheter was inverted so that it could be maneuvered into the supra-aortic vessels. The catheter was carefully withdrawn under fluoroscopic control until it entered the origin of a supra-aortic artery. Contrast injection under fluoroscopic control confirmed that the tip of the catheter was in the brachiocephalic trunk. From that position the Terumo guidewire was advanced into a cervical vascular branch. The guidewire was removed. Catheter placement was checked by manual injection of 2–3 mL of contrast medium (iohexol, Accupaque,

GE Healthcare, concentration 300 mg/mL), which confirmed that the right vertebral artery had been catheterized. At that moment the patient complained of severe nausea. She turned her head to the left side and vomited several times. Both radiologists interpreted this event as an allergic reaction to the iodinated contrast medium. The catheter was withdrawn into the aortic arch, whereupon 50 mg of Ranitic (ranitidine, Hexal), 4 mg of Fenistil (dimethindene maleate, Novartis), 250 mg of Prednisolut (prednisolone-21-hydrogen succinate, Mibe GmbH), and 1 ampoule of Vomex (62 mg, dimenhydrinate, Astellas Pharma) were administered intravenously. Several minutes later the patient's clinical status had improved, and the right vertebral artery was again catheterized. Fluoroscopically guided contrast injection confirmed correct catheter placement with the tip approximately 2 cm cranial to the origin of the vertebral artery. As indicated by the electronic clock of the angiography system (Allura Xper FD 20, Philips Healthcare), the first series of sagittal angiographic images was taken at 11:03 following the manual injection of 6 mL undiluted contrast medium (**Fig. 7.2**). A second, lateral series was obtained at 11:06. Because the patient had moved during acquisition of the second series, the sequence was repeated at 11:07 (**Fig. 7.3**). At that point in the examination, the patient became unresponsive to verbal commands. Inspection revealed ptosis of the right eye.

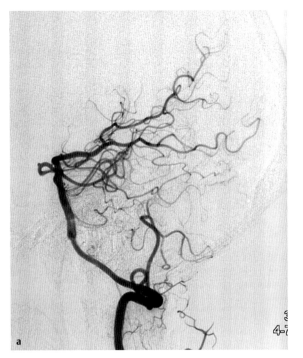

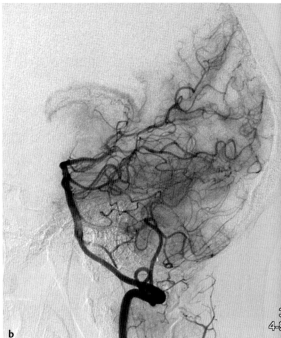

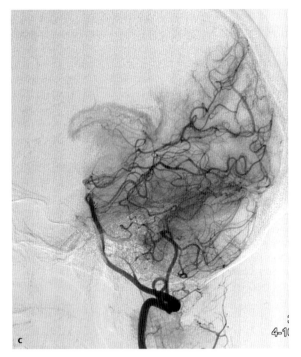

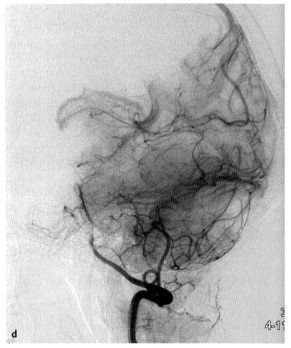

Fig. 7.3 a–d Chronologically third angiographic series in the lateral projection, taken at 11:07.

a Chronologically first image documented in the series.
b Chronologically second image documented in the series.
c Chronologically third image documented in the series.
d Chronologically fourth image documented in the series.

Further Case Summary

When neurologic symptoms arose, the chief radiologist entered the room and terminated the examination. The catheter and sheath were removed. The supervising neurologist was summoned by telephone to the angiography suite. The catheter and sheath were removed. The puncture site in the right femoral artery was occluded with Angioseal STS Plus (St. Jude Medical). Scrutiny of both angiographic series showed that blood flow was already diminished during acquisition of the first image series. Initially the contrast bolus drained normally through the hypoplastic right vertebral artery (**Fig. 7.2 a**), but later in the series the caliber of the vessel decreased and perfusion was delayed. By the end of the series, some opacified blood was still present in the right vertebral artery (**Fig. 7.2 e**). Filling defects were not seen initially, suggesting that a vasospasm was the most likely diagnosis.

Subsequent CT angiography of the cerebral supply arteries (at 11:23) revealed segmental occlusions of both vertebral arteries and a thrombus at the junction of the vertebral arteries with the basilar artery (**Fig. 7.4**). A vasospasm with spasm-induced thrombus formation at the confluence of the vertebral arteries was still considered to be the most likely diagnosis. Management options were discussed with the senior neurologist and a neuroradiologist. The consensus was to initiate intravenous thrombolytic therapy with Actilyse (alteplase, Boehringer Ingelheim) in order to avoid future thrombus formation induced by the spasm-induced disturbances of blood flow. Intra-arterial thrombolysis was withheld because by the time of the intra-arterial angiography, no thrombembolus had been visualized. The spasmolytic agent Nimodipin (nimodipine, Carinopharm) was also administered intravenously. The neurologist and neuroradiologist also recommended heparinization.

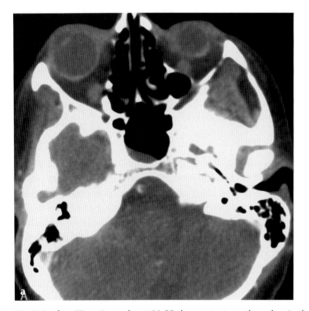 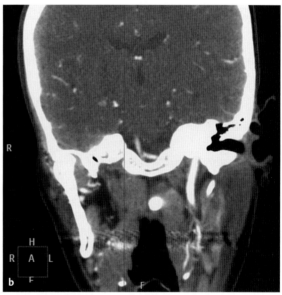

Fig. 7.4 a, b CT angiography at 11:23 demonstrates a thrombus in the right vertebral artery and thrombotic occlusion of the left vertebral artery (**a**). A thrombus is also detected at the confluence of the vertebral arteries just proximal to the basilar artery (**b**).

The patient was transferred to the stroke unit. MRI was performed 5 hours later (**Fig. 7.5**). Diffusion-weighted sequences showed ischemia-induced diffusion changes in both cerebellar hemispheres (right > left), in the cerebellar vermis, in the right mesencephalon, and in the territory of the right posterior cerebral artery. By this time both vertebral arteries were freely perfused. Long segmental hypoplasia of the right vertebral artery, predominantly affecting segments 3 and 4, was still present and was unchanged relative to preangiographic MRI. The white-matter lesions also appeared unchanged. Computed tomography confirmed a cerebellar infarction. Perifocal

edema had led to the development of internal hydrocephalus (**Fig. 7.6**). A decompressive occipital craniectomy was performed the same evening.

Three months after the intervention, the patient still suffered from predominantly left-sided spastic tetraparesis and aphasia. Her vigilance had improved. She was now able to sit up for 3 hours a day and could communicate with her environment through eye movements and grunts. Dysphagia and myoclonic spasms were regressive. While the attending neurologists believed that further improvement was likely, they agreed that the patient would have severe disabilities for the rest of her life.

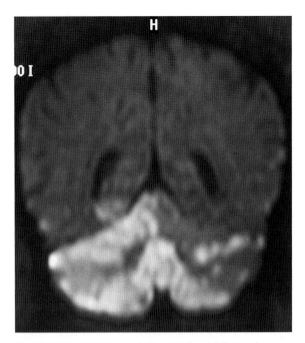

Fig. 7.5 MRI at 16:15 shows ischemia-induced diffusion abnormalities in both cerebellar hemispheres, the vermis, the right mesencephalon, and the territory of the right posterior cerebral artery. At this time both vertebral arteries are freely perfused as proven by an MR-angiographic sequence not visualized.

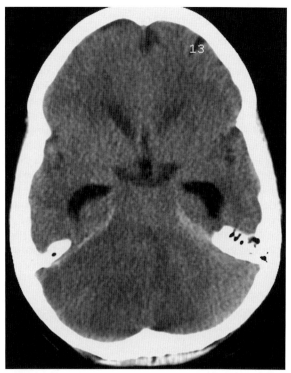

Fig. 7.6 CT at 23:13 displays a fresh cerebellar infarction. Internal hydrocephalus has developed due to compression of the aqueduct by edema.

Error Analysis and Strategy for Error Prevention

The following errors were made during diagnostic angiography of the cerebral arteries related to the indication for performing the examination, the examination technique that was used, and misinterpretation of the symptoms that arose during angiography, and the management of the complicaton.

- There was only a relative medical indication for intra-arterial DSA of the cerebral arteries. It is true, of course, that conventional angiography is better than magnetic resonance angiography for detecting slight caliber variations and microaneurysms of the small cerebral arteries in the setting of vasculitis because of its superior spatial and contrast resolution. But when it comes to patient selection, the potential therapeutic benefit of intra-arterial DSA should always be weighed against the facilities available in the particular situation and risk of complications.

  According to published data (review in Morris 2007), between 0.3% and 6.8% of patients who undergo cerebral arteriography develop new, sometimes transient neurologic symptoms referable to angiography within 72 hours after undergoing the procedure. Studies that included all patients undergoing angiography for suspected brain ischemia and all new neurologic symptoms put the rate of all neurologic sequelae at 9–12%

and the rate of permanent neurologic deficits at 5%. According to the American College of Radiology (ACR), the reported rates of arterial occlusion requiring surgical thrombectomy or thrombolysis range between 0.0% and 0.4%, and the rates of reversible neurologic deficits and permanent neurologic deficits should not exceed 2.5% and 1.0%, respectively.

The patient in this case was a 36-year-old woman with mild neurologic symptoms that were noted only as incidental findings. Her Crohn disease had been asymptomatic for years. She was hospitalized for dizzy spells following a chiropractic manipulation of the cervical spine. Duplex ultrasound, MRI, and MR angiography had excluded a vertebral artery dissection as a possible complication of the treatment. While she was hospitalized, she experienced hypertensive episodes which, like the dizzy spells, were not causally related to the findings of the neurologic examination. The differential diagnosis of cerebral vasculitis was based on the white-matter lesions that had been detected incidentally by MRI, although the inflammatory serum and liquor parameters were not significantly elevated. Morphologically, the MRI changes were consistent with the sequelae of microangiopathy secondary to hypertensive disease or atherosclerosis. Given their distance from the corpus callosum, circumscribed nature, and subcortical location, they were not consistent with multiple sclerosis. Florid vasculitis was excluded by the lack of enhancement after IV contrast administration. Moreover, areas of cerebral vasculitis caused by a variety of pathogenic organisms and mechanisms tend to appear on MRI as larger enhancing areas with ill-defined margins. MR angiography had shown no evidence of vascular changes typical of vasculitis (stenoses, pseudoaneurysms of the small cerebral arteries). In retrospect, even a positive DSA result would not have justified corticosteroid therapy in this situation, and so the sole purpose of intra-arterial DSA was to confirm the diagnosis and not to direct therapeutic decisions.

- Recognized risk factors for complications are patient age >70 years, the angiographic investigation of strokes or TIAs, the angiographic detection of ≥50% or ≥70% stenoses, procedure times longer than 60 minutes, the use of multiple catheters, and the experience of the radiologists/neuroradiologists in performing the examination. In a multicenter analysis of 5000 catheter cerebral angiographic procedures, the rate of severe permanent neurologic sequelae and deaths was found to be 3.9% in training hospitals and 0.9% in nontraining hospitals (Mani et al. 1978). Willinsky et al. (2003) obtained very similar results (1.3% vs. 0.5%) in their analysis of 2899 cerebral angiograms. For this reason, it would have been desirable for a specialist experienced in angiographic techniques to have been present from the start of the procedure in this patient. When the first neurologic symptoms appeared, the specialist could have quickly intervened and terminated the examination.

- From a procedural standpoint, the carotid arteries should have been catheterized first for anatomical reasons. Also, they supply brain areas that are less critical than those supplied by the vertebral arteries. Another factor is that, in the case presented here, the white-matter lesions requiring etiologic investigation were located in the territory of the anterior and middle cerebral arteries. Hence it would have been sufficient to detect or exclude vasculitic changes in the anterior circulation.

- In view of the poor prognosis, intra-arterial thrombolytic therapy using rt-PA (recombinant tissue plasminogen activator) would have been warranted either directly after the onset of the neurologic symptoms or at least after the visualization of thrombotic material in both vertebral arteries in CT angiography carried out 20–30 minutes thereafter. According to current literature this would have been a more promising approach to achieve a quick re-vascularization than the intravenous thrombolytic therapy favored in this case. However, whether intra-arterial rt-PA-therapy would have prevented the unfortunate course remains unknown.

- In the present case the pathologic cause of the complication remains uncertain. Most likely it resulted from vasospasms induced by the intra-arterially applied contrast medium and/or the catheter manipulation as assumed during the complication management phase of the intervention, the thrombemboli CT angiographically visualized in both vertebral arteries 20–30 minutes after the onset of the symptoms being due to the disturbances of blood flow secondarily induced by the vasospasms. A systemic allergic reaction to intra-arterial contrast administration is another possible explanation for vasospastic reactions of the cerebral vasculature despite the high physiological tolerance of modern iodinated contrast media. A local vasomotor reaction of the vertebral artery to intra-arterial contrast administration is another possibility. Local vasomotor reactions to intra-arterial contrast media were first described in the 1980s, mainly in association with cardiac catheterizations. With advances in the pharmacological development of contrast media, this type of complication is no longer reported in the literature and thus seems to berare in clinical routine. Thrombembolism induced by catheter manipulation is another possible cause. Lastly, a thrombus that had formed in the distal catheter lumen during the time when the guidewire had been withdrawn into the catheter and the distal lumen was occupied not by the guidewire but by stagnant blood might have been be embolized into the cerebral arteries by injection of contrast medium via the catheter.

Complication Management in Angiography and Interventional Radiology

A complication during angiography is an emergency that requires instantaneous therapeutic reaction. This is especially true for procedurally induced ischemic neurologic deficits. Timely recanalization of the occluded artery is the only effective treatment for acute ischemic stroke. The appropriate management depends entirely on the pathological cause of the complication. An immediate analysis of the clinical situation and the underlying pathology thus is warranted. Also, the radiologist/neuroradiologist must be experienced in the endovascular procedures that are required and must have available all the technical and pharmacological requirements for carrying out the endovascular interventions. For this reason, all international guidelines on the performance of angiography and interven-

tional radiology put high emphasis on the competence of the radiologists/neuroradiologists and the radiology technicians as well as on the quality of the angiographic facilities and equipment, the physiologic monitoring, the resuscitation system, and the procedural care. To the authors' knowledge there are no official or approved international guidelines on the appropriate management of complications. The further therapeutic approach rather has to follow the guidelines of the underlying pathology. Thus it is possible that different radiologist/neuroradiologists will assess the pathomechanism of an acute complication differently and consequently advise different therapeutic approaches. Moreover, it must be borne in mind that all endovascular techniques discussed below are associated with considerable risks, which must be traded off against the poor prognosis of acute cerebral ischemia of the posterior cerebral vasculature in each individual patient.

In vasospasms, as is often the case following aneurysmal rupture and subarachnoid hemorrhage, the most frequently used therapeutic techniques aim to achieve arterial vessel dilatation by means of intra-arterial local administration of vessel-dilating substances such as calcium channel blockers (nimodipine, verapamil), by mechanical balloon angioplasty, or by a combination of both approaches. Whereas balloon angioplasty is applicable only in the proximal cerebral arteries, intra-arterial pharmacological dilatation has the advantage of also acting on smaller distal arterial branches and diffuse vasospasms. Calcium antagonists such as nimodipine reduce the influx of calcium in the smooth-muscle cells through blockage of the voltage-operated calcium channels. This may lead to reduced vascular smooth-muscle constriction and a decrease in the release of vasoactive substances from endothelium and platelets. Clinical studies are ongoing on the clinical effectiveness of intra-arterial endovascular therapy and its potential superiority to intravenous medical management for symptomatic cerebral vasospasms.

In acute thrombembolic ischemia, intravenous administration of fibrinolytic substances such as the recombinant tissue plasminogen activator (rt-PA) within 3 hours of symptom onset is the only US FDA-approved treatment. Innovative intravenous pharmacological reperfusion strategies such as the use of novel fibrinolytic agents (tenecteplase, reteplase, desmeteplase, plasmin, microplasmin), glycoprotein (GP) IIb/IIIa antagonists with platelet disaggregating effects (abciximab and tirofiban), and combination therapies potentially improve the efficacy of clot lysis (fibrinolytics and GP IIb/IIIa agents, fibrinolytics and direct thrombin inhibitors), increase the time window for clot lysis (fibrinolytics and neuroprotectants), and reduce the frequency of hemorrhagic complications (fibrinolytics and vasoprotectants). Recently, new mechanical neuroendovascular devices have shown high recanalization rates with acceptable safety in early studies. Multimodal reperfusion therapy including intra-arterial infusion of thrombolytics (mainly rt-PA) and/or antiplatelet agents (tirofiban), mechanical clot disruption and retrieval, and balloon angioplasty with stent placement are emerging endovascular mechanical reperfusion strategies for the management of major acute thrombembolic vessel occlusions. Recent results suggest that the multimodal endovascular approach results in greater chance of both recanalization of the occluded artery and reperfusion of the ischemic tissue than does intravenous therapy.

References and Further Reading

American College of Radiology (ACR). Practice Guideline for the Performance of Cervicocerebral Angiographies in Adults. http://www.acr.org/SecondaryMainMenuCategories/quality_safety/guidelines/iv/cervicocerebral_angio.aspx (accessed January 16, 2011)

Berguer R. Vertebrobasilar ischemia: indications, techniques and results of surgical repair. In: Rutherford RB, ed. Vascular Surgery. 5th ed. Philadelphia: WB Saunders; 2000:1823–1837

Biondi A, Ricciardi GK, Louis Puybasset L, et al. Intra-arterial nimodipine for the treatment of symptomatic cerebral vasospasm after aneurysmal subarachnoid hemorrhage: Preliminary results. AJNR 2004; 25:1067–1076

Bishop N, Rees MR. Idiosyncratic reaction to intracoronary injection of nonionic contrast media. Clin Radiol 1988; 39: 396–397

Cohen JE, Itshayek E, Moskovici S, et al. State-of-the-art reperfusion strategies for acute ischemic stroke. J Clin Neurosci 2011 [Epub ahead of print]. http://www.ncbi.nlm.nih.gov/pubmed/21256755 (accessed January 25, 2011)

Earnest IV F, Forbes G, Sandok BA, et al. Complications of cerebral angiography: prospective assessment of risk. AJR 1984; 142: 247–253

Fleming G, Shanes JG. Left ventriculography induced coronary artery spasm. Clin Cardiol 1984; 7: 560–562

LeVeen RF, Wolf GL, Biery D. Angioplasty-induced vasospasm in rabbit model. Mechanisms and treatment. Invest Radiol 1985; 20: 938–944

Limbruno U, Petronio AS, Amoroso G, et al. The impact of coronary artery disease on the coronary vasomotor response to nonionic contrast media. Circulation 2000; 101: 491–497

Mani RL, Eisenberg RL, McDonald jr EJ, Pollock JA, Mani RJ. Complications of catheter cerebral arteriography: analysis of 5,000 procedures. I. Criteria and incidence. AJR 1978; 131: 861–865

Mani RL, Eisenberg RL. Complications of catheter cerebral arteriography: analysis of 5,000 procedures. III. Assessment of arteries injected, contrast medium used, duration of procedure, and age of patient. AJR 1978; 131: 871–874

Molina CA, Saver JL. Extending reperfusion therapy for acute ischemic stroke: emerging pharmacological, mechanical, and imaging strategies. Stroke 2005; 36: 2311–2320

Morris PP. Practical Neuroangiography. 2nd ed. Philadelphia: Lippincott Williams & Wilkins; 2007

Satoh A, Matsuda Y, Sakai H, et al. Coronary artery spasm during cardiac angiography. Clin Cardiol 1990; 13: 55–58

Tountopoulou A, Ahl B, Weissenborn K, Becker H, Goetz F. Intra-arterial thrombolysis using rt-PA in patients with acute stroke due to vessel occlusion of anterior and/or posterior cerebral circulation. Neuroradiology 2008; 50: 75–83

Williams M, Patil S, Toledo EG, et al. Management of acute ischemic stroke: current status of pharmacological and mechanical endovascular methods. Neurol Res 2009; 31: 807–815

Willinsky RA, Taylor SM, terBrugge K, Farb RI, Tomlinson G, Montanera W. Neurologic complications of cerebral angiography: prospective analysis of 2,899 procedures and review of the literature. Radiology 2003; 227: 522–528

Complication of Embolization

History and Clinical Findings

A healthy 9-year-old boy experienced sudden weakness on the left side of his body. Cranial CT revealed a hemorrhage in the right hemisphere with intraventricular rupture caused by a bleeding arteriovenous (AV) malformation (**Fig. 7.7**). Ventricular dilatation was consistent with grade 1 hydrocephalus due to obstruction of CSF flow by blood clots in the aqueduct. Pressure was relieved by establishing CSF drainage through a right frontal bur hole. Diagnostic angiography of the cerebral arteries confirmed an AV malformation (**Fig. 7.8**). Since angiography showed only one large-caliber feeder from the right pericallosal artery, it was decided to occlude the AV malformation by endovascular embolization.

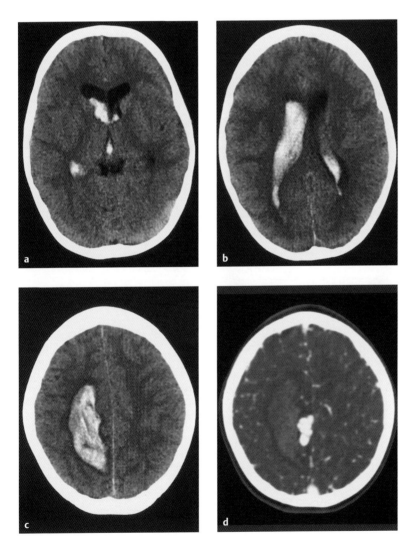

Fig. 7.7 a–d   CT demonstrates a hematoma with intraventricular rupture high in the right parietal white matter (**a–c**) due to bleeding from an AV malformation (**d**).
a–c   CT scans without contrast medium.
d   CT angiography.

Following superselective catheterization of the feeder vessel, a mixture of Ethibloc and lipiodol was injected under fluoroscopic guidance. When the result was checked by angiography, it was found that an estimated 1 mL of the embolic material had passed through the high-flow angioma and into the superior sagittal sinus (**Fig. 7.9**). At that point the embolization mixture was made more viscous by altering the mixing ratio, and the embolization was continued. The final angiogram showed a smaller perfused residual nidus.

CT scans the day after the intervention confirmed virtually complete occlusion of the AV malformation (**Fig. 7.10**).

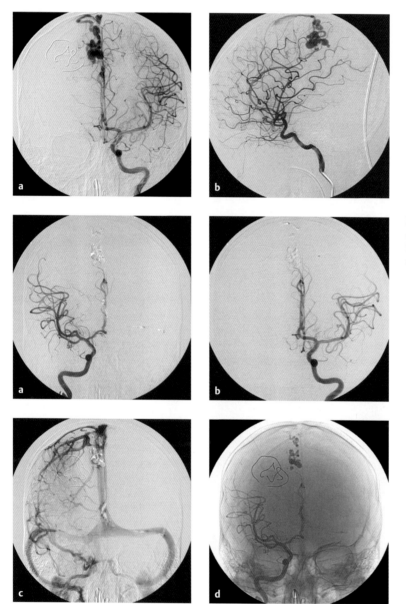

Fig. 7.8 a, b Angiography of the left internal carotid artery shows an AV malformation fed by the right pericallosal artery with a patent anterior communicating artery. Dressing material is projected over the right frontal bone after placement of a CSF drain.

Fig. 7.9 a–d Angiography immediately after embolization. Embolic material is visible in the superior sagittal sinus and left sigmoid sinus.

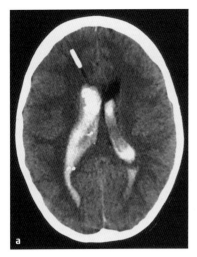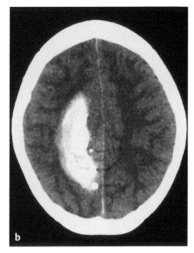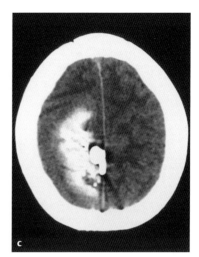

Fig. 7.10 a–c Noncontrast CT scans the day after the intervention. The vascular malformation is filled with embolic material (see **Fig. 7.7 d**). A ventricular drain has been placed through a right frontal bur hole. The hematoma appears unchanged relative to earlier images.

Further Case Summary

Two days after the intervention, clinical and laboratory parameters indicated the development of pleuropneumonia (**Fig. 7.11**) and hepatitis. The patient was moved to the ICU and placed on positive-pressure ventilation. At times his pulmonary status was classified as life-threatening. Chest radiographs showed embolic material projected over both lower lung zones. Based on experience with pulmonary emboli, the degree of embolization of terminal pulmonary artery branches was not considered sufficient to explain the patient's condition. Since laboratory inflammatory markers were elevated, the embolic injury was obviously accompanied by a toxic component, and the patient was treated accordingly. One week later the patient was transferred from the ICU to general in-patient care. He showed subsequent improvement of left-sided hemiparesis.

Arteriovenous Malformations (AV Angiomas)

An AV malformation (AVM) is an angiodysplasia of the brain with an estimated prevalence and incidence of 1–10/100 000 population per year. Asymptomatic AVMs are probably more prevalent than symptomatic AV angiomas. The latter usually present between 20 and 50 years of age with intracerebral hemorrhage and, less commonly, headaches or seizures. Two-thirds of hemorrhages involve the brain parenchyma. Subarachnoid and intraventricular hemorrhages are less common. The bleeding risk is estimated at 2–4% per year and is increased 2- to 4-fold after a previous bleed. AVMs are characterized by their location as cortical AVMs that drain into the superior sagittal sinus or as deep, central AVMs.

In planning the embolization of an AVM, it is important to identify the transit arteries because they supply the nidus as well as the surrounding healthy brain tissue. Most AVMs have a high arteriovenous shunt volume (high-flow angiomas), but low-flow lesions are also encountered. A high shunt volume may produce a steal effect that diverts blood away from other brain regions into the angioma. This may lead to cerebral ischemia in extreme cases. The actual collection of tangled vessels, called the nidus, consists of enlarged, densely packed capillaries with an abnormal structure. The nidus is the site where arterial blood flows directly into the veins, by-passing normal capillary pathways. The goal of embolization, then, is to permanently occlude the nidus and its arteriovenous connections. It is common to find drainage patterns involving multiple veins.

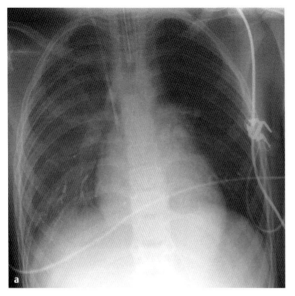

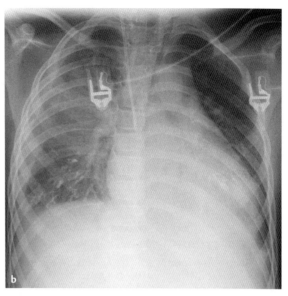

Fig. 7.11 a, b Chest radiographs taken during treatment in the ICU for bilateral toxic pleuropneumonia.

a Radiograph 2 days after embolization shows embolic material in both lower lung zones, predominantly on the right side. Other findings are early infiltrates in the right lower lobe and a small pleural effusion on the right side.

b Radiograph 6 days after embolization shows progression of right lung infiltration and the right pleural effusion. New infiltrates have appeared in the left lower lobe. The patient has been extubated.

Error Analysis and Strategy for Error Prevention

The embolic material had passed through the sigmoid sinuses, internal jugular veins, superior vena cava, and right atrium and ventricle and had entered the pulmonary artery. Some of the material had lodged in peripheral branches of the pulmonary artery. The lower lobes were predominantly affected due to the relatively high blood flow in those regions. Toxic inflammation also developed in the lungs and liver.

Anaphylactoid reactions have been described in patients undergoing lymphography with the oily contrast agent lipiodol, an ethyl ester of iodized fatty acids derived from poppy seed oil. Ethibloc, on the other hand, is a bioinert occluding emulsion composed mainly of amidotrizoic acid, zein, oleum papaveris, propylene glycol, and ethanol.

The relatively large diameter of the feeder artery and the high blood flow in the AV malformation led to technical problems during the embolization procedure. Other al-ternative embolic materials such as starch or Gelfoam particles would also have been carried by the bloodstream across the arteriovenous shunt and into the draining veins and pulmonary circulation. Modern, more advanced embolic agents were not available at the time of the intervention. Open ligation of the pathologic vessels would have been associated with a high surgical risk and a significant risk of potential complications (paralysis).

Endovascular embolization also carries a risk of occluding normal vessels that supply healthy brain parenchyma. Increasing occlusion of the pathologic vessels may cause a redistribution of blood flow, resulting in the undesired embolization of nutrient vessels.

References and Further Reading

Hurst RW, Rosenwasser RH, eds. Interventional Neuroradiology. New York: Informa Healthcare; 2008

Morris PP, ed. Practical Neuroangiography. 2nd ed. Philadelphia: Lippincott Williams & Wilkins; 2007

Complication of an Interventional Procedure

History and Clinical Findings

A 55-year-old woman complained of severe headache, dizziness, and nausea of sudden onset. She was verbally responsive when hospitalized but later showed a diminished level of consciousness. She was subsequently sedated, intubated, and placed on mechanical ventilation. Cranial CT revealed a subarachnoid hemorrhage (SAH), an apparent ruptured aneurysm of the left middle cerebral artery (MCA), signs of increased intracranial pressure, and compression of the ventricular system predominantly on the left side (**Fig. 7.12**). The severity of the SAH was classified as Hunt and Hess grade 4 based on level of consciousness before intubation (see **Table 1.3**, p. 17).

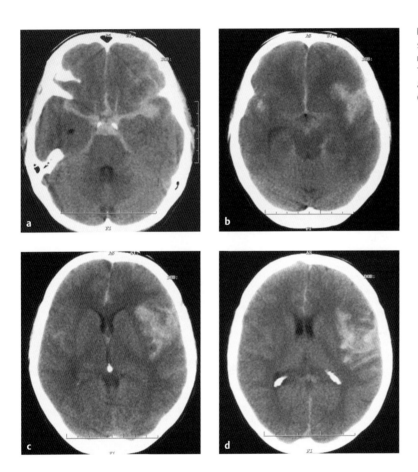

Fig. 7.12 a–d Noncontrast cranial CT scans taken on admission show a predominantly left-sided Fischer grade 4 SAH (see **Table 1.4**) originating from a perforated aneurysm at the bifurcation of the MCA. Cerebral edema is also present.

Based on a consultation between neurosurgery and radiology, it was decided to proceed with emergency angiography of the cerebral supply arteries. The principal finding was an aneurysm at the bifurcation of the left MCA, which was ruptured by angiographic criteria and was therefore responsible for the SAH detected by computed tomography (**Fig. 7.13**). An incidental aneurysm was also noted at the bifurcation of the right MCA, and the terminal segment of the basilar artery was dilated.

Given the severity of the SAH, the frequency of rebleeding during the initial hours after an aneurysm rupture, the configuration of the perforated aneurysm, local vascular topography, and the potential complications and complication rates of endovascular and neurosurgical procedures, it was decided to proceed with endovascular treatment in the same sitting (**Fig. 7.14**).

A microcatheter was advanced into the left MCA aneurysm through a coaxial catheter system. A 3D coil (length 15 cm, diameter 6 mm) was introduced into the aneurysm lumen under fluoroscopic guidance (**Fig. 7.15**). Fluoroscopy did not show the marker alignment indicat-

ing that the coil was fully deployed and ready for detachment. The peripheral end of the coil extended slightly into the main branch of the MCA. It was then decided to retract and reposition the coil, but the operator could only retract approximately 5 cm of the coil from the aneurysm back into the catheter. Further coil removal was not possible because the loops of the coil had become entangled within the aneurysm lumen. On repeated attempts to pack the platinum coil completely into the aneurysm, the coil broke off near the solder joint with the pusher. At that point, part of the coil was inside the aneurysm, while a straight portion remained within the MCA and the terminal segment of the carotid artery. A retriever system was advanced through the guide catheter and into the internal carotid artery to the site of the coil. Due to the adherent surface of the platinum coil, however, the end of the coil could not be captured with the retrieval snare (**Fig. 7.16**). These maneuvers were accompanied by a rapidly progressive thrombosis of the left internal carotid artery extending into the MCA. After interdisciplinary consultation, it was decided to schedule the patient for surgical retrieval of the

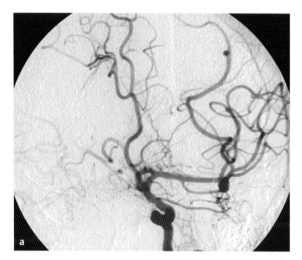

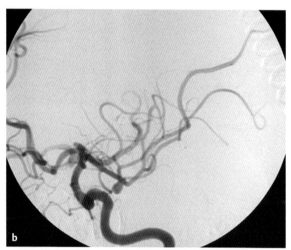

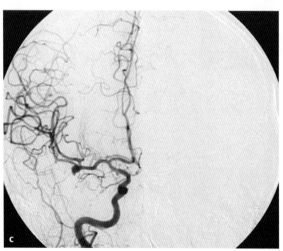

Fig. 7.13 a–c Approximately 6-mm aneurysm at the bifurcation of the MCA (**a, b**). A second aneurysm is noted at an identical site on the right side (**c**).
a, b Selective angiography of the left internal carotid artery.
c Selective angiography of the right internal carotid artery.

detached and displaced coil and surgical resection of the aneurysm. Postinterventional findings included the detection of spasms and thrombi in the left internal carotid artery, a thrombus at the origin of the left anterior cerebral artery, and an occlusion of the main trunk of the left MCA.

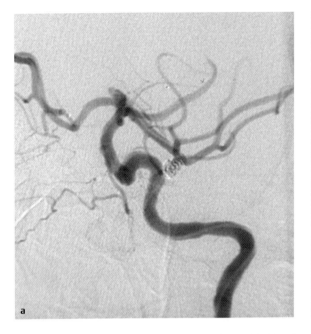

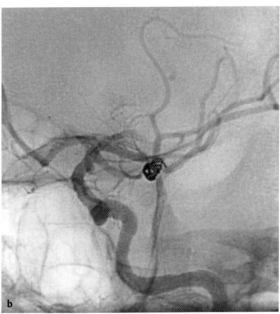

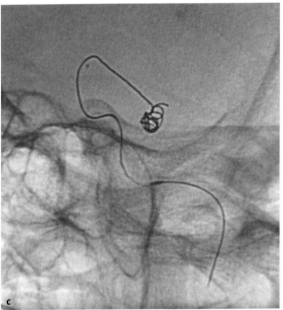

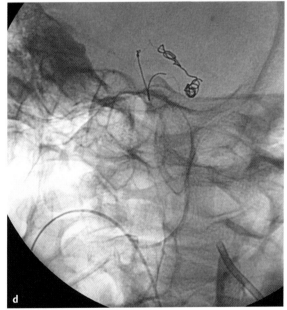

Fig. 7.14 a–d Coil occlusion of an aneurysm of the left MCA.
a The platinum coil has been partially deployed into the aneurysm lumen.
b The end of the platinum coil extends slightly into the MCA.

c Incomplete retraction of the coil. The end of the coil lies within the main trunk of the MCA and the terminal segment of the internal carotid artery.
d At the end of the intervention, a large portion of the coil is in the left MCA and induces acute thrombosis.

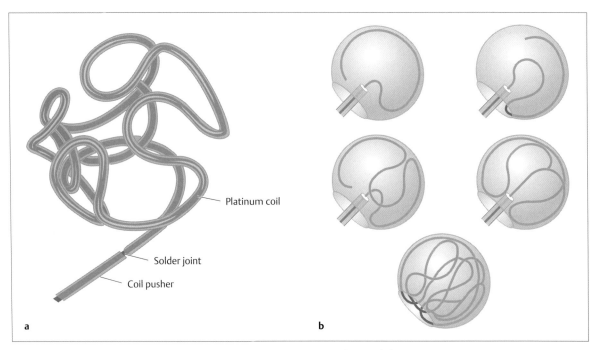

Fig. 7.15 a, b   Technique of 3D endovascular coiling.

a 3D coil, unraveled.
b Diagrammatic representation of the endovascular occlusion of an aneurysm with a platinum coil.

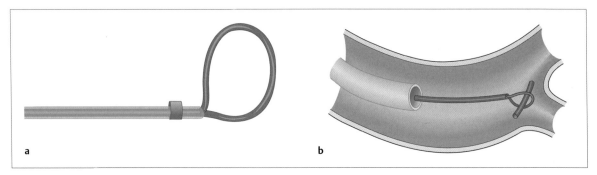

Fig. 7.16 a, b   Snare principle for the retrieval of an intravascular foreign body.

a Retrieval snare.
b Retrieval of an intravascular foreign body.

Further Case Summary

At operation, it was confirmed that the platinum coil was located partly within the aneurysm lumen and partly in the MCA and the terminal segment of the internal carotid artery. There was one site where it had perforated the wall of the aneurysm sac. The coil was retrieved, the aneurysm was resected, the blood clots were removed, and the vessel wall defect was closed with sutures. Transcranial Doppler scans detected blood flow in the main trunk and distal branches of the MCA, confirming that the operation had improved the blood supply to the brain. One day later a hematoma was evacuated and a decompressive craniotomy was performed (**Fig. 7.17**).

CT follow-up 1 month later showed infarctions in the territories of the left middle and anterior cerebral arteries and edema of the left cerebral hemisphere, which gradually diminished in its intensity and extent. The bone flap was reimplanted 5 months later, and MRI at that time showed a left MCA infarction with compensatory dilatation of the left lateral ventricle (**Fig. 7.18**).

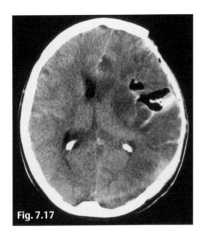

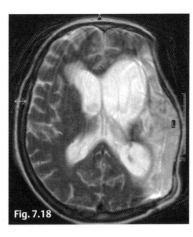

Fig. 7.17 Noncontrast cranial CT on the first postinterventional day. The hematoma has been evacuated and a decompressive craniectomy has been performed. Increasing ischemia is noted in the left white matter along with predominantly left-sided brain edema.

Fig. 7.18 MRI 5 months after the intervention shows a parenchymal defect and gliosis in the left hemisphere with dilatation of the left lateral ventricle.

Error Analysis and Strategy for Error Prevention

A ruptured aneurysm of the left MCA caused a subarachnoid hemorrhage that was classified as Hunt and Hess grade 4 and Fisher grade 4 (see **Table 1.4**, p. 18). Diagnostic angiography confirmed the CT suspicion of a ruptured aneurysm at the bifurcation of the left MCA. Based on its location and configuration, the aneurysm was considered accessible to endovascular treatment. Surgical clipping would have been more hazardous due to the brain edema detected by CT and the consequent higher risk of vasospasms.

The complications that arose (coil could not be placed fully within the aneurysm, coil disconnected from pusher wire, failed extraction attempt) have all been described in previously published reports on the endovascular occlusion of ruptured aneurysms with electrolytically detachable platinum coils. Ordinarily, a coil improperly placed in the aneurysm can be retracted into the microcatheter while still attached to the delivery wire. But in this case the coil could not be fully advanced into the aneurysm and could not be withdrawn into the catheter because loops of the coil had become entangled within the aneurysm. As the delivery wire was alternately pulled and pushed in an effort to maneuver the coil into the aneurysm, the solder joint between the pusher and coil was broken. Several possible solutions were available in this situation, but none has been evaluated for safety and efficacy in treatment studies or according to the principles of evidence-based medicine. Thus, the solution applied in any given case is always an individual decision made in an emergency situation, and its efficacy can be evaluated only in retrospect:

- One option is to leave the coil in the parent vessel, followed by anticoagulant therapy with the plasma coagulation inhibitor heparin and/or the platelet aggregation inhibitor acetysalycil acid and/or tirofiban. Since the aneurysm was only partly filled by the platinum coil, this option would have increased the risk of rebleeding. Another problem was that angiography after coil placement showed that thrombi had already formed.
- Another option is to use greater force in an effort to pack the coil into the aneurysm. This maneuver could have caused an additional aneurysm rupture. There was also a risk of dislodging the thrombi (embolic stroke), so this approach was rejected.
- Endovascular retrieval of the detached coil was tried unsuccessfully at the end of the intervention. More intensive manipulations were withheld to avoid prolonged ischemia since thrombosis had already commenced in the parent vessel.
- Open surgical removal of the intravascular and intra-aneurysmal coil was finally performed as a last resort.

Interventional Radiology in the Treatment of Subarachnoid Hemorrhage

Indications

The incidence of SAH is 7–10 per 100 000 population per year. The cause of the hemorrhage in 65–85% of patients is the rupture of an intradural arterial aneurysm. One-third of patients die before reaching the hospital. Another one-third survive with disability despite adequate treatment, and one-third survive without life-altering disability. The peak age incidence is from the fourth through sixth decades.

Rebleeding occurs in approximately 20% of patients during the initial hours after a SAH. Another 20% bleed within the next 2 weeks, and 35% within the first month. The incidence of rebleeding by 6 months after a SAH is greater than 50%. The mortality rate of each rebleed is approximately 50%. The incidence of rerupture thereafter is approximately 3% per year.

The basic treatment goal is to occlude the aneurysm as soon as possible. The main options are surgical clipping and endovascular coiling using an electrolytically detachable platinum coil. Endovascular treatment, introduced clinically in the early 1990s, has proven superior to the surgical techniques practiced for more than 40 years and has increasingly become the treatment of first choice for aneurysmal SAH. The goal of endovascular treatment is to occlude the aneurysm while maintaining the patency of the parent artery by advancing a platinum coil into the aneurysm through a transfemoral approach. Once deployed within the aneurysm, the coil is electrolytically detached from the delivery wire.

The superiority of endovascular treatment over surgery has been documented by two prospective, randomized two-arm studies that involved 109 patients (Vanninen et al. 1999) and 2143 patients (Molyneux et al. 2002). In the Vanninen study, endovascular treatment had a mortality rate of 1% compared with 4% for surgical treatment. In the Molyneux study, the patients treated by endovascular coiling had such better clinical results than surgically treated patients that the trial was discontinued after the interim evaluation. By 1 year after treatment, 24% of the patients in the endovascular treatment group and 31% of the patients in the surgery group had died or had developed serious disability.

Severity of the SAH as a Prognostic Factor

The severity of the SAH critically affects the prognosis. The causes of a poor outcome after a severe SAH include rebleeding and vasospasms leading to ischemia and increased intracranial pressure with compromise of microcirculation. In a multicenter study by Gallas et al. (2005) involving 650 patients with 705 ruptured aneurysms, the mortality rate was only 1% in patients with a Hunt and Hess grade 1 SAH and 2% in patients with a Fisher score of 1. By contrast, the mortality rates were 22% in patients with a Hunt and Hess score of 4 and 21% in patients with a Fisher score of 4. Weir et al. (2003) reported on 27 consecutive patients that had been treated for a Hunt and Hess grade 4 or 5 aneurysmal SAH by detachable coil embolization. Only 4 of 16 patients with a Hunt and Hess score of 4 (25%) and 3 of 11 patients with a Hunt and Hess score of 5 (27%) had a long-term outcome compatible with a normal life. In 73% and 75% of these cases, respectively, the SAH and subsequent treatment were followed by severe neurologic deficits, an apallic syndrome (7%), or death (59% of the patients died during the first 30 days, 70% within 1 year). Henkes et al. (2004) described a severe neurologic deficit in 27% of 216 patients with a Hunt and Hess grade 4 or 5 SAH. There was a 32% incidence of apallic syndrome or death following coil embolization. In 163 consecutive patients who underwent endovascular treatment of a ruptured intradural aneurysm, Sluzewski et al. (2003) found that a high Hunt and Hess grade of SAH was the most important risk factor for a clinically adverse or fatal outcome (relative risk factor 4.1), followed by technical complications (relative risk factor 3.4), patient age (relative risk factor 1.8), and an aneurysm more than 15 mm in diameter (relative risk factor 1.2).

Complications

To date only a few reports have been published on technical complications during the endovascular treatment of ruptured intracranial aneurysms. These complications have an average reported incidence of 20%. The range from 8% to 63% is explained by small patient groups, different study designs (prospective vs. retrospective, different inclusion criteria), and varying definitions of complications. Coil fragmentation is observed in 1–2% of the procedures. Coil misplacement with protrusion into the parent vessel is reported in 2–6% of cases. The average reported incidence of ischemia (vasospasm, thrombosis, thromboembolism) is 16% (ranging from 4% to 58%).

To the authors' knowledge, there have been 12 reported cases of coil fragmentation, although the number of unpublished cases is certainly higher (Standard et al. 1994; Kremer et al. 1999; Baltsavias et al. 2000; Raftopoulos et al. 2002; Schumacher and Berlis 2003; Gallas et al. 2005; Schütz et al. 2005). Five fragmentations resulted from an attempt to extract the protruding end of the coil from the parent vessel (Standard et al. 1994; Schumacher and Berlis 2003; Schütz et al. 2005). Raftopoulos et al. (2002) attributed their coil fracture to pressure and shear forces acting on the last coil advanced into an aneurysm lumen that had already been packed with other coils. Four of the 12 fragmentations were successfully treated by endovascular retrieval, resulting in a favorable long-term neurologic outcome in 2 of the 4 patients.

References and Further Reading

Baltsavias GS, Byrne JV, Molyneux AJ, Coley SC, Sohn MJ. Effects of timing of coil embolization after aneurysmal subarachnoid hemorrhage on procedural morbidity and outcomes. Neurosurgery 2000; 47; 1320–1331

Berenstein A, Lasjaunias P, Ter Brugge KG. Surgical Neuroangiography. 2nd ed. Berlin: Springer; 2004

Brilstra EH, Rinkel GJ, Algra A, Van Gijn J. Rebleeding, secondary ischemia, and timing of operation in patients with subarachnoid hemorrhage. Neurology 2000; 55; 1656–1660

Brisman JL, Niimi Y, Song JK, Berenstein A. Aneurysmal rupture during coiling: low incidence and good outcome at a single large-volume center. Neurosurgery 2005; 57: 1103–1109

Cloft HJ, Kallmes DF. Cerebral aneurysm perforations complicating therapy with Guglielmi detachable coils: a meta-analysis. AJNR 2002; 23: 1706–1709

Deng J, Zhao Z, Gao G. Periprocedural complications associated with endovascular embolisation of intracranial ruptured aneurysms with matrix coils. Singapore Med J 2007; 48: 429–433

Fessler RD, Ringer AJ, Qureshi AI, Guterman LR, Hopkins LN. Intracranial stent placement to trap an extruded coil during endovascular aneurysm treatment: technical note. Neurosurgery 2000; 46: 248–253

Gallas S, Pasco A, Cottier J-P, et al. A multicenter study of 705 ruptured intracranial aneurysms treated with Guglielmi detachable coils. AJNR 2005; 26: 1723–1731

Graves VB, Strother CM, Duff TA, Perl J. Early treatment of ruptured aneurysms with Guglielmi detachable coils: effect on subsequent bleeding. Neurosurgery 1995; 37: 640–647

Henkes H, Fischer S, Weber W, et al. Endovascular coil occlusion of 1811 intracranial aneurysms: early angiographic and clinical results. Neurosurgery 2004; 54: 268–285

Henkes H, Lowens S, Preiss H, et al. A new device for endovascular coil retrieval from intracranial vessels: alligator retrieval device. Am J Neuroradiol 2006; 27: 327–329

Hunt WE, Hess RM. Surgical risk as related to time of intervention in the repair of intracranial aneurysms. J Neurosurg 1968; 28: 14–20

Koivisto T, Vanninen R, Hurskainen H, Saari T, Hernesniemi J, Vapalahti M. Outcomes of early endovascular versus surgical treatment of ruptured cerebral aneurysms. A prospective randomized study. Stroke 2000; 31; 2369–2377

Kremer C, Grodon C, Hansen HC, Grzyska U, Zeumer H. Outcome after endovascular treatment of Hunt & Hess grade IV und V aneurysms. Stroke 1999; 30: 2617–2622

Molyneux A, Kerr R, Stratton I, et al. International Subarachnoid Aneurysm Trial (ISAT) Collaborative Group. International Subarachnoid Aneurysm Trial (ISAT) of neurosurgical clipping versus endovascular coiling in 2143 patients with ruptured intracranial aneurysms: a randomised trial. Lancet 2002; 360; 1267–1274

Raftopoulos Ch, Goffette P, Billa RF, et al. Transvascular coil hooking procedure to retrieve an unraveled Guglielmi detachable coil: technical note. Neurosurgery 2002; 50: 912–915

Schumacher M, Berlis A. The balloon retriever technique. Neuroradiology 2003; 45: 267–269

Schütz A, Solymosi L, Vince GH, Bendszus M. Proximal stent fixation of fractured coil: technical note. Neuroradiology 2005; 47: 874–878

Shin YS, Lee KC, Kim DI, Lee KS, Huh SK. Emergency surgical recanalisation of A1 segment occluded by Guglielmi detachable coil. J Clin Neurosience 2000; 7: 259–262

Sluzewski M, Bosch JA, van Rooij WJ, Nijssen PC, Wijnalda D. Rupture of intracranial aneurysms during treatment with Guglielmi detachable coils: incidence, outcome, and risk factors. J Neurosurg 2001; 94; 238–240

Sluzewski M, van Rooij WJ, Rinkel GJE, Wijnalda D. Endovascular treatment of ruptured intracranial aneurysms with detachable coils: long-term clinical and serial angiographic results. Radiology 2003; 227; 720–724

Standard SC, Tamerla C, Wakhloo AJ, et al. Retrieval of a Guglielmi detachable coil after unraveling and fracture: case report and experimental results. Neurosurgery 1994; 35: 994–999

Thornton J, Dovey Z, Alazzaz A, et al. Surgery following endovascular coiling of intracranial aneurysms. Surg Neurol 2000; 54: 352–360

van Loon J, Waerzeggers Y, Wilms G, Van Calenbergh F, Goffin J, Plets C. Early endovascular treatment of ruptured cerebral aneurysms in patients in very poor neurological condition. Neurosurgery 2002; 50; 457–464

van Rooij WJ, Sluzewski M, Beute GN, Nijssen PC. Procedural complications of coiling of ruptured intracranial aneurysms: incidence and risk factors in a consecutive series of 681 patients. Am J Neuroradiol 2006; 27: 1498–1501

Vanninen R, Koivisto T, Saari T, et al. Ruptured intracranial aneurysms. Acute endovascular treatment with electrolytically detachable coils—a prospective randomized study. Radiology 1999; 211; 325–336

Vora N, Thomas A, Germanwala A, Jovin, T. and Horowitz, M. Retrieval of a displaced detachable coil and intracranial stent with an L5 Merci retriever during endovascular embolization of an intracranial artery. J Neuroimaging 2008; 18: 81–84

Weir RU, Marcellus ML, Do HM, Steinberg GK, Marks MP. Aneurysmal subarachnoid hemorrhage in patients with Hunt and Hess grade 4 or 5: treatment using the Guglielmi detachable coil system. AJNR 2003; 24: 585–590

Zoarski GH, Bear HM, Clouston JC, Ragheb J. Endovascular extraction of malpositioned fibered platinum microcoils from the aneurysm sac during endovascular therapy. Am J Neuroradiol 1997; 18: 691–695

Internal Carotid Artery Aneurysm/Infundibular Origin of the Posterior Communicating Artery

History and Clinical Findings

A 52-year-old man with a subarachnoid hemorrhage underwent cerebral angiography (**Fig. 7.19**). The images showed no abnormalities other than a broad-based protrusion from the inferior surface of the left internal carotid artery in proximity to the posterior communicating artery. The protrusion was interpreted as an aneurysm of the internal carotid artery.

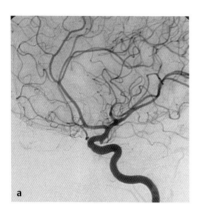
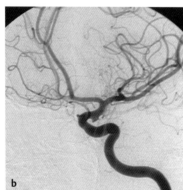
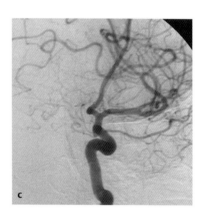

Fig. 7.19a–c Angiography of the left internal carotid artery. The study was described as showing an aneurysm of the internal carotid artery.

Further Case Summary

The next morning a craniotomy was performed to allow surgical clipping of the aneurysm. The exposure revealed a small, funnel-shaped dilatation of the proximal posterior communicating artery, but there was no aneurysm. The source of the subarachnoid hemorrhage was not identified.

Error Analysis and Strategy for Error Prevention

An infundibulum at the origin of the posterior communicating artery (**Fig. 7.20**) frequently resembles a saccular aneurysm in the terminal segment of the internal carotid artery on angiograms. An infundibulum is defined as a tunnel- or funnel-shaped vascular dilatation caused by the incomplete regression of a fetal artery. The origin of the posterior communicating artery is most commonly affected. Infundibula are occasionally found at the origin of the anterior choroidal artery. The pathognomonic angiographic appearance is that of a rounded or conical ex-

pansion of the vessel diameter (up to 3 mm) at its origin from the internal carotid artery, with the distal portion of the posterior communicating artery arising from the center of the dilatation. Infundibular diameters greater than 3 mm have been reported in isolated cases. By contrast, the majority of aneurysms are larger than 3 mm in diameter and are often lobulated. If the distal posterior communicating artery arises eccentrically from a vascular dilatation, an aneurysm should be suspected.

In the case shown, the relationship of the posterior communicating artery to the presumed aneurysm was misinterpreted as a superimposed vessel (**Fig. 7.21**). This problem may have been solved by taking additional angiograms at different projection angles to define the vascular relationships more clearly. Rotational angiography would have been an even better option. In this technique the C-arm is rotated 180° around the region of interest during contrast injection and image acquisition, providing a complete cine sequence that allows the vascular territory to be viewed from arbitrary angles in the rotational plane.

In German medical malpractice law, the misinterpretation of angiograms is considered a "diagnostic error." This

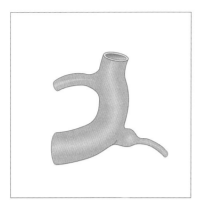

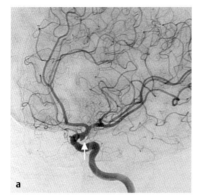

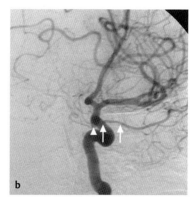

Fig. 7.20 Infundibular dilatation at the origin of the posterior communicating artery.

Fig. 7.21 a, b Relationship of the infundibular origin of the posterior communicating artery (arrowhead in **b**), which was misinterpreted as a carotid aneurysm, to the distal portion of the posterior communicating artery (arrows).

denotes an error in the diagnostic interpretation of an imaging procedure. In itself, an objectively wrong diagnosis is not considered to be a *treatment error* or *misinterpretation of findings* because radiologists are allowed some leeway in making diagnostic interpretations and decisions. If the interpretation would be considered unreasonable by an expert in the field, the law would define this situation as a *simple* misinterpretation of findings. If the interpretation is not only unreasonable but is also considered to be an error that a competent physician absolutely would not make and that clearly violates established medical standards, this would justify the assumption of a *gross* misinterpretation of findings. In the case of a simple misinterpretation, the burden of proof lies with the patient, who must prove that the injury to his or her health would not have occurred, or would have been less severe, if the correct diagnosis had been made. It is often difficult to meet this standard of proof. But if the court decides that a gross treatment error has taken place, the burden of proof lies with the physician.

References and Further Reading

Morris PP, ed. Practical Neuroangiography. 2nd ed. Philadelphia: Lippincott Williams & Wilkins; 2007

Osborn AG. Diagnostic Cerebral Angiography. 2nd ed. Philadelphia: Lippincott Williams & Wilkins; 1999

Osborn AG, Blaser SI, Salzmann KL, Katzman GL, Provenzale J, Castillo M. Diagnostic Imaging: Brain. Salt Lake City: Amyrsis; 2004

Cause of Death: Cerebral Ischemia/ Pulmonary Embolism/ Myocardial Infarction

History and Clinical Findings

A 64-year-old man was hospitalized for operative treatment of hypopharyngeal carcinoma. CT and MRI showed that the tumor had infiltrated the right internal carotid artery (ICA), so that the vessel would have to be sacrificed at operation. Angiography with a balloon test occlusion of the right ICA was performed to determine whether sacri-

fice of the ICA would cause cerebral ischemia and whether collateral flow via the circle of Willis could compensate for the occlusion (**Fig. 7.22**). Coagulation tests were within normal limits. Angiography was performed using standard technique. Heparin 12 000 IU was administered through the balloon-tipped catheter before the artery was occluded. Next the balloon was inflated for 30 minutes to occlude all blood flow in the right ICA. Somatic evoked potentials (SEPs) were simultaneously recorded under the supervision of a neurologist to evaluate brain function.

The extra- and intracranial portions of both carotid arteries were well defined by angiography and appeared normal. The anterior communicating artery and left posterior communicating artery were patent. Pathologic tumor vessels were not detected. The balloon occlusion was well tolerated by the patient. When the occlusion was released, the completion angiogram continued to show normal blood flow in the right ICA.

At the end of the procedure the needle tract was closed by placing manual pressure on the inguinal puncture site for 30 minutes. Next a pressure dressing was applied, and the patient was placed on 24 hours' bed rest.

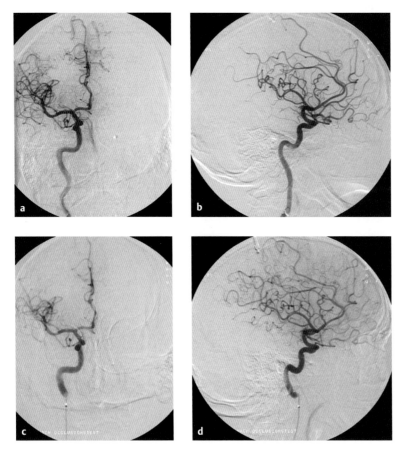

Fig. 7.22 a–d Angiographic test occlusion of the right internal carotid artery. Simultaneous EEG traces are recorded to evaluate brain function during the period of ischemia. The angiograms document normal vascular anatomy.
a, b   Preocclusion series.
c, d   Postocclusion series.

Further Case Summary

According to statements from the patient's family, ward nurses, and ward physician, the patient did well during the 24 hours of prescribed bed rest. In particular, the patient showed no evidence of dyspnea, pain, or leg edema. Routine subcutaneous low-dose heparin was administered for prevention of thrombosis. The ward nurse removed the pressure dressing the following morning. Immediately afterward the patient rose from bed and walked to a nearby sink. At that point he collapsed with manifestations of right heart decompensation (distended neck veins, respiratory distress, gestures consistent with retrosternal chest pain). Resuscitation was unsuccessful. Autopsy was withheld at the request of the family.

Error Analysis and Strategy for Error Prevention

Without an autopsy, a definitive cause of death could not be established. Because venous return was diminished due to the pressure dressing, prolonged bed rest (which compromised the muscle pump), and apparent signs of acute right heart decompensation, it is reasonable to assume that the patient suffered a severe pulmonary embolism secondary to asymptomatic deep lower-extremity venous thrombosis. Evidently the hypopharyngeal cancer had caused a paraneoplastic syndrome, promoting the development of deep iliofemoral venous thrombosis that embolized to the lung.

The results of meta-analyses indicate that the prophylactic subcutaneous administration of unfractionated heparin, low–molecular-weight fractionated heparin, and heparinoids does reduce the incidence of deep lower-extremity venous thrombosis and pulmonary embolism. A residual risk of thrombosis and pulmonary embolism still exists, however. Meta-analyses do not show a mortality benefit from pharmacologic thromboprophylaxis. There is always a risk of venous compression from pressure dressings applied after an arterial puncture in the groin because the arterial blood pressure is higher than the venous pressure and because the arterial and venous vessels are in close proximity to one another.

References and Further Reading

Kaanan AO, Silva MA, Donovan JL, Roy T, Al-Homsi AS. Meta-analysis of venous thromboembolism prophylaxis in medically ill patients. Clin Ther 2007; 29: 2395–2405

Wein L, Haas SJ, Shaw J, Krum H. Pharmacological venous thromboembolism prophylaxis in hospitalized medical patients. Arch Intern Med 2007; 167: 1476–1486

Evoked Potentials

Evoked potentials are useful for testing the conductivity of nerve pathways. The test consists of stimulating a sensory organ (eye, ear) or peripheral nerve and then taking EEG readings to measure the electrical potential that is evoked in the brain region processing the stimulus. Evoked potentials have much smaller amplitudes than spontaneously occurring EEG signals ($1–15\,\mu V$ versus $50–100\,\mu V$). While the spontaneous signals are independent of applied stimuli, evoked potentials occur in direct response to the applied stimuli. A stimulus is repeatedly presented and the subsequent EEG segments are averaged together to sum the stimulus-evoked potentials while leveling out the spontaneous potentials. In the case of somatically evoked potentials, a stimulating electrode is placed close to a sensory nerve and electrical stimuli are repeatedly applied to evaluate the central somatosensory conduction pathways and peripheral sensory nerves.

Renal Artery Stenosis?

History and Clinical Findings

A 55-year-old woman with known peripheral arterial occlusive disease (PAOD) presented with an acute decrease in pain-free walking distance. She was diagnosed clinically with Fontaine stage IIb PAOD on the right side (**Table 7.1**). Three years earlier the patient had an occlusion of the right common iliac artery that had been treated by intra-arterial thrombolytic therapy and percutaneous transluminal angioplasty (PTA) with stenting. The patient suffered from arterial hypertension with pressures of 200/90 mm Hg.

The clinical and duplex findings were suspicious for a thromboembolic occlusion of the stent in the right common iliac artery, and this impression was confirmed by angiography (**Fig. 7.23**). Angiograms were also described as showing a new, high-grade fusiform stenosis of the right renal artery approximately 6 mm distal to its origin from the aorta and a hemodynamically insignificant stenosis of the left renal artery. The reocclusion of the right iliac artery was successfully treated by intra-arterial thrombolytic therapy with urokinase and repeat PTA with the placement of a new stent.

Because the patient had arterial hypertension, it was recommended that she be rehospitalized for elective angiography and stent-assisted PTA of the renal artery stenosis in the same sitting.

Table 7.1 Fontaine classification of peripheral arterial occlusive disease (PAOD)

Stage	Symptoms
I	Asymptomatic peripheral arterial occlusive disease
II	Intermittent claudication
IIa	Walking distance > 200 m
IIb	Walking distance < 200 m
III	Rest pain
IV	Necrosis, gangrene

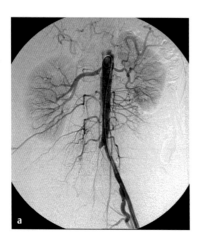
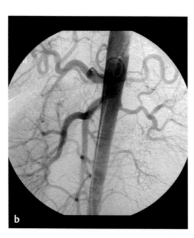

Fig. 7.23 a, b Diagnostic angiography. The images were interpreted as showing reocclusion of the right common iliac artery in the area treated 3 years earlier by PTA with stent insertion (**a**) and a high-grade stenosis of the right renal artery approximately 6 cm distal to its origin from the aorta (**b**). Moderate ostial stenosis of the left renal artery was also diagnosed.

Further Case Summary

Four months later the patient was hospitalized for elective interventional treatment of the right renal artery stenosis. However, angiography showed that the patient did not have a significant renal artery stenosis requiring treatment (**Fig. 7.25**). The initial angiographic findings had been misinterpreted because the superimposed segments of the right renal artery and superior mesenteric artery created the false impression of a renal artery stenosis (**Fig. 7.26**).

Error Analysis and Strategy for Error Prevention

The following errors led to a false-positive diagnosis of renal artery stenosis:

- Neither the aortic survey view (**Fig. 7.23 a**) nor the spot view of the right renal artery (**Fig. 7.23 b**) gave a clear projection of the proximal right renal artery (**Fig. 7.24**). In the survey view, the aorta was superimposed over the origin of the renal artery; in the spot view, the superior mesenteric artery was projected over the vessel origin. A clear projection of the renal artery origin would have enabled a correct diagnosis (**Fig. 7.25**).

- The x-ray absorption of the two superimposed arterial segments added together, creating the appearance of a stenosis (**Fig. 7.26**). Since the arteries had roughly equal diameters, the x-ray absorption was approximately twice that in the adjacent, nonsuperimposed segments of the superior mesenteric artery (proximal) and renal artery (distal).

- The survey aortogram showed that the right kidney was larger than the left kidney (**Fig. 7.23 a**). That finding would not be consistent with a long-standing, hemodynamically significant stenosis of the right renal artery.

The angiographic projection angle should be matched to the individual vascular anatomy of the patient (**Fig. 7.24**).

References and Further Reading

Kadir S. Diagnostic Angiography. Philadelphia: WB Saunders; 1986

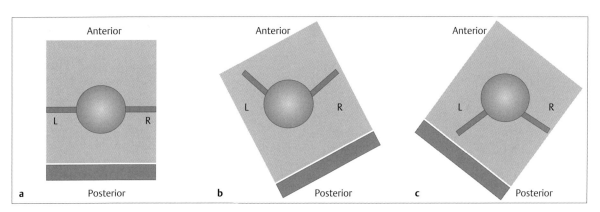

Fig. 7.24 a–c Angled views may be necessary to obtain a clear projection of the right renal artery, depending on its angle of origin from the aorta.

a True lateral origin of the renal arteries from the aorta. Prevalence: approximately 50 % on the right side, 70 % on the left side.

b Anterolateral origin of the renal arteries. Prevalence: approximately 50 % on the right side, 25 % on the left side.

c Posterolateral origin of the renal arteries. Prevalence: < 1 % on the right side, < 5 % on the left side.

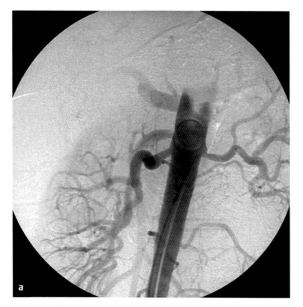

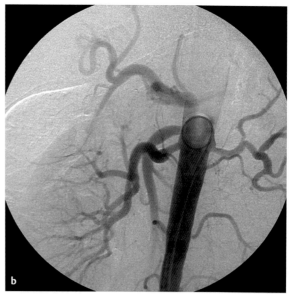

Fig. 7.25 a, b   Supplemental angiograms of the renal arteries 4 months after the previous examination give a nonsuperimposed view of the origins of the renal arteries. The images show only slight ostial stenosis that is not hemodynamically significant.

a LAO projection at approximately 30°.
b LAO projection at approximately 40°.

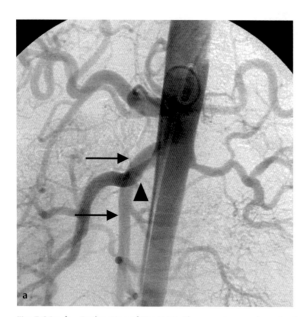

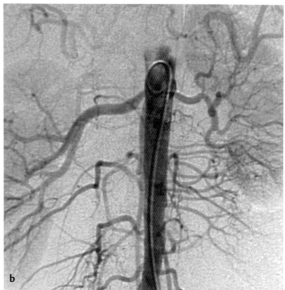

Fig. 7.26 a, b   Explanation of **Fig. 7.23**. The superimposed proximal portions of the superior mesenteric artery (arrows) and right renal artery (arrowhead) create the appearance of a hemodynamically significant renal artery stenosis.

Complication of PTA and Stenting of the Renal Artery

History and Clinical Findings

A 67-year-old woman with a single functioning kidney and compensated renal failure (serum creatinine 2 mg/dL) was referred for the interventional treatment of a hemodynamically significant renal artery stenosis. Her left kidney was small and atrophic due to an unknown cause. Systemic blood pressure was normal. Angiography before the intervention confirmed a high-grade stenosis of the right renal artery, occlusion of the left renal artery, and atherosclerotic irregularities in the aortic wall (**Fig. 7.27**). The stenosis of the right renal artery was treated by percutaneous transluminal angioplasty (PTA) with stent insertion. The intervention was uneventful. Postinterventional angiography confirmed proper stent placement and a normal luminal size of the renal artery. The puncture site in the groin appeared normal on final physical examination.

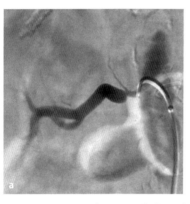 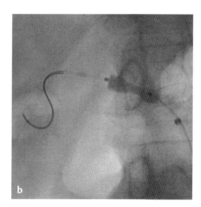 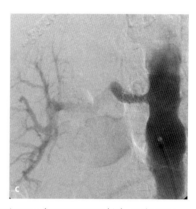

Fig. 7.27 a–c PTA and stenting of a hemodynamically significant right renal artery stenosis.

a Preinterventional angiogram demonstrates a high-grade stenosis of the right renal artery.
b Stent-assisted PTA of the right renal artery.
c Postinterventional angiogram.

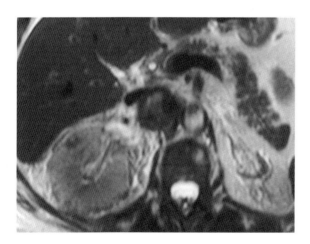

Fig. 7.28 MRI 3 weeks after the intervention. T2-weighted sequence shows a new retrocaval hypointensity next to the stent, along with a small left kidney. The hypointensity was interpreted as an intramural hematoma in the setting of a confined perforation.

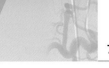
Three days after the intervention, the patient was hospitalized with nausea, vomiting, diarrhea, and a fever of 40 °C. The clinical diagnosis was gastritis. Laboratory tests showed elevated serum CRP and renal retention values. Her blood culture was positive for *Staphylococcus aureus*. The right kidney and renal artery were normal by duplex ultrasound. Clinical complaints and CRP level responded well to symptomatic therapy.

Later in her hospital stay the patient developed right flank pain and dyspnea. Serum CRP was elevated to 180 mg/L (< 8 mg/L is normal), serum creatinine to 8.7 mg/dL (0.5–0.9 mg/dL is normal). When anuria developed, the patient was placed in the ICU. Color duplex ultrasound showed arterial flow signals in the renal parenchyma. The findings prompted a clinical diagnosis of prerenal renal failure secondary to *Staphylococcus aureus* sepsis.

MR angiography 3 weeks after the intervention showed a typical stent-induced signal void in the proximal renal artery (**Fig. 7.28**). Perfusion of the peripheral renal artery and the segmental and subsegmental arteries was normal. The renal parenchyma was abnormally thickened. Postinterventional MRI demonstrated a new structure approximately 3 cm in diameter with predominantly low T2-weighted signal intensity and central hyperintensity located adjacent to the stent. Interpreted as a hematoma, the process was displacing and compressing the renal vein and inferior vena cava but did not cause stagnation of venous blood flow.

MRI follow-up 2 weeks later showed enlargement of the pseudotumor next to the right renal artery (**Fig. 7.29**). An intramural hematoma of the renal artery/aorta in the setting of a confined perforation was considered in the differential diagnosis. Swelling of the renal parenchyma and the presence of small infarctions were unchanged relative to previous images.

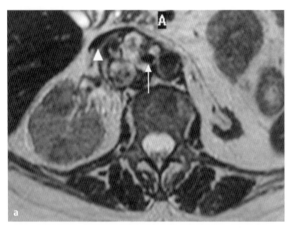

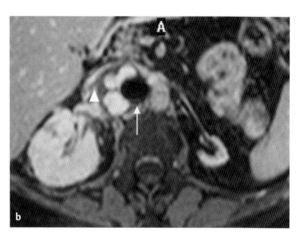

Fig. 7.29 a, b MRI 2 weeks after **Fig. 7.28** shows enlargement of the perivascular inflammatory pseudotumor. The arrow points to the signal void caused by the stent, and the arrowhead points to the displaced inferior vena cava. The larger stent-induced signal void in **b** is based on greater susceptibility disturbances in the MR angiographic sequence.

a T2-weighted sequence.
b T1-weighted MR angiographic sequence after IV contrast administration.

Further Case Summary

Selective angiography of the right kidney showed a new false aneurysm of the right renal artery in addition to the known fusiform aortic aneurysm (**Fig. 7.30**). A normal renal artery caliber was seen only in the area of the renal hilum.

The mycotic renal artery aneurysm was treated surgically by creating a bypass from the right iliac artery to the right renal artery distal to the aneurysm at the level of the renal hilum and inserting a Dacron-coated aortic endostent to seal off the origin of the right renal artery. Inflammatory changes were noted in the soft tissues surrounding the false aneurysm and were debrided as thoroughly as possible.

The postoperative course was uneventful. Renal function returned to preinterventional values by approximately 8 weeks. While interventional treatment of the mycotic aneurysm would have been technically possible by implanting a coated endostent into the renal artery, this treatment was withheld because it would not have eliminated the inflammatory focus. Clinical experience has shown that, even if an excellent primary clinical result had been achieved, there would still have been a risk of sepsis developing months or even years after obliteration of the mycotic aneurysm.

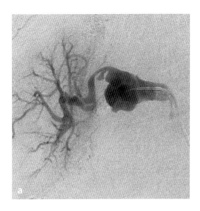 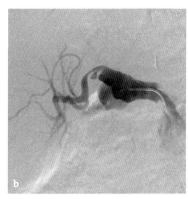

Fig. 7.30 a, b Selective renal angiography shows a mycotic aneurysm of the renal artery after the stent-assisted PTA in **Fig. 7.29**. The stent is projected over the proximal part of the aneurysm.

Error Analysis and Strategy for Error Prevention

The mycotic aneurysm developed because *Staphylococcus aureus* had colonized the stent in the setting of bacteremia and sepsis. This incited an inflammation of the renal artery wall, which had been damaged somewhat by the transluminal stent insertion, leading in turn to the development of a mycotic aneurysm and the inflammatory changes in the surrounding soft tissues that were noted at operation. The following portals of entry may have been available:

- Staphylococci probably entered the bloodstream during the intervention. This is indicated by the high degree of colonization of the groin skin by *Staphylococcus aureus*, the difficulty of disinfecting the puncture site in the groin, and the fact that sepsis coincided with the interventional procedure. The bacteria were introduced into the bloodstream despite aseptic protocols (personnel: sterile masks, caps, gloves, and gowns; patient: groin shaved without nicking the skin, complete removal of the shaved hairs, repeated wetting of the groin with alcohol allowing 10-minute exposure time, sterile draping). Despite these precautions, bacteria may still enter the blood. The incidence of sepsis by this route is estimated at approximately 1 in 1000 angiography sessions and angiographic interventions. Prophylactic antibiotics are generally withheld because of their potential side effects (anaphylaxis, induction of resistance) and the extremely low incidence of septic complications.

- A less likely scenario is that bacteremia was already present before the intervention, having originated from a clinically occult focus (skin inflammation, minor injury, etc.). In this case the bacteria would also have colonized the stent and caused a superinfection of the damaged renal artery wall.

- The portal of entry could not have been the gastrointestinal tract. Staphylococcal enteritis is caused by the endotoxins produced by certain bacterial strains. The bacteria themselves do not enter the bloodstream during gastrointestinal transit.

The enhancing mass with high T2-weighted signal intensity seen on MRI (**Figs. 7.28, 7.29**) consisted of inflammatory granulation tissue. Hematoma would have been a reasonable differential diagnosis only if the blood had undergone fibrous organization.

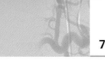

Staphylococcus aureus

Staphylococcus aureus is a ubiquitous Gram-positive coccus that often colonizes the skin and mucous membranes as a commensal organism. It is present in approximately 30% of the normal population and more than 90% of hospital staff. A normal component of the skin flora, *Staphylococcus aureus* is commonly found in smears taken from the ear, nose, throat, and groin. On entering the bloodstream, *Staphylococcus aureus* becomes pathogenetic and may incite a variety of inflammatory conditions (furuncles, carbuncles, puerperal fever, endocarditis, inflammatory hepatic abscess, osteomyelitis, bacterial arthritis, sepsis).

This is particularly true in immunocompromised patients. *Staphylococcus aureus* is among the principal causative organisms of hospital-acquired nosocomial infections. The incubation period ranges from several days to months in invasive staphylococcal infections. Treatment consists of antibiotic therapy. The development of antibiotic resistance (multidrug-resistant *Staphylococcus aureus*) is an increasingly common problems in hospitals with potentially serious medical and economic implications.

References and Further Reading

Chambers CE, Eisenhauer MD, McNicol LB, et al. and the Members of the Catheterization Lab Performance Standards Committee for the Society for Cardiovascular Angiography and Interventions. Infection control guidelines for the cardiac catheterization laboratory: society guidelines revisited. Catheter Cardiovasc Interv 2006; 67: 78–86

Chen C, Tsan YM, Hsueh PR, et al. Bacterial infections associated with hepatic angiography and transarterial embolization for hepatocellular carcinoma: a prospective study. Clin Infect Dis 1999; 29: 161–166

Cooper CL, Miller A. Infectious complications related to the use of the Angio-Seal hemostatic puncture closure device. Catheter Cardiovasc Interv 1999; 48: 301–303

Wagner HJ, Feeken T, Mutters R, Klose KJ. Bacteremia in intra-arterial angiography, percutaneous transluminal angioplasty and percutaneous transhepatic cholangiodrainage. RoFo 1998; 169: 402–407

Vascular Perforation during Subintimal PTA and Stenting

History and Clinical Findings

A 53-year-old overweight woman presented with Fontaine stage IIb peripheral arterial occlusive disease (walking distance < 200 m; see **Table 7.1**, p. 332). Diagnostic angiography through a right femoral approach mainly demonstrated an occlusion of the left common iliac artery and a high-grade stenosis of the right common iliac artery (**Fig. 7.31a, b**). Based on interdisciplinary consultation with a vascular surgeon, it was decided to schedule the patient for interventional radiology treatment.

The stenosis in the right common iliac artery was treated by stent-assisted PTA (**Fig. 7.31c, d**). A self-expanding uncoated stent was advanced into the stenosis and dilated with a balloon catheter. No residual stenosis was detected.

The occlusion of the left common iliac artery was also treated by stent-assisted PTA (**Fig. 7.31e–k**). Retrograde catheterization of the occluded segment was attempted first, but the catheter and guidewire could not be advanced into the aortic lumen. A crossover technique was then used in which a sidewinder catheter was advanced into the occlusion from the right side. Similarly, a guidewire and catheter could not be passed into the femoral artery in the antegrade direction, but a crossover technique was used to grasp the guidewire passed into the occlusion with a goose-neck snare (see **Fig. 7.16**, p. 324) and pull it into the femoral artery on the left side. This established a secure connection between the left external iliac artery and the aorta. It is likely that the catheter was partially subendothelial at this stage of the procedure (see **Fig. 7.33**). Next a self-expanding stent was introduced over the guidewire to recanalize the occlusion of the left common iliac artery. After the occlusion had been dilated, the patient complained of severe pain and anxiety. Angiography showed contrast extravasation originating from the common iliac artery (**Fig. 7.31l**). At this point in the procedure, the angiography machine abruptly shut down and the patient lost consciousness. She had no palpable peripheral pulses and no measurable blood pressure.

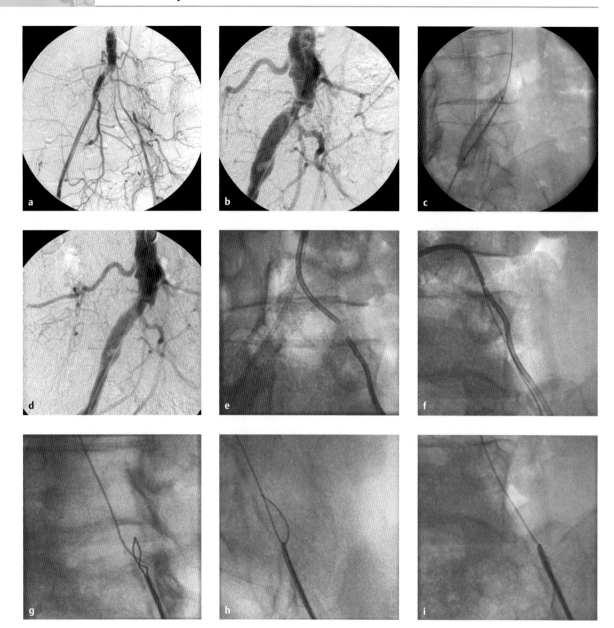

Fig. 7.31 a–o   Recanalization of the common iliac arteries.

a Survey angiography through a right transfemoral approach.

b Detailed view of the stenosis in the right common iliac artery.

c Stent-assisted PTA of the right common iliac artery.

d Result after stent-assisted PTA of the right common iliac artery.

e A retrograde catheter advanced to the occlusion through a left femoral approach meets an antegrade catheter passed down the aortic bifurcation.

f A hydrophilic-coated guidewire is introduced through the proximal antegrade catheter and advanced distally into the true vessel lumen after passing through a subintimal channel.

g The guidewire is extracted with a wire loop via the left femoral approach.

h The guide catheter is pulled into the left femoral catheter with a retriever.

i A subintimal channel has been fully developed past the occlusion.

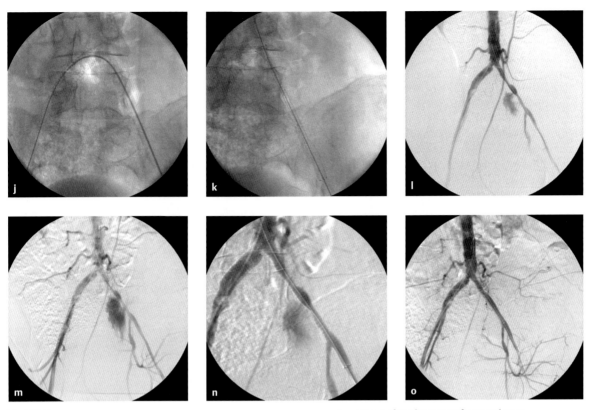

Fig. 7.31 j–o

j   Bitransfemoral passage of the guidewire.

k   Status following stent-assisted PTA of the iliac occlusion (with an uncoated stent).

l, m   Vessel wall injury and contrast extravasation from the left common iliac artery after stent-assisted PTA.

n   Appearance after placement of a coated stent.

o   Completion angiogram.

Further Case Summary

The angiography unit shut down automatically due to overheating of the cathode (length and rapid succession of interventions the previous day, plus an unusually high mA·s product in the current intervention due to the patient's body weight). The unit had an emergency backup system that provided a very limited fluoroscopic view with a maximum image intensifier input format (poor spatial resolution) and a very low tube current (poor image contrast).

Aided by this fluoroscopic option, a second PTA maneuver was performed and a coated stent was placed to seal the leak. The patient reacted to the dilatation pain. Her blood pressure was again measurable and returned to a normal range, and she regained consciousness. By 7 minutes after the shutdown, the x-ray cathode had cooled enough to allow continued operation of the system. Diagnostic angiography showed that the coated stent was correctly positioned and had effectively sealed the perforation (**Fig. 7.31n, o**). The extent of the hematoma was defined by computed tomography (**Fig. 7.32**).

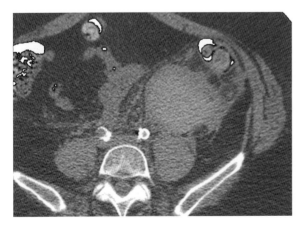

Fig. 7.32 Abdominal CT after the intervention shows a retroperitoneal hematoma anterior to the left psoas muscle. Stents have been placed in both common iliac arteries.

Error Analysis and Strategy for Error Prevention

Vascular perforation is a rare complication of interventional recanalization. To date, few reliable data have been published on the incidence of perforations in different vascular regions. Possible causes include perforation with the guidewire and by the balloon PTA maneuver. Most perforations are small and self-limiting, at least in the femoropopliteal arteries. Larger leaks can generally be managed at interventional radiology by deploying a coated stent at the level of the defect. Perforations are more likely to occur in the recanalization of vascular occlusions than stenoses. This particularly applies to older, long-segment occlusions, which may require subintimal catheterization.

The occurrence of a perforation depends on various factors that include:

- Preexisting damage to the treated vessels (e.g., atherosclerosis)
- The age of the occlusion
- The vascular region (smaller vessels are at higher risk for perforation, but the effects are less severe)
- Overstretching of the vessel wall by a balloon catheter of improper size
- Catheterization errors

The only alternative treatments to be considered were the laparoscopic or open surgical placement of a bifurcation prosthesis. Published reports indicate that this option has a 30-day morbidity of 12–30% and a mortality rate of 3–4%. When indications were discussed in an interdisciplinary meeting, the individual surgical risk due to morbid obesity was correctly judged to be higher than the risk of interventional radiology. Surgery would have been available as a second-line option after the primary or secondary failure of interventional radiology treatment.

References and Further Reading

AbuRahma AF, Hayes JD, Flaherty SK, Peery W. Primary iliac stenting versus transluminal angioplasty with selective stenting. J Vasc Surg 2007; 46: 965–970

Coggia M, Javerliat I, Di Centa I, et al. Total laparoscopic bypass for aortoiliac occlusive disease: 93-case experience. J Vasc Surg 2004; 40: 899–906

DeRoeck A, Hendriks JM, Delrue F, et al. Long-term results of primary stenting for long and complex iliac artery occlusions. Acta Chir Belg 2006; 106: 187–192

Dimick JB, Cowan JA Jr, Henke PK, et al. Hospital volume-related differences in aortobifemoral bypass operative mortality in the United States. J Vasc Surg 2003; 37: 970–975

Liapis CD, Balzer IK, Benedetti-Valentini F, Fernandes e Fernandes J, eds. Vascular Surgery. European Manual of Medicine. Berlin: Springer; 2007

Ragg JC, Biamino G. Perforations in recanalization of arterial occlusions in the femoropopliteal area. Zentralbl Chir 2000; 125: 34–41

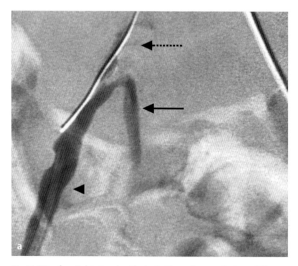
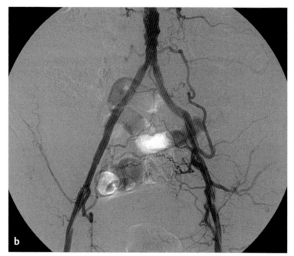

Fig. 7.33 a, b Subintimal catheterization of an occlusion of the right common iliac artery in a different patient. As in the principal case study, this occlusion was recanalized with a partial subintimal dissection from the proximal side (dotted arrow). An ipsilateral catheter was advanced into the occlusion from the distal side (arrowhead). Solid arrow = internal iliac artery.

a Subintimal catheterization.
b Completion angiogram.

Complication of Intra-Arterial Thrombolytic Therapy?

History and Clinical Findings

A 72-year-old woman presented with ischemia of the right lower leg, which was cold to the touch on physical examination. The patient was underweight (height 155 cm, weight 35 kg) and in a debilitated condition. Cachexia, a goiter, an enlarged liver, and peripheral edema were also noted on physical examination. The skin of the right lower leg and foot was marbled, and the toes were numb and showed bluish discoloration. Peripheral pedal pulses could not be palpated, and Doppler wedge pressures were not measurable. The left leg was clinically normal. Intra-arterial digital subtraction angiography (DSA) of the right leg revealed long, poorly collateralized occlusions of the superficial femoral artery from the femoral bifurcation to the adductor canal, and of the distal popliteal artery extending to the tibioperoneal trunk and tibial arteries (**Fig. 7.34**). The large arteries of the abdomen, pelvis, and left lower limb appeared normal except for atherosclerotic wall irregularities.

The fresh thromboembolism was treated by initiating intra-arterial thrombolytic therapy with urokinase in the same sitting (**Fig. 7.35**). The occlusions of the right femoropopliteal and crural arteries were catheterized through a sheath placed in the left common femoral artery using crossover technique. A bolus of 200 000 IU urokinase was injected into the distal popliteal artery from that catheter position. The catheter was then withdrawn into the proximal superficial femoral artery while 200 000 IU urokinase was administered by fractioned injection. Afterward the thrombolytic therapy was continued by infusing 100 000 IU urokinase per hour while the patient was heparinized to 2.5 times the baseline PTT (normal value of 38 seconds is prolonged by heparin therapy). Angiography following the administration of 800 000 IU urokinase showed recanalization of the right lower-extremity arteries down to the lower leg. The residual occlusion of the distal posterior tibial artery was catheterized to the level of the ankle joint. After another bolus injection of 200 000 IU urokinase, the catheter was withdrawn into the popliteal artery and the urokinase infusion was continued with the catheter in that position. Completion angiography following the total infusion of 3 450 000 IU urokinase 28 hours after the start of thrombolytic therapy showed residual thrombi in the proximal superficial femoral artery, atherosclerotic wall changes in the distal superficial femoral artery, and a collateralized occlusion of the distal posterior tibial artery and distal peroneal artery (**Fig. 7.35**).

After coagulation times returned to normal, the sheath was removed from the left common femoral artery. The puncture tract was manually compressed. When hemostasis was achieved, a pressure dressing was placed on the groin. Shortly thereafter the patient complained of rest pain in the left leg. Color duplex scans showed a fresh occlusion of the common femoral artery and superficial femoral artery on the left side.

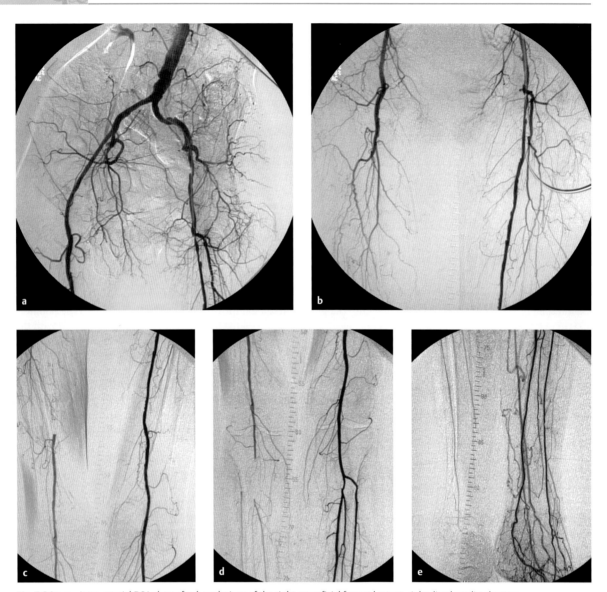

Fig. 7.34 a–e Intra-arterial DSA shows fresh occlusions of the right superficial femoral artery, right distal popliteal artery, and tibioperoneal trunk.

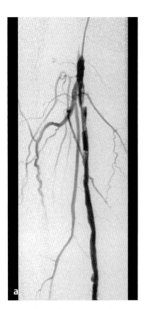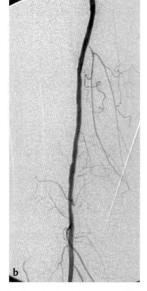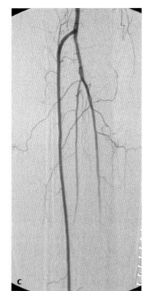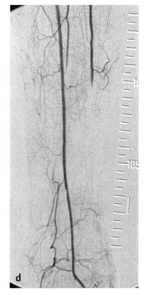

Fig. 7.35 a–d Final angiograms following the local intra-arterial infusion of 3 450 000 IU of urokinase over a 28-hour period show patency of the right superficial femoral artery, popliteal artery, and tibioperoneal trunk. The images also show recurrent stenosis of the proximal superficial femoral artery and peripheral occlusions of the distal posterior tibial artery and peroneal artery.

Further Case Summary

The new arterial thromboembolism on the left side was treated by thrombectomy and patch grafting of the left common femoral artery. Despite full heparinization, reocclusions of the left femoral arteries occurred on the first and second postoperative days and necessitated surgical reintervention. Meanwhile the patient's platelet count fell from 250 000 to 135 000. This was initially interpreted as heparin-induced thrombocytopenia, but corresponding antibody tests were negative. Anticoagulation was switched from heparin to lepirudin (Refludan). The patient's general condition deteriorated during the next few days, and she required intensive care. Laboratory tests showed a steady rise of retention values, transaminases, bilirubin, and creatine kinase. CT findings were suspicious for cystic pancreatic carcinoma, diffuse hepatic metastasis, and necrotizing bowel ischemia (**Fig. 7.36**). Diagnostic laparotomy confirmed the diagnoses. Intraoperative frozen section histology of a liver biopsy yielded a diagnosis of undifferentiated adenocarcinoma of the biliary tract or exocrine pancreas. Due to the grave prognosis, the operation was concluded as a diagnostic laparotomy. The patient died several hours later on a regular ward.

Error Analysis and Strategy for Error Prevention

Viewed in retrospect, this case ran an inevitable clinical course. The cachexia and hepatomegaly should have suggested the possibility of a malignant underlying disease on initial presentation and during selection for intra-arterial thrombolytic therapy. Because metastatic lesions would have contraindicated intra-arterial thrombolytic therapy due to the bleeding risk, the therapy should have been preceded by chest x-rays and abdominal ultrasound. Since the right leg was severely ischemic and the hypercoagulability of the blood due to paraneoplastic syndrome was not known to be present when treatment was planned, it was decided to proceed with thrombolytic therapy in the present case.

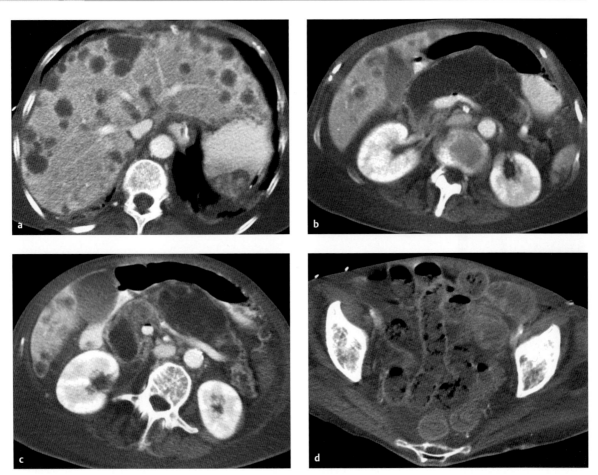

Fig. 7.36 a–d CT demonstrates hepatic metastases (**a–c**) and a malignant cystic mass in the head of the pancreas (**b, c**). Air in the superior mesenteric vein (**b, c**) and thick-walled loops of small bowel (**d**) are secondary to segmental occlusion of the superior mesenteric artery.

Complication of Peripheral Intra-Arterial Thrombolytic Therapy

History and Clinical Findings

An 89-year-old man was hospitalized with acute ischemia of the left leg diagnosed as Fontaine stage III disease (see **Table 7.1**, p. 332). He had age-related dementia and had suffered a stroke several years before that resolved without clinical deficits. Years earlier he had undergone surgical treatment of a femoral neck fracture. He had no other known preexisting or coexisting illnesses. Clinical examination showed a general deterioration of health status and raised suspicion of a fresh thromboembolic occlusion of the left lower extremity arteries.

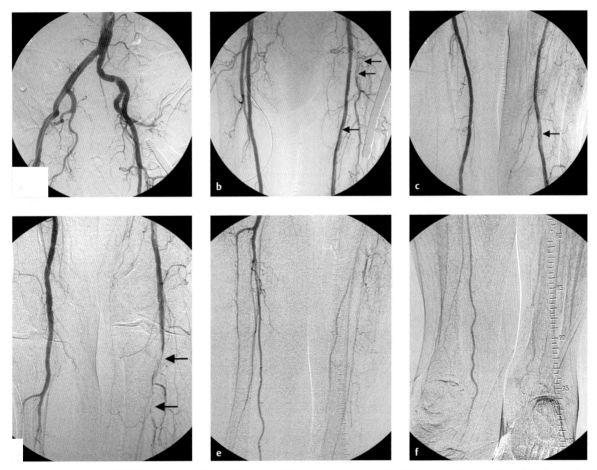

Fig. 7.37 a–f Intra-arterial DSA. Thromboembolism has caused filling defects (arrows) in the left profunda femoris artery (**b**), left superficial femoral artery (**b, c**), left popliteal artery (**d**) and left crural arteries (**d–f**).

Since the patient complained of rest pain, the limb was evaluated by angiography with facilities ready for interventional treatment if needed. Angiograms confirmed a fresh thromboembolism of the left superficial femoral artery and left profunda femoris artery (**Fig. 7.37**). The thromboembolus in the superficial femoral artery extended from the femoral bifurcation past the popliteal segment and into the proximal crural arteries. After consultation with the vascular surgeon, the left superficial femoral artery and left profunda femoris artery were catheterized through a right femoral approach using a crossover technique (**Fig. 7.38**). The catheter was also advanced into the posterior tibial artery and peroneal artery.

As the catheter was withdrawn, 400 000 IU of urokinase was injected into the partially occluded vessels. Next, with the patient heparinized to 2.5 times the baseline PTT and the catheter placed with its tip in the popliteal artery, urokinase was infused through the catheter at a rate of 100 000 IU/h. Angiography performed through the catheter in the popliteal artery 13 hours after the start of thrombolytic therapy (i.e., after the total intra-arterial infusion of 1 700 000 IU urokinase) showed incipient dissolution of the thrombi (**Fig. 7.39**), so the therapy was continued. Approximately 4 hours later the patient became obtunded and hypotensive and developed the clinical manifestations of an acute abdomen.

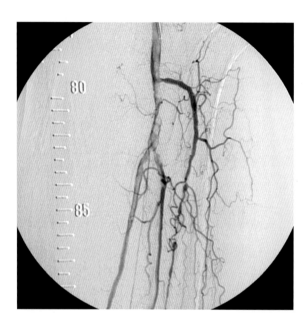

Fig. 7.38   Intra-arterial thrombolytic therapy. Visualization of the thrombus during urokinase infusion.

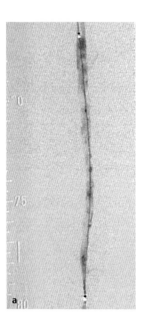 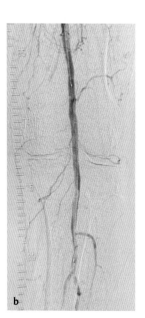

Fig. 7.39 a, b   Intra-arterial thrombolytic therapy. Residual thrombosis following the administration of 1.7 million IU urokinase.

Further Case Summary

Intra-arterial thrombolytic therapy was discontinued. The patient's blood pressure stabilized after the administration of packed red blood cells. CT revealed fresh hematomas in the psoas muscle, mesenteric root, and anterior abdominal wall (**Fig. 7.40**). Unenhanced cranial CT confirmed the old left hemispheric infarction (**Fig. 7.41**). Intracerebral hemorrhage and acute cerebral ischemia were initially excluded. Selective DSA of the visceral arter-

ies showed displacement of the small bowel by the hematoma in the mesenteric root (**Fig. 7.42**). A bleeding site could not be identified on images or at endoscopy. Meanwhile, new thrombi had formed in the left superficial femoral artery and left profunda femoris artery (**Fig. 7.43**). Since they threatened the vitality of the limb, they were surgically removed by thromboembolectomy. When respiratory failure ensued, a tracheostomy was performed and the patient was placed on mechanical ventilation. The patient subsequently developed a pulmonary embolism

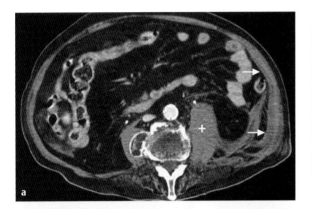

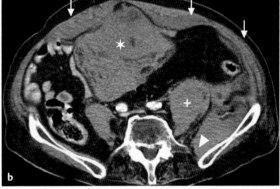

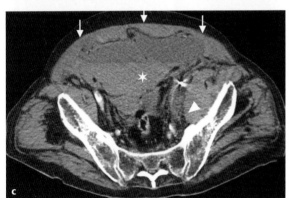

Fig. 7.40 a–c Abdominal CT scans one day after **Fig. 7.37** show fresh hemorrhagic areas in the psoas muscle (+ in **a** and **b**), iliacus muscle (arrowhead in **b** and **c**), mesentery (✱ in **b** and **c**) and abdominal wall (arrows).

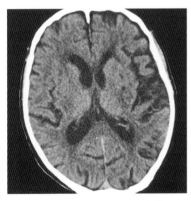

Fig. 7.41 CT detection of an old left middle cerebral artery infarction. There is no evidence of recent bleeding.

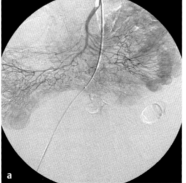

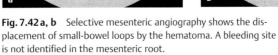

Fig. 7.42 a, b Selective mesenteric angiography shows the displacement of small-bowel loops by the hematoma. A bleeding site is not identified in the mesenteric root.

a Arterial perfusion phase.

b Venous perfusion phase.

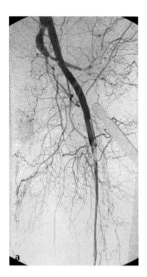

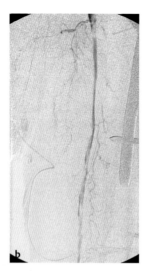

Fig. 7.43 a, b Selective angiography of the left lower-extremity arteries the day after intra-arterial thrombolytic therapy demonstrates new thrombi in the profunda femoris and superficial femoral arteries.

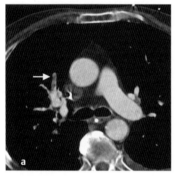

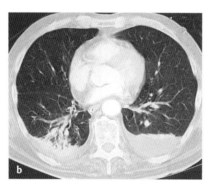

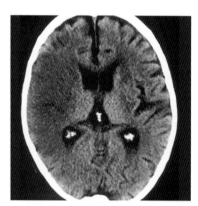

Fig. 7.44 a, b Thoracic CT scans 3 weeks after intra-arterial thrombolytic therapy.
a Thromboembolus in a segmental branch of the right pulmonary artery (arrow).
b Dystelectasis in both lower lobes and bilateral pleural effusions.

Fig. 7.45 Noncontrast cranial CT scan 3 weeks after intra-arterial thrombolytic therapy displays an extensive right hemispheric infarction.

(**Fig. 7.44**) and suffered another infarction in the right MCA territory (**Fig. 7.45**). He died 3 weeks after the conclusion of thrombolytic therapy.

Error Analysis and Strategy for Error Prevention

Without interventional revascularization or surgical recanalization, the patient would have had a grave prognosis due to lower-extremity ischemia. Thus, the indication for intra-arterial thrombolytic therapy was weighed against the relative bleeding risks (*relative contraindications:* advanced age, old cerebral infarction, senile dementia, general debilitation) as well as the anesthesia and surgical risks. None of these risks is an absolute contraindication to intra-arterial thrombolysis. The following would be considered *absolute contraindications* to that procedure: fresh

cerebral infarction, arterial puncture, muscular injection or surgery in the previous 2 weeks, gastrointestinal ulcers, aneurysms, metastatic tumors, hematologic bleeding diathesis, renal failure, severe liver disease, or thrombi in the left atrium. Studies have reported success rates of approximately 70–90% for intra-arterial thrombolytic therapy. The primary patency rates at 1 month, 30-day morbidity, and 30-day mortality have been reported as 55%, <30%, and <3%, respectively. Surgical revascularization has alleged 30-day morbidity rates of up to 4% and 30-day mortality rates of <3% (range 0.9%–7.8%). A Cochrane meta-analysis summarized all randomized studies on the treatment of lower extremity ischemia that met the criteria of evidence-based medicine. In the 1283 cases analyzed, there was no statistically significant difference between intra-arterial thrombolytic therapy and surgery regarding the rates of limb loss or patient death at 30 days, 6 months, and 1 year. The group treated by intra-arterial thrombolysis had a higher incidence of strokes at 30 days than the surgically treated group (8 of 840 patients vs. 0 of 540 patients). They also had higher rates of bleeding complications (52/588 vs. 16/482) and distal embolization (42/340 vs. 0/338). The overall survival rates were the same in both groups, however. Initial intra-arterial thrombolysis tended to be followed by fewer serious reinterventions and operations during the further course of the disease.

In the case presented here, interventional radiology treatment was initially a sound and reasonable choice. All laboratory tests showed that the coagulation parameters were within the desired therapeutic range. But given the risk profile for bleeding (see relative contraindications) and the poor angiographic results after the administration of 1.7 million IU urokinase (**Fig. 7.39**), intra-arterial thrombolytic therapy should have been discontinued at an earlier time. Angiographic response should have been checked after the administration of 1.2–1.5 million IU urokinase; experience has shown that this should be sufficient to produce a systemically effective urokinase level. When lack of response had been promptly confirmed, it would have been appropriate to discontinue intra-arterial thrombolysis without further delay.

References and Further Reading

Berridge DC, Kessel D, Robertson I. Surgery vs. thrombolysis for acute ischemic limb ischemia: initial management. Cochrane Database Syst Rev 2002; (3): CD002784

Korn P, Khilnani NM, Fellers JC, et al. Thrombolysis for native arterial occlusions of the lower extremities: clinical outcome and costs. J Vasc Surg 2001; 33: 1148–1157

Liapis CD, Balzer IK, Benedetti-Valentini F, Fernandes E, Fernandes J, eds. Vascular Surgery. European Manual of Medicine. Berlin: Springer; 2007

Wholey MH, Maynar MA, Wholey MH, et al. Comparison of thrombolytic therapy of lower-extremity acute, subacute, and chronic arterial occlusions. Cathet Cardiovasc Diagn 1998; 44: 159–169

Vertebrogenic Back Pain/ Retroperitoneal Hematoma

History and Clinical Findings

A 56-year-old man underwent coronary angiography for the investigation of suspected coronary heart disease. The ward physician was requested to perform a color duplex scan of the groin the next morning for a "complicated" puncture of the right femoral artery. Shortly after the cardiac catheterization, the patient developed severe back pain. When his blood pressure also fell, a noncontrast abdominal CT examination was performed 5 hours after the procedure. The CT scans showed a retroperitoneal hematoma that contained contrast medium (**Fig. 7.46**).

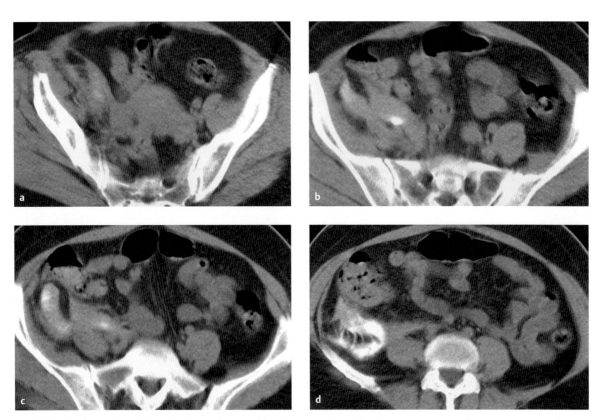

Fig. 7.46 a–d Noncontrast abdominal CT scans show a right-sided retroperitoneal hematoma containing radiopaque contrast medium.

Further Case Summary

The contrast medium was present in a concentration sufficient to produce attenuation values of approximately 120 HU. This could only have resulted from a perforation of the artery wall during cardiac catheterization. A review of the images documenting the coronary angiography showed that a significant volume of contrast medium had extravasated into the retroperitoneum through a perforation in the right iliac artery (**Fig. 7.47**). The contrast extravasation was treated conservatively.

Error Analysis and Strategy for Error Prevention

The risk of perforating the iliac artery was underestimated. While arterial injuries caused by femoral artery puncture below the inguinal ligament can be controlled by compressing the artery wall defect owing to counterpressure from the underlying bones and muscles of the thigh, punctures or injuries above the inguinal ligament cannot be controlled in this manner. Blood spurting from the iliac artery into the extraperitoneal fibrofatty tissue can spread freely along myofascial planes up into the retroperitoneum and down into the soft tissues of the thigh. The hemorrhage may reach a volume of several liters. Approximately 50% of these retroperitoneal hematomas will require operative treatment. There have been isolated reports of fatal outcomes.

The nature and incidence of serious complications of angiography and angiocardiography are listed in **Table 7.2**. The use of large-bore sheaths and catheters, a high ingui-

Table 7.2 Meta-analysis of local complications of femoral vascular punctures in 61 859 diagnostic cardiac catheterizations and percutaneous coronary interventions reported in the list of references.

Type of complication	Incidence (%)	
	Mean value	Range of values
False aneurysm	0.2	0.1–0.6
Retroperitoneal hematoma (blood transfusion, surgery)	0.5	0.1–0.7
Arteriovenous fistulas	0.1	0.1
Arterial dissection	0.1	0.1
Local vascular occlusion	0.5	0.1–0.8
Peripheral thromboembolism	0.2	0.1–0.6
Infections	0.2	0.1–0.3

nal puncture, systemic anticoagulation, thrombocytopenia or coagulopathies, and peripheral arterial occlusive disease promote the occurrence of complications. Swelling and muscular rigidity of the abdomen on the side of the puncture (100%), abdominal, back and groin pain (23–64%), bradycardia (31%), a fall in blood pressure (92%), and a fall in the hematocrit are clinical signs of retroperitoneal hematoma.

References and Further Reading

Farouque HM, Tremmel JA, Raissi Shabari F, et al. Risk factors for the development of retroperitoneal hematoma after percutaneous coronary intervention in the era of glycoprotein IIb/IIIa inhibitors and vascular closure devices. J Am Coll Cardiol 2005; 45: 363–368

Fransson SG, Nylander E. Vascular injury following cardiac catheterization, coronary angiography, and coronary angioplasty. Eur Heart J 1994; 15: 232–235

Fruhwirth J, Pascher O, Hauser H, Amman W. [Local vascular complications after iatrogenic femoral artery puncture.] Wien Klin Wochenschr 1996; 108: 196–200

Heintzen MP, Schumacher T, Rath J, et al. Incidence and therapy of peripheral arterial vascular complications after heart catheter examinations. Z Kardiol 1997; 86: 264–272

Hirano Y, Ikuta S, Uehara H, et al. Diagnosis of vascular complications at the puncture site after cardiac catheterization. J Cardiol 2004; 43: 259–265

Kaufmann J, Moglia R, Lacy C, Dinerstein C, Moreyra A. Peripheral vascular complications from percutaneous transluminal coronary angioplasty: a comparison with transfemoral cardiac catheterization. Am J Med Sci 1989; 297: 22–25

Kent KVC, Moscucci M, Mansour KA, et al. Retroperitoneal hematoma after cardiac catheterization: prevalence, risk factors, and optimal management. J Vasc Surg 1994; 20: 905–910

Ricci MA, Trevisani GT, Pilcher DB. Vascular complications of cardiac catheterization. Am J Surg 1994; 167: 375–378

Sreeram S, Lumsden AB, Miller JS, Salam AA, Dodson TF, Smith RB. Retroperitoneal hematoma following femoral arterial catheterization: a serious and often fatal complication. Am Surg 1993; 59: 94–98

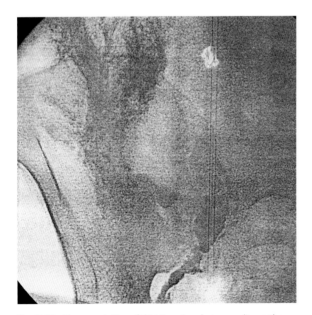

Fig. 7.47 Documentation of DSA imaging during cardiac catheterization. This thermoprint from the patient's chart shows that contrast medium extravasated from the right iliac artery and diffused into retroperitoneal fibrofatty tissues.

Complication of a Transjugular Intrahepatic Portosystemic Shunt?

History and Clinical Findings

A 68-year-old woman suffered from refractory ascites due to hepatic cirrhosis secondary to chronic hepatitis C. She was placed on the waiting list for a liver transplant. Her serum GOT was 70 U/L ($<$ 35 U/L is normal); GPT was 41 U/L ($<$ 35 U/L is normal); γ-GT was 58 U/L ($<$ 40 U/L is normal); total bilirubin was 2.1 mg/dL ($<$ 1.1 mg/dL is normal); platelet count was 90000/L (normal range is 150000–400000); and the Quick PT was 67. A transjugular intrahepatic portosystemic shunt (TIPS) was inserted (**Fig. 7.48**). This is an interventional procedure in which a communication is created between the right or middle hepatic vein and the intrahepatic portal vein in the right or left lobe of the liver and is maintained by inserting a stent. Blood from the portal vein is mainly shunted along the pressure gradient into the hepatic vein and thence to the inferior vena cava. The reduction of portal venous pressure by the TIPS procedure improves the abnormal hemodynamics in the splanchnic bed, thereby reducing or preventing the development of ascites in many patients.

During the intervention a catheter was advanced into the middle hepatic vein via the right internal jugular vein (**Fig. 7.49**). A main branch of the portal vein in the right lobe of the liver was punctured under ultrasound guidance via the catheter in the middle hepatic vein. After the catheter was advanced into the portal vein, a portosystemic pressure gradient of 21 mm Hg was measured, indicating that the patient was a good candidate for the TIPS procedure. The parenchymal tract between the middle hepatic vein and portal vein was dilated. The wall of the portal vein was found to be so rigid that it could be dilated only with a cutting balloon (special catheter with microsurgical blades on the balloon that cut longitudinal slits in the vessel wall). This was followed by the implantation of a balloon-expandable stent. Luminal narrowing at the junction with the hepatic vein was managed by the overlapping insertion of a balloon-expandable stent. Angiography immediately after stent placement showed thrombi in the distal portion of the TIPS stent with sluggish perfusion of the stent, so the entire TIPS tract was dilated to a diameter of 10 mm. The completion angiogram showed brisk perfusion of the TIPS stent and faint opacification of the intrahepatic portal vein branches. The measured portosystemic pressure gradient was 10 mm Hg. Long segmental narrowing of the portal vein due to an unknown cause persisted at its junction with the stent. Following the intervention, the patient was moved to the gastroenterology ward.

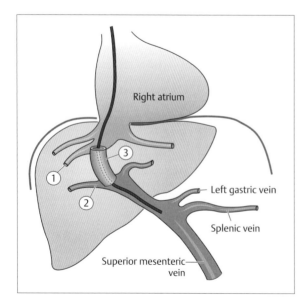

Fig. 7.48 Diagrammatic representation of the TIPS procedure. Percutaneous access is established through the internal jugular vein, and a catheter is advanced through the vena cava and right atrium into the right or middle hepatic vein (1) under fluoroscopic guidance. A needle is advanced through the wall of the hepatic vein and into an intrahepatic portal vein branch (2), aided if necessary by ultrasound guidance. The parenchymal tract between the liver and portal vein branch is dilated with a balloon catheter (8–10 mm) and then stabilized with stents of the desired luminal size (3). While a mean pretherapeutic pressure gradient of 20–40 mm Hg is measured between the portal vein and vena cava in portal hypertension, the treatment goal is to achieve a residual gradient of approximately 10 mm Hg after stent insertion. This residual gradient will ensure that the liver is not completely isolated from the portal circulation (risk of encephalopathy).

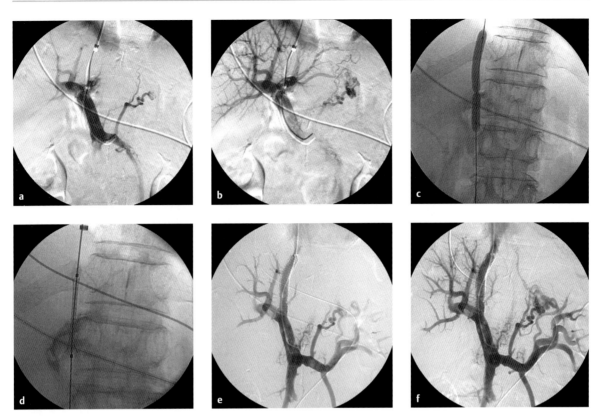

Fig. 7.49 a–f Image documentation of TIPS placement, performed as described in the legend to **Fig. 7.48**.
a Puncture of the portal vein, early perfusion phase.
b Puncture of the portal vein, late perfusion phase.
c Balloon dilatation of the junction of the parenchymal tract and portal vein.

d Stent expansion along the parenchymal tract.
e Completion angiogram in the early perfusion phase shows good stent perfusion with normal residual perfusion of the intrahepatic portal vein branches.
f Completion angiogram in the late perfusion phase.

Further Case Summary

The patient died a few hours after the intervention without showing any clinical abnormalities and without calling for help. The postmortem needle aspiration of ascites confirmed the presence of intraperitoneal hemorrhage. Autopsy revealed a perforation in the surface of the liver, which was considered the cause of the fatal hemorrhage. The liver may be injured during the intrahepatic puncture of a portal vein branch if the needle is advanced too far and pierces the surface of the organ. This risk is greater in patients with a shrunken liver.

Error Analysis and Strategy for Error Prevention

The intervention-associated mortality rate of the TIPS procedure is approximately 1 % based on published studies. Many of these deaths are caused by intraperitoneal hemorrhage due to puncture of the extrahepatic portion of the portal vein (**Fig. 7.50**). It has been recommended, therefore, that the right branch of the portal vein be punctured at least 1–2 cm distal to the bifurcation, as only the relatively peripheral portal vein segments are definitely intrahepatic and surrounded by liver parenchyma. This is a particularly good precaution in patients with hepatic cirrhosis, because shrinkage of the right lobe has the effect of lengthening the extrahepatic portal vein segments. The bifurcation is often extrahepatic in patients with hepatic cirrhosis. In the case presented here, the portal vein was punctured in the area where the main trunk divides into the right and left portal vein branches. This suggested that the puncture had injured the extrahepatic portal vein, but autopsy showed that only the surface of the liver had been injured. Since a slow intraperitoneal hemorrhage causes few symptoms, it would have been appropriate to place the patient in the ICU for observation. The puncture site in the liver surface found at autopsy resulted from the intervention.

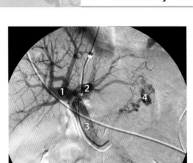
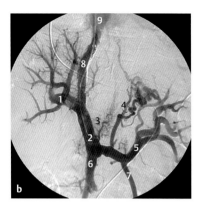

Fig. 7.50 a, b Keys to images in **Fig. 7.49 b** and **f**.

a Key to **Fig. 7.49 b**.
- 1 = Intrahepatic branches of the right portal vein
- 2 = Intrahepatic branches of the left portal vein
- 3 = Extrahepatic portal vein
- 4 = Coronary vein of the stomach and varices supplied by it

b Key to **Fig. 7.49 f**.
- 1 = Intrahepatic branches of right portal vein branch
- 2 = Extrahepatic portal vein
- 3 = Left gastric vein with varices
- 4 = Coronary vein of the stomach and varices supplied by it
- 5 = Splenic vein
- 6 = Superior mesenteric vein
- 7 = Inferior mesenteric vein
- 8 = TIPS
- 9 = Right atrium

Ascites in Hepatic Cirrhosis

Ascites in patients with hepatic cirrhosis develops as a result of decompensated liver dysfunction and is an unfavorable prognostic sign. The average survival time in patients with refractory ascites is less than 5 years.

Pathophysiology. Several factors are involved in the pathophysiology of ascites in hepatic cirrhosis. As the synthetic function of the liver declines, blood albumin levels fall, leading to a decreased colloid osmotic pressure in the blood vessels. This is accompanied by vasodilation in the splanchnic bed. As peripheral resistance declines in the splanchnic bed, the peripheral resistance in the rest of the systemic circulation (kidneys, muscles, brain) remains normal or elevated, leading to local hyperperfusion. The high blood flow in the microcirculation raises the hydrostatic pressure, resulting in an increased production of lymph. When lymph production exceeds the capacity for lymph drainage, the fluid enters the peritoneal cavity and ascites develops. The hyperperfusion of the splanchnic vessels leads to a regulatory hypoperfusion of the kidneys. With activation of the renin–angiotensin system, the kidneys retain greater amounts of sodium and water, leading to further deterioration in the circulatory status of the liver, small bowel, and colon.

Treatment. If conservative measures such as a low-sodium diet and diuretic therapy are insufficient to control ascites ("refractory ascites"), the treatment methods of choice are paracentesis and TIPS placement. Several randomized prospective studies have shown that TIPS is superior to paracentesis in the control of ascites. A meta-analysis of four studies found that the transplant-free 2-year survival rate was 49% in TIPS patients compared with 35% in paracentesis patients. TIPS placement did not affect average survival time, however. Since the procedure routes blood past the liver, the TIPS patients were more likely to experience further deterioration of liver function and chronic hepatic encephalopathy, resulting in no overall difference in survival times between the groups.

The clinical manifestations of an intra-abdominal hemorrhage tend to be subtle. Generally they involve a slow, continuous bleed based on abnormal coagulation (liver dysfunction) combined with the residual pressure gradient in the portal venous system after the TIPS placement and the increased splanchnic blood volume that occurs in hepatic cirrhosis.

References and Further Reading

Arroyo V. Pathophysiology, diagnosis and treatment of ascites in cirrhosis. Ann Hepatol 2002; 1: 72–79

Boyer TD. Transjugular intrahepatic portosystemic shunt: current status. Gastroenterology 2003; 124: 1700–1710

Boyer TD. Transjugular intrahepatic portosystemic shunt in the management of complications of portal hypertension. Curr Gastroenterol Rep 2008; 10: 30–35

Brountzos EN, Alexopoulou E, Koskinas I, Thanos L, Papathanasiou MA, Kelekis DA. Intraperitoneal portal vein bleeding during transjugular intrahepatic portosystemic shunt. AJR 2000; 174: 132–134

Gore RM. Ascites and peritoneal fluid collections. In: Gore RM, Levine MS, Laufer I, eds. Gastrointestinal Radiology. Philadelphia: WB Saunders; 1994: 2352–2366

Hassoun Z, Pomier-Layrargues G. The transjugular intrahepatic portosystemic shunt in the treatment of portal hypertension. Eur J Gastroenterol Hepatol 2004; 16: 9–18

Owen RJT, Rose JDG. Endovascular treatment of a portal vein tear during TIPS. Cardiovasc Intervent Radiol 2000; 23: 230–232

Rossle M, Haag K, Ochs A, et al. The transjugular intrahepatic portosystemic stent-shunt procedure for variceal bleeding. N Engl J Med 1994; 330: 165–171

Tripathi D, Helmy A, Macbeth K, et al. Ten year's follow-up of 472 patients following transjugular intrahepatic portosystemic stent-shunt insertion at a single centre. Eur J Gastroenterol Hepatol 2004; 16: 9–18

Hepatic Metastases from Colon Cancer: Complication of Transarterial Chemoembolization

History and Clinical Findings

A 38-year-old woman underwent a left hemicolectomy for sigmoid cancer. Three months later, CT detected metastases in multiple segments of the liver. The lesions were considered inoperable because of their distribution (**Table 7.3**, see p. 358).

Transarterial chemoembolization (TACE) of the liver was undertaken as a palliative treatment. The chemoembolic mixture was a suspension of degradable starch microspheres (Spherex), mitomycin C (15 mg/m^2 body surface area), and the oily contrast agent lipiodol. The starch microspheres, measuring approximately 40 μm in diameter, served to temporarily occlude the precapillary arte-

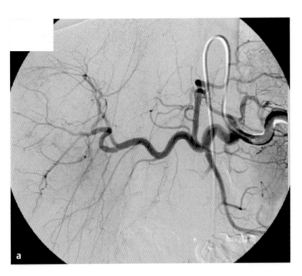

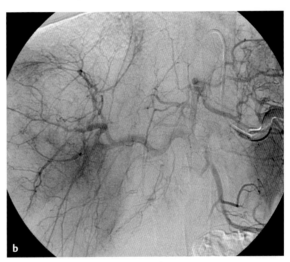

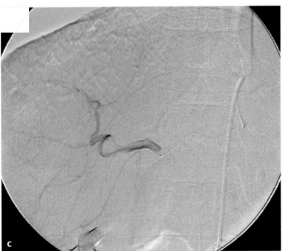

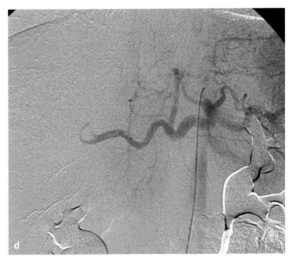

Fig. 7.51 a–d   Transarterial chemoembolization of the liver (TACE), initial treatment. Hyperperfused masses are projected over the right lobe of the liver (**a, b**). Chemoembolic material is injected from a superselective catheter position into the right hepatic artery (**c**). Normal, transient vascular occlusion is confirmed at the end of the procedure (**d**).

a Indirect splenoportography, arterial phase.
b Indirect splenoportography, parenchymal phase.
c Superselective catheterization of the right hepatic artery.
d Completion angiogram.

Table 7.3 Patient selection criteria for the TACE of hepatic metastases

- Resection of the primary colorectal tumor
- No extrahepatic metastases
- Tumors permeating < 75 % of the liver
- Karnofsky index > 50 %
- Inoperable liver tumors
- Patent portal vein with antegrade perfusion
- Bilirubin < 2.5 mg/dL
- Cholinesterase > 1 kU/L
- Quick PT > 50 %
- Creatinine < 2.5 mg/dL
- Platelets > 100 000/μL
- WBC > 2000/L
- Hemoglobin (Hb) > 10 g/dL

rioles of the hepatic artery. Mitomycin C is a chemotherapeutic drug that is active against metastases from colon carcinoma under hypoxic conditions. It has a high liver extraction rate and a short plasma half-life. The chemoembolization mixture was infused while its flow was monitored by fluoroscopy.

The first chemoembolization was performed without complications (**Fig. 7.51**). The second chemoembolization was performed 5 weeks later (**Fig. 7.52**), and immediately afterward the patient complained of back pain. The pain improved during the further hospital stay, and the patient was discharged 2 days later. On the same night she was discharged, the patient was readmitted with new, girdling upper abdominal pain. Her ECG was normal. Laboratory tests showed WBC elevated to 16 200/μL and CRP elevated to 187 mg/L. Pancreatic enzymes were within normal limits.

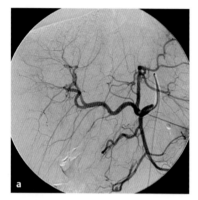 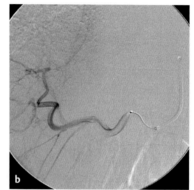 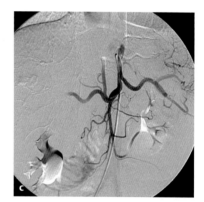

Fig. 7.52 a–c   Second TACE 5 weeks after the initial treatment. The peripheral branches of the right hepatic artery are somewhat thinned compared with the first intervention (**a**). Chemoembolization from a superselective catheter placement in the right hepatic artery (**b**). Normal, transient vascular occlusion is seen at the end of the second procedure (**c**).

a Selective angiography of the hepatic artery and its branches.
b Superselective catheterization of the right hepatic artery.
c Completion angiogram.

Further Case Summary

Abdominal CT scans after readmission mainly showed thickening of the gallbladder wall, which also displayed contour irregularities and abnormal contrast enhancement. A small pericholecystic fluid collection was also found (**Fig. 7.53**). Ischemic necrotizing cholecystitis was suspected, and surgical cholecystectomy was performed the same evening. The presumptive diagnosis was confirmed at operation. Histology revealed suppurative ulcerating cholecystitis.

Error Analysis and Strategy for Error Prevention

The development of ischemic cholecystitis in the setting of TACE results from improper positioning of the catheter during infusion of the chemoembolic material. The following situations may arise:

- The tip of the catheter is proximal to the origin of the cystic artery from the proper hepatic artery during embolization, so that absorbable starch particles and the cytostatic drug are delivered not only to the intrahepatic target but also to the cystic artery and its side branches, causing the occlusion of those vessels. When the position of the microcatheter was checked before

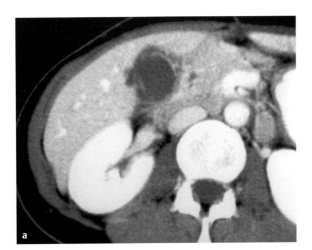

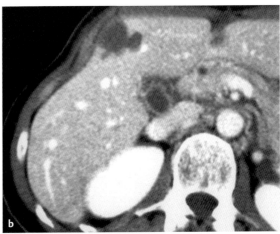

Fig. 7.53 a, b Abdominal CT on the third day after the second TACE shows cholecystitis with discontinuities, thickening, and abnormal enhancement of the gallbladder wall, accompanied by fluid in the gallbladder bed. The smooth-bordered hypodense masses in the hepatic parenchyma are necrotic metastases that were shrunk relative to the first CT examination as a result of the second TACE procedure.

chemoembolization, the catheter tip occupied a position that was several centimeters more proximal than during the first TACE (**Fig. 7.54** and **7.55**). This mechanism could account for the cholecystitis in the case under review.

- In another scenario the tip of the catheter is just distal to the origin of the cystic artery, which supplies the gallbladder and cystic duct. But the high injection pressure or peripheral vascular occlusion cause the starch microspheres and cytostatic agent to reflux into the cystic artery.

Ischemic cholecystitis has a reported incidence of up to 2%, depending on the underlying disease (metastases, hepatocellular carcinoma) and on the chemotherapeutic agent and embolic material that are used.

Transarterial Chemoembolization (TACE)

TACE is a special form of intra-arterial embolization used in the treatment of primary and secondary hepatic tumors. One advantage of TACE compared with other treatment options (surgery, radiofrequency ablation, cryotherapy) is that it can be used in patients with extensive tumor involvement (>5 lesions) and tumors >5 cm in diameter. Cases must meet the selection criteria listed in **Table 7.3**.

Principle. The liver has a dual blood supply from the hepatic artery and portal vein, but hepatic malignancies, unlike normal liver, receive most of their blood from the hepatic artery. Embolization of the tumor-feeding vessels by local intra-arterial cytostatic therapy deprives the tumor of oxygen, and the stasis of blood flow also prolongs exposure of the tumor tissue to the cytostatic drug. This increases the concentration that is delivered to the tumor compared with systemic chemotherapy. Because the drug concentration in the extrahepatic vascular system is lower than with systemic chemotherapy, systemic side-effects are relatively mild in most cases.

Materials and technique. Various techniques and formulations are available for TACE. The most commonly used embolic materials are starch particles (Spherex), which cause transient occlusion of the targeted hepatic artery segments and are broken down by serum amylase within approximately 30 minutes, and polyvinyl alcohol particles. Lipiodol is generally used as the contrast agent. The mixture of the cytostatic drug, starch particles, and lipiodol is administered through selective or coaxial microcatheter systems under fluoroscopic guidance.

Complications. When the criteria listed in **Table 7.3** are followed, the most likely complication is postembolization syndrome. This condition is characterized by fever, pain, and vomiting resulting from extensive tumor necrosis (reactive hepatic swelling causing tension on the liver capsule).

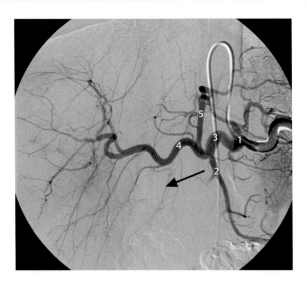

Fig. 7.54   Vascular anatomy, second TACE. 1 = Celiac trunk; 2 = gastroduodenal artery; 3 = common hepatic artery; 4 = right hepatic artery; 5 = left hepatic artery; arrow = cystic artery.

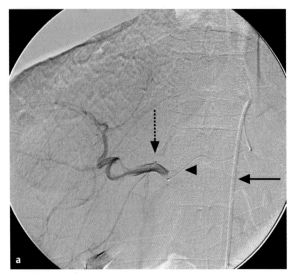

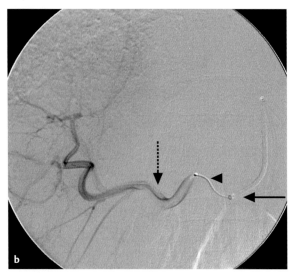

Fig. 7.55 a, b   Comparison of the superselective catheter positions in the first and second TACE procedures. Solid arrow = guide catheter; arrowhead = microcatheter; dotted arrow = right hepatic artery.

a   Catheter position for the first TACE.
b   Catheter position for the second TACE.

References and Further Reading

Kim HK, Chung YH, Song BC, et al. Ischemic bile duct injury as a serious complication after transarterial chemoembolization in patients with hepatic carcinoma. J Clin Gastroenterol 2001; 32: 423–427

Tarazov PG, Polysalov VN, Prozorovskij KV, Grishchenkova IV, Rozengauz EV. Ischemic complications of transcatheter arterial chemoembolization in liver malignancies. Acta Radiol 2000; 41: 156–160

Hepatic Rupture, Intrahepatic vs. Extrahepatic Hematoma/ Hemangioma

History and Clinical Findings

A 45-year-old woman was delivered by an emergency physician at 21:00 on a Friday. She had been seriously injured falling from a horse. Her abdomen appeared normal by inspection and palpation. Her arterial blood pressure and hemoglobin level were normal. Spiral CT scans of the skull, chest, and abdomen taken immediately after admission showed a traumatic subarachnoid hemorrhage, a fracture of the left anterior arch of the atlas, a fracture of the left clavicle, multiple rib fractures on the left side, and contusions of the left lung. The written CT report also described a 6- to 8-cm hematoma in the epigastrium (**Fig. 7.56**). The source of the hemorrhage could not be positively identified on CT scans. Bleeding from the left portal vein branch or left hepatic vein and diffuse arterial bleeding were considered as possibilities.

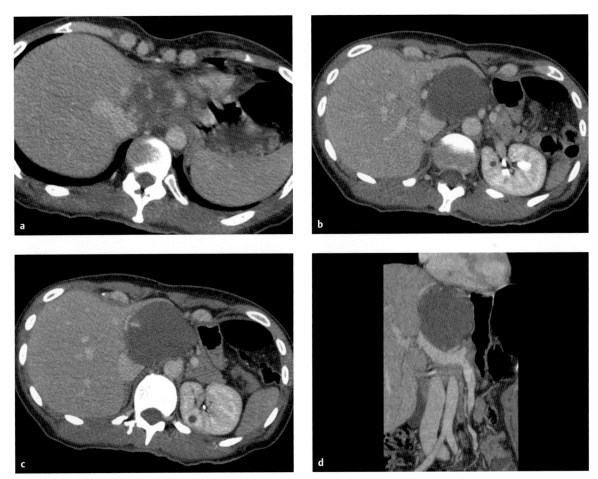

Fig. 7.56 a–d Abdominal CT after IV contrast injection showed a well-circumscribed mass in the left lobe of the liver (maximum dimensions 6 cm × 8 cm × 6 cm). The mass showed circumscribed zones of peripheral enhancement after contrast administration.

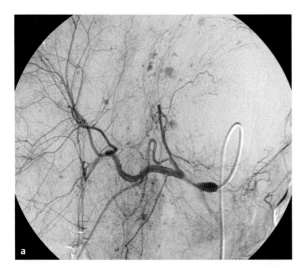

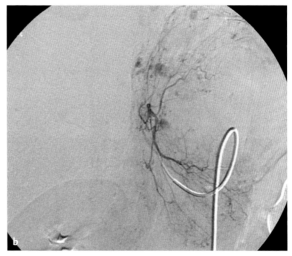

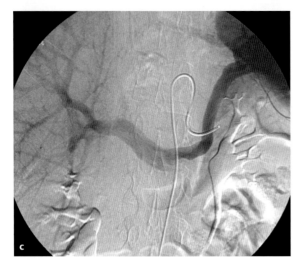

Fig. 7.57 a–c Intra-arterial DSA. A mass arising from the left lobe of the liver contains hyperperfused areas ("cotton-wool spots").
a Selective angiography of the proper hepatic artery.
b Superselective angiography of the left hepatic artery.
c Splenoportography demonstrates the splenic vein and portal vein after contrast injection into the splenic artery.

Intra-arterial DSA of the hepatic arteries was performed the next day (**Fig. 7.57**). Selective visualization of the common hepatic artery showed diffuse enhancement in the territory of the left hepatic artery that matched the location of the CT finding and was interpreted as active arterial bleeding from the left hepatic artery. This prompted selective embolization of the left hepatic artery with a mixture of histoacryl and lipiodol (**Fig. 7.58**). The intervention was performed without complications. The completion angiogram showed normal arteries in the right lobe of the liver and dearterialization of the left lobe.

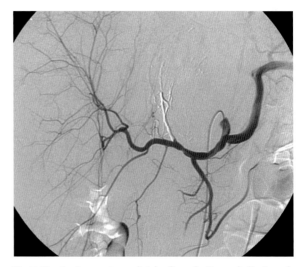

Fig. 7.58 Angiogram immediately after selective embolization of the left hepatic artery confirms occlusion of the artery with a histoacryl-lipiodol mixture.

Further Case Summary

The patient was hospitalized for several more weeks due to her subarachnoid hemorrhage and atlas fracture. Even after the intervention, abdominal findings remained normal throughout the observation period. On the Monday after admission, the weekend interventions were discussed at a meeting of interventional radiologists. It was noted that the CT findings in this patient were typical of a cavernous hemangioma. Angiography also showed cotton-wool spots that were typical of a hemangioma rather than arterial bleeding. Asymptomatic patients with a hepatic hemangioma do not require treatment and may be scheduled for ultrasound follow-ups.

Error Analysis and Strategy for Error Prevention

The diagnosis of a cavernous hemangioma was missed for the following reasons:

- The case was an emergency situation in which spiral CT was performed from the calvaria to the pelvic floor in the late perfusion phase after IV contrast administration to permit the detection of life-threatening injuries. Data acquisition in the early perfusion phase, while routinely added in elective liver examinations, was correctly omitted in this case because the patient required intensive care. The possibility of data acquisition in an even later perfusion phase (in the absence of immediately life-threatening findings) and the option of sequential CT scanning of the upper abdomen were not considered. The series of superselective diagnostic angiograms was misinterpreted because a hepatic hemangioma is no longer considered an indication for diagnostic angiography, and so its features are not widely known or recognized.
- The hemangioma had attenuation values of 33 to 39 HU, which are consistent with liquid or clotted blood. The peripheral oval hyperdensities were ectatic cavernous spaces that were enhanced by the entry of opacified blood.
- During evaluation of the CT images, the proximity of the changes to the left portal vein branch was misinterpreted as a possible rupture site, despite the absence of visible contrast extravasation arising from the left portal vein branch.
- The patient had no clinical manifestations of a ruptured liver or ruptured hemangioma. That type of injury would necessarily cause a hemoperitoneum, which was excluded by computed tomography.

Surgical resection of hepatic hemangioma is indicated only if there is a significant risk of rupture ($>$ 4–7 cm in diameter, growth) or there is a compression syndrome (gastric complaints, cholestasis, etc.) that cannot be managed by other means. There have been only sporadic reports on the embolization of hematomas by interventional radiology. The indications are the same as for surgery. Published results indicate low complication rates and high recurrence rates.

The present case also confirms that even severe trauma does not necessarily lead to rupture and bleeding from a hepatic hemangioma. From data in the literature, there is no compelling need for preventive embolization or surgical resection in asymptomatic patients.

References and Further Reading

Althaus S, Ashdown B, Coldwell D, Helton WS, Freeney P. Transcatheter arterial embolization of two symptomatic giant cavernous hemangiomas of the liver. Cardiovasc Intervent Radiol 1996; 19: 364–367

Di Carlo I, Sofia M, Toro A. Does the psychological request of the patient justify surgery for hepatic hemangioma? Hepatogastroenterology 2005; 52: 657–661

Giavroglu C, Economou H, Ioannidis I. Arterial embolization of giant hepatic hemangiomas. Cardiovasc Intervent Radiol 2003; 26: 92–96

Herman P, Costa ML, Machado MA, et al. Management of hepatic hemangiomas: a 14-year experience. J Gastrointest Surg 2005; 9: 853–859

Hosokawa A, Maeda T, Tateishi U, et al. Hepatic hemangioma presenting atypical radiologic findings: a case report. Radiat Med 2005; 23: 371–375

Masui T, Katayama M, Nakagarawa M, et al. Exophytic giant cavernous hemangioma of the liver with growing tendency. Radiat Med 2005; 23: 121–124

Moreno EA, Del Pozo RM, Vicente CM, Abellan AJ. Indications for surgery in the treatment of hepatic hemangiomas. Hepatogastroenterology 1996; 43: 422–426

Srivastava DN, Gandhi D, Seith A, et al. Transcatheter arterial embolization in the treatment of symptomatic cavernous hemangiomas of the liver: a prospective study. Abdom Imaging 2001; 26: 510–514

Yoon SS, Charny CK, Fong Y, et al. Diagnosis, management, and outcome of 115 patients with hepatic hemangioma. J Am Coll Surg 2003; 197: 392–402

Hepatocellular Carcinoma: Complication of Transarterial Chemoembolization

History and Clinical Findings

A 61-year-old woman had a 20-year history of refractory hepatic cirrhosis secondary to chronic hepatitis C. Multifocal hepatocellular carcinoma had developed in both lobes of the liver (**Fig. 7.59**). The diagnosis was confirmed histologically by percutaneous core needle biopsy. Enlarged lymph nodes up to 1 cm in diameter detected by CT in the porta hepatis were initially interpreted as reactive lymphadenitis. The tumor was inoperable due to the involvement of both hepatic lobes. To exhaust all treatment options, chemoembolization of the liver was initiated. The first two TACE treatments with a doxorubicin–lipiodol mixture were limited to the left hepatic artery, which supplied the largest tumors (**Figs. 7.60, 7.61**), in order to preserve healthy liver parenchyma. The tumors in the left lobe of the liver responded to both treatments. CT scans before the third TACE showed progression in the size and number of liver tumors (**Fig. 7.62 a**). The enlarged lymph nodes in the porta hepatis and upper retroperitoneum had

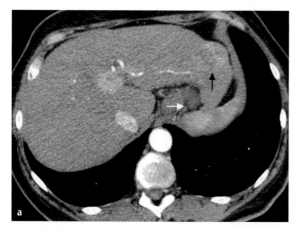

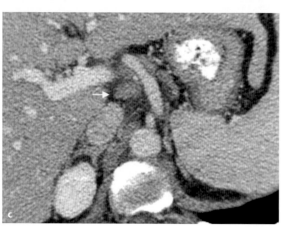

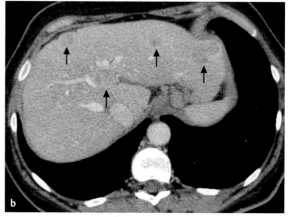

Fig. 7.59 a–c Multifocal hepatocellular carcinoma. CT before the first chemoembolization with selective treatment of the left hepatic artery shows enlarged retroperitoneal lymph nodes (white arrows).
a CT in the early arterial phase after IV contrast administration shows hyperperfused tumor elements (black arrow).
b The tumors show inhomogeneous enhancement with high peripheral density and hypodense centers (black arrows).
c Enlarged lymph nodes in the porta hepatis.

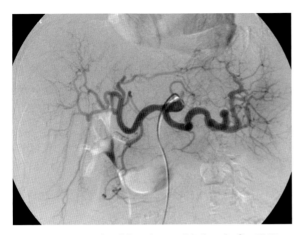

Fig. 7.60 Angiography of the celiac trunk before the first TACE procedure.

become larger and more numerous (**Fig. 7.62 b, c**). This finding was interpreted as evidence of tumor progression and of progressive lymph node metastasis. Perihepatic ascites was present. For the first time in the course of the disease, abnormalities were found in the following laboratory parameters: GOT 173 U/L (< 35 is normal), GPT 135 U/L (< 35 is normal), γ-GT 142 U/L (< 40 is normal), cholinesterase 1.3 kU/L (5.3–12.9 is normal), total bilirubin 1.7 mg/dL (< 1.1 is normal), Quick PT 66 % (normal range is 70–120 %), and platelets 60 000/µL (normal range is 150 000–400 000). TACE treatment of the right and left hepatic arteries was performed the next day using standard technique and 50 mg of a doxorubicin–lipiodol mixture (**Fig. 7.63 a, b**). The intervention was performed without complications. The patient was released from the hospital the following day.

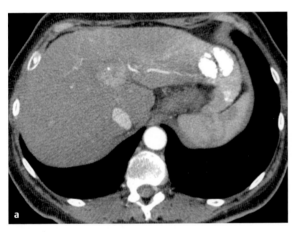

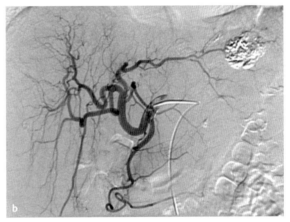

Fig. 7.61 a, b Second chemotherapy cycle.

a CT before the second TACE shows lipiodol uptake by the tumors in the left lobe of the liver. The hepatocellular carcinoma at the center of the right lobe appears unchanged.

b Angiography of the common hepatic artery before the second TACE shows lipiodol uptake in the hepatocellular carcinomas in the left lobe of the liver.

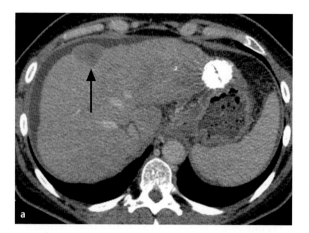

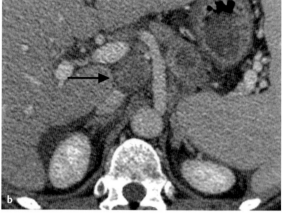

Fig. 7.62 a–c Third chemotherapy cycle. Axial CT shows increased volume of an HCC (hepatocellular carcinoma) in the right lobe of the liver (arrow in **a**) and lipiodol uptake in the right and left lobes after the second TACE. Progressive lymph node metastasis is noted in the porta hepatis and retroperitoneum (**b, c**). Ascites is also present.

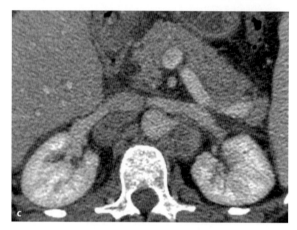

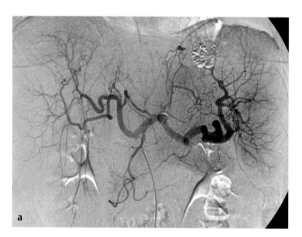

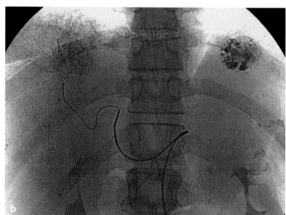

Fig. 7.63 a, b Third chemotherapy cycle.
a Selective angiography of the common hepatic artery before the third TACE.

b Selective angiography of the right hepatic artery after the third TACE.

Further Case Summary

Six days after her last TACE, the patient was hospitalized for a recurrence of ascites and for deterioration of liver and renal function, which continued to decline on subsequent days. The ascites increased, and peripheral edema developed. Seventeen days after the last TACE, the patient was transferred to the ICU with drowsiness and an acute fall in blood pressure. Her hemoglobin was 5.8 mg/dL. Bleeding esophageal varices were treated by gastroscopic ligation. A hepatorenal syndrome subsequently developed, however. The liver failed first, and the patient died of multiple organ failure 19 days after the last TACE.

Error Analysis and Strategy for Error Prevention

The enlarged lymph nodes in the porta hepatis detected by CT during the first two chemotherapy cycles were misinterpreted as reactive lymphadenitis. Due to the lack of tissue discrimination by CT, it would have been correct to include a postinflammatory change (hepatitis C) and metastasis (multifocal HCC) in the differential diagnosis.

The last hepatic chemoembolization was contraindicated for the following reasons:

- Because they were extrahepatic, the lymph node metastases were a relative contraindication for TACE. They showed progressive enlargement during the course of the TACE treatments.
- Some of the liver tumors did not respond to the previous chemoembolizations, despite appropriate interventional technique, and intrahepatic tumor elements showing no lipiodol uptake had enlarged since the last chemoembolization. This meant that there was no sound rationale for repeating the same therapeutic procedure.
- The abnormal liver function values and ascites before the last chemoembolization indicated that the liver, already damaged by cirrhosis and multifocal HCC, sustained further diffuse parenchymal damage from the previous chemoembolizations. It is true that the cholinesterase level of 1.3 kU/L (contraindication < 1 kU/L), the total bilirubin of 1.7 mg/dL (contraindication > 2.5 mg/dL), and the Quick PT of 66% (contraindication < 50%) were within acceptable limits, but the low platelet count of 60000/μL was an absolute contraindication for TACE.

Intravascular Foreign Body?

History and Clinical Findings

A 75-year-old woman suffered from urolithiasis. A urinary tract obstruction on the right side with incipient urosepsis had been successfully treated 4 weeks earlier by the placement of a ureteral stent. During her current hospitalization, the stones in both pelvicaliceal systems were disintegrated by extracorporeal shockwave lithotripsy (ESWL) so that they could pass in the urine. Routine chest radiographs mainly showed an S-shaped curvature of the spine and an "indeterminate" threadlike foreign body of metallic density projected over the mediastinum and upper abdomen (**Fig. 7.64**).

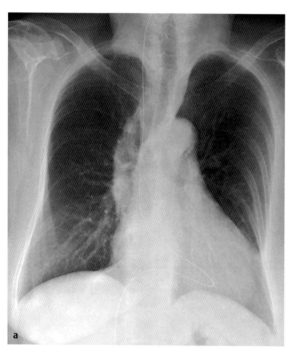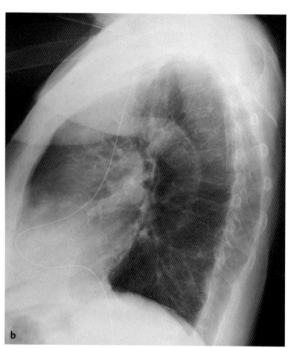

Fig. 7.64 a, b Chest radiographs show thoracic scoliosis and an indeterminate foreign body of metallic density projected over the mediastinum and upper abdomen.

Further Case Summary

Four weeks later, a second chest radiographic examination was performed following a myocardial infarction. This time the report correctly described the foreign body as a guidewire fragment that extended from the right cervical region down the superior vena cava and right atrium into the inferior vena cava that presumably had been "lost" during the attempt to place a central venous catheter. The patient recovered from the myocardial infarction and was referred 3 weeks later for interventional retrieval of the foreign body. The radiographs of the cervical spine and abdomen taken for catheter localization are shown in **Fig. 7.65**. Consistent with the radiology report, a guidewire 1.5 m long was extracted through the right common femoral vein without complications (**Fig. 7.66**).

Error Analysis and Strategy for Error Prevention

The anatomic relationships of the foreign body were disregarded when the initial radiographs were interpreted. The foreign body was located in the superior vena cava, formed a loop in the right atrium and ventricle, and extended into the inferior vena cava. The fact that the patient was discharged with an unidentified foreign body was due mainly to the vague wording of the radiology report. Whenever an unexplained foreign body is seen on radiographic films, the referring physician should be contacted for further clinical information and the ward physician should be notified of the findings. Often this is the only way to make an accurate differential diagnosis, determine the risk to the patient, and institute appropriate treatment.

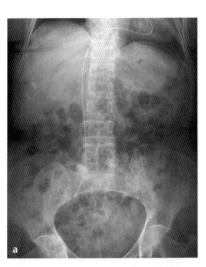
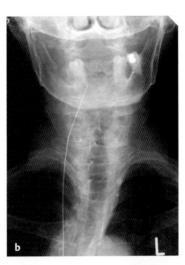

Fig. 7.65 a, b Radiographs for planning the foreign body extraction.

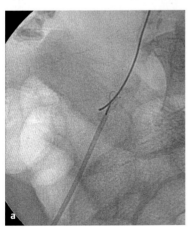
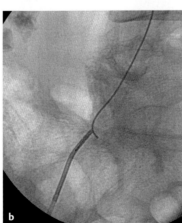

Fig. 7.66 a, b Percutaneous extraction of the intravascular foreign body with a wire loop. The foreign body is snared with the wire loop (**a**) and removed with a retrieval catheter (**b**).

Pneumothorax/ Mediastinal Hematoma/ Pulmonary Embolism

History and Clinical Findings

A 54-year-old woman with breast cancer had undergone a left breast-conserving lumpectomy and axillary dissection 3 days earlier and presented now for portacath implantation in preparation for chemotherapy. The catheter was inserted into the subclavian vein under ultrasound guidance. The patient felt faint after the procedure and was placed on a stretcher for observation. When her complaints improved, an expiratory chest radiograph was taken in the standing position to exclude pneumothorax and was interpreted as normal (**Fig. 7.67**). During the next hour the patient developed respiratory problems and complained of stabbing paravertebral pain behind the right scapula. When an attempt was made to take another standing chest radiograph, the patient collapsed. A critical care physician was summoned as a safety precaution. Breath sounds were not audible on the right side, prompting a clinical diagnosis of pneumothorax. When the patient's vital signs were stable, a supine chest radiograph was obtained and showed widening of the mediastinum relative to the previous film (**Fig. 7.68**). The radiologist interpreted this finding as a mediastinal hematoma. A pneumothorax could not be identified on the supine film. Pulmonary embolism was considered as a possible cause of the complaints, and CT scans were obtained (**Fig. 7.69**).

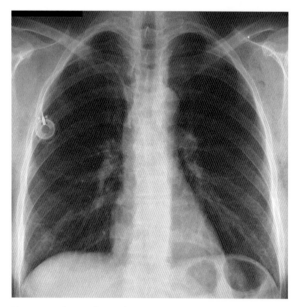

Fig. 7.67 Chest radiograph, upright expiratory view after port implantation. Soft-tissue emphysema is present following an axillary dissection on the left side.

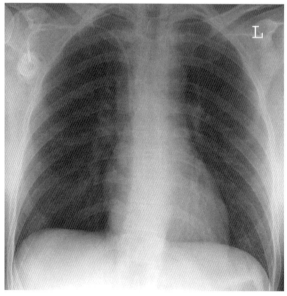

Fig. 7.68 Chest radiograph, expiratory view in the supine position. The upper mediastinum appears widened relative to the previous radiograph. This was interpreted as evidence of a mediastinal hematoma.

Further Case Summary

CT showed an anterior pneumothorax on the right side (**Fig. 7.69**). The catheter was correctly positioned. Mediastinal hemorrhage and pulmonary embolism were excluded.

The pneumothorax was treated by the placement of a suction drain. The further course was uneventful, and the patient was discharged 3 days later.

Error Analysis and Strategy for Error Prevention

Pneumothorax is a very rare complication of port implantation. In a retrospective study of 802 patients who underwent port implantation at the Radiology Department of Cologne University Hospital between December 1, 2004, and January 23, 2009, only two of the patients (0.3%) developed a pneumothorax that required treatment with a thoracostomy tube (see **Table 7.4**). The diagnostic and therapeutic management of this complication was medically appropriate in the present case. Two errors of interpretation occurred during the diagnostic process, however:

- A vertical line in the right lateral lower lung zone was missed during interpretation of the supine radiograph (**Fig. 7.70**). This line was formed by the visceral pleura, which had been separated from the parietal pleura by air in the pleural space. No lung markings were visible lateral to the line. The portion of the diaphragm lateral to the line was defined more sharply than other portions because of air outlining.
- The apparent widening of the upper mediastinum in **Fig. 7.68** is explained by the supine body position. The hydrostatic pressure gradient in the mediastinal veins is higher in the standing position than in the supine position. Because of this pressure gradient, the veins in the upper mediastinum are less engorged with blood when the patient stands upright.
- Supine radiographs with a tangential beam may be helpful in detecting or excluding an anterior pneumothorax (**Fig. 7.71**).

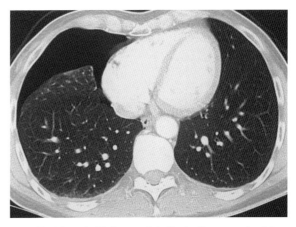

Fig. 7.69   Thoracic CT shows a clinically significant anterior right pneumothorax with no signs of tension.

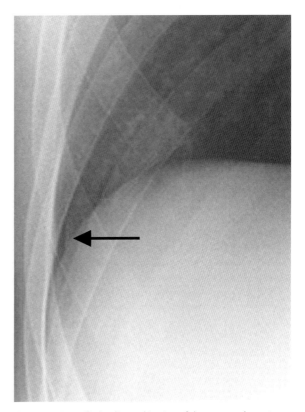

Fig. 7.70   Magnified radiographic view of the pneumothorax in **Fig. 7.68**. The CT-confirmed anterior pneumothorax is manifested on the supine chest radiograph only by a vertical pleural line (arrow). Lung markings are not visible lateral to the line, causing that portion of the diaphragm to appear more sharply outlined than the medial portions.

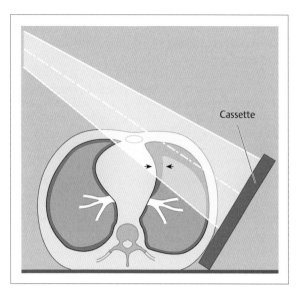

Fig. 7.71 Supine chest radiograph. The x-ray cassette is positioned at an oblique angle for detection of anterior pneumothorax.

Cassette

References and Further Reading

Zähringer M, Hilgers J, Krüger K, et al. [Ultrasound guided implantation of chest port systems via the lateral subclavian vein]. RoFo 2006: 178; 324–329

Iatrogenic Pneumothorax

Pneumothorax results from an abnormal communication between the pleural space and atmosphere, causing loss of the negative intrapleural pressure. The communication may be caused by an injury to the chest wall or lung parenchyma that involves the visceral pleura. Most traumatic cases have an iatrogenic cause. The cardinal symptoms are chest pain and dyspnea. Smaller pneumothoraces undergo spontaneous resorption.

Direct and indirect signs. A pneumothorax may present the following direct radiographic signs:
- Because of air in the pleural space, the visceral pleura appears as a hairline shadow that is separate from the parietal pleura.
- Pulmonary vascular markings do not extend to the chest wall.

Indirect radiographic signs of pneumothorax:
- The costal pleura, mediastinum, and diaphragm have sharper-than-normal outlines due to the high contrast between the soft tissues and the air in the pleural cavity.
- Air in the posterior costophrenic recess makes the upper abdominal quadrants appear more radiolucent.

Expiratory radiograph. There are several reasons why a pneumothorax is easier to detect on expiratory radiographs than on inspiratory views. The volume of the chest is smaller in expiration than inspiration. Air expulsion from the alveoli and airways increases the density of the lungs. Because the pneumothorax maintains a constant air volume in the pleural space, the absorption difference between the intrapleural air and the lung is increased during expiration.

Supine radiograph. Smaller pneumothoraces are not visible on supine radiographs because the air rises into the higher portions of the pleural space. When the x-rays pass through the patient, they traverse the air in the pleural space as well as the lung, resulting in an absence of visible absorption differences. Larger anterior pneumothoraces are detectable as rounded lucencies with smooth margins that are not localized in relation to key pulmonary or mediastinal structures.

Supine Chest Radiographs

Upright radiographs provide better physiologic and geometric imaging conditions than supine radiographs and are therefore preferred in patients who are able to stand erect. Supine radiographs differ from upright radiographs in several key respects:
- The film–focus distance is 1 m instead of 2 m. This alters the beam geometry and creates a magnification effect.
- The film cassette is placed behind the patient's back, resulting in an AP projection. This causes a geometric magnification of the anterior mediastinum compared with upright radiographs taken in the PA projection.

- The supine position restricts inspiration, causing the diaphragm to be superimposed over the basal lung zones. The supine position also decreases the aeration of the upper lobes and causes the mediastinum to appear wider than in the standing position due to relatively greater venous distension in the upper mediastinum.
- A low-voltage technique (tube voltage < 100 kV) is generally used for bedside radiographs to improve contrast.

Complication of Minimally Invasive Placement of a Central Venous Port Catheter?

History and Clinical Findings

A 51-year-old woman with breast cancer had a port catheter implanted in preparation for chemotherapy. The insertion was done as a minimally invasive procedure in an angiography suite using local anesthesia and aseptic technique. The subclavian vein was punctured under ultrasound guidance, and the central venous limb of the port system was advanced by guidewire into the superior vena cava. At the end of the intervention, an expiratory chest radiograph was taken to exclude a postintervention pneumothorax (**Fig. 7.72**). The radiograph was interpreted as normal.

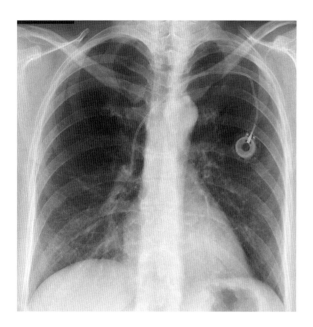

Fig. 7.72   Expiratory chest radiograph after port implantation was interpreted as normal.

Further Case Summary

Five weeks later the patient was referred for an angiographic assessment of port patency, as it had been difficult to aspirate blood from the port and the patient had developed retrosternal pain after her initial chemotherapy (**Fig. 7.73**). Angiography showed that the central venous limb of the port was in the internal thoracic vein. The chemotherapy had led to thrombophlebitic occlusion of the internal thoracic vein, necessitating removal of the port. At the request of the patient, a new central venous port was placed for the continuation of chemotherapy.

Error Analysis and Strategy for Error Prevention

Although the chest radiograph was interpreted as normal, it actually showed that the catheter segment projected over the upper mediastinum did not follow a convex arc along the course of the superior vena cava (vertical arrow in **Fig. 7.74**) while its lower portion was projected outside the mediastinum over the lung (horizontal arrow in **Fig. 7.74**). This meant that the catheter did not occupy the lumen of the superior vena cava, which forms the right border of the upper mediastinal shadow.

As a rule, ultrasound can display the subclavian vein only as far as its confluence with the jugular vein. When transcutaneous color duplex scanning is performed

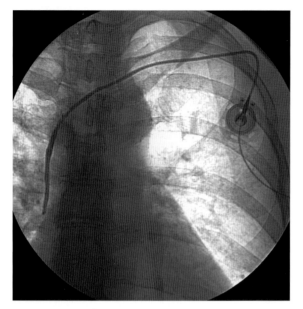

Fig. 7.73 Image after contrast injection into the port documents incorrect placement of the port in the thrombosed right internal thoracic vein.

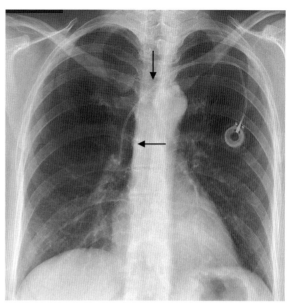

Fig. 7.74 Explanation of **Fig. 7.72**. The vertical arrow marks the catheter position, which did not follow the course of the vena cava (horizontal arrow).

Table 7.4 Retrospective analysis of all 802 patients who underwent port implantation at the Cologne University Radiology Department between December 1, 2004, and January 23, 2009 (Boecker et al. 2007; Zähringer et al. 2006). The technical success rate was 98.3%

Type of complication	Patients (n)	Patients (%)
Unsuccessful venipuncture	8	1.0
Acute complications	11	1.4
■ Pneumothorax, total	4	0.5
– Pneumothorax requiring drainage	2	0.3
■ Inadvertent arterial puncture	1	0.1
■ Postoperative bleeding, total	4	0.5
– Postoperative bleeding requiring revision	2	0.3
■ Foreign bodies left in situ	2	0.3
Infections	1	0.1
■ Allergic skin eruption	1	0.1

through a parasternal approach, air in the upper lobe of the lung prevents visualization of the middle mediastinum. During the intervention the catheter was introduced under fluoroscopic guidance, and the catheter malposition was not detected. The only goal in interpreting the chest radiograph was to exclude a pneumothorax (**Table 7.4**).

References and Further Reading

Boecker J, Bovenschulte H, Schröer V, et al. Die sonographisch gesteuerte Implantation von Portkathetersystemen über die laterale Vena subclavia. Fortschr Röntgenstr 2007; 179: VO 401.6 www.DRG.de

Zähringer M, Hilgers J, Krüger K, et al. [Ultrasound guided implantation of chest port systems via the lateral subclavian vein]. RoFo 2006: 178; 324–329

Complication of Tumor Embolization

History and Clinical Findings

A 35-year-old woman complained of thoracolumbar back pain of recent onset. On orthopedic examination, tenderness to percussion was noted in that area. Neurologic findings were normal. Radiographs of the thoracic spine showed extensive osteolytic destruction of the T12 vertebral body (**Fig. 7.75**). MRI (**Fig. 7.76**) and CT (**Fig. 7.77**) revealed an extraosseous soft-tissue tumor that had almost completely destroyed the left pillar of the vertebral segment and the central and left portions of the vertebral body. The tumor extended into the spinal canal, displacing the cord to the right, and had infiltrated the erector trunci muscle. Disseminated pulmonary nodules up to 1.5 cm in diameter were detected in both lungs.

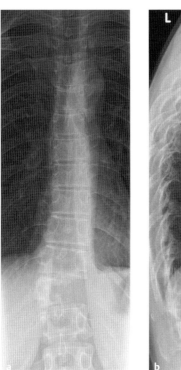
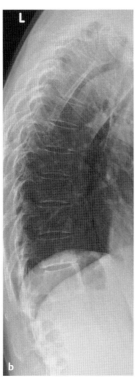

Fig. 7.75 a, b Osteolytic destruction of the T12 vertebral body.

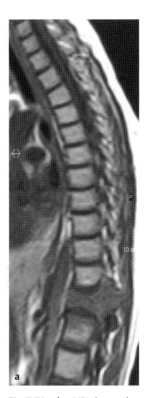
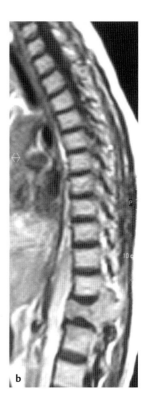

Fig. 7.76 a, b MRI shows a hypovascular mass spreading from the T12 to L1 vertebral body with an intraspinal component.
a Unenhanced T1-weighted image.
b T1-weighted image after IV contrast administration.

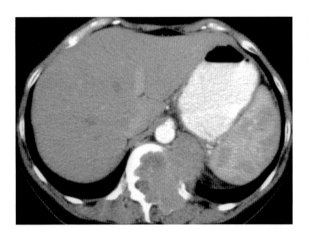

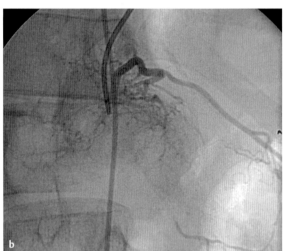

Fig. 7.77 Axial CT scan shows T12 vertebral body destruction by an extensive spinal and paravertebral soft-tissue mass. The tumor has displaced the spinal cord to the right and infiltrated the left erector trunci muscle.

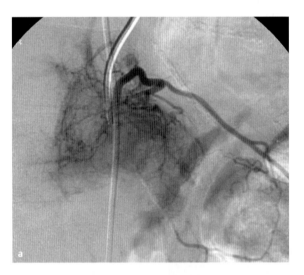

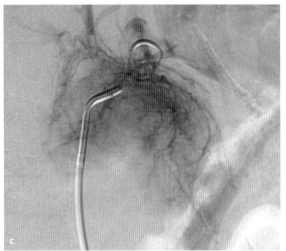

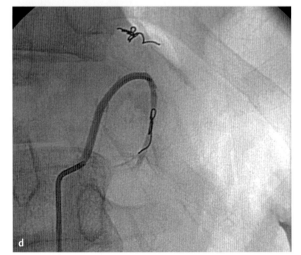

Fig. 7.78 a–d Superselective embolization of the tumor-feeding intercostal and lumbar arterial branches with hydrophilic, nonabsorbable acrylic-copolymer microparticles impregnated with gelatin (Embospheres, BioSphere Medical) 40–120 μm in diameter, followed by proximal vascular occlusion with complex helical-fibered platinum coils (Boston Scientific).

a Superselective angiography of the left intercostal artery at level T12 before embolization.

b Superselective angiography of the left intercostal artery at level T12 after embolization.

c Superselective angiography of the left lumbar artery at level L1 before embolization.

d Superselective angiography of the left lumbar artery at level L1 after embolization.

A tumorectomy with vertebral corporectomy was proposed to stabilize the spinal column and reduce the tumor volume. Since experience has shown that these tumors have a rich blood supply, surgery is often complicated or even prevented by heavy bleeding. Surgical complications may range from a prolonged operating time or ischemia-induced transverse cord symptoms to a fatal hemorrhage. For this reason, the tumor was embolized by interventional radiology one day before the planned operation (**Fig. 7.78**). The procedure began with selective diagnostic angiography of the two intercostal arteries arising cranial to the T12 vertebral body and the two lumbar arteries arising caudal to T12. The tumor was supplied chiefly by the left intercostal and lumbar arteries. The right intercostal and lumbar arteries appeared normal. This was followed by superselective catheterization of the tumor-feeding arteries with a microcatheter. Contrast runoff to the anterior spinal artery was not observed. Both arteries were embolized with microspheres (Embospheres, BioSphere Medical) 40–120 µm in diameter, followed by proximal vascular occlusion with platinum coils (complex helical-fibered platinum coils, Boston Scientific). Postinterventional angiography confirmed effective dearterialization of the tumor.

Further Case Summary

Shortly after the intervention the patient complained of sensory deficits on the lateral sides of both thighs, which increased rapidly over time. Motor paralysis also developed. In the belief that the neurologic symptoms were caused by cord compression brought on by sudden swelling of the soft-tissue tumor due to ischemic edema, a left-sided laminectomy was performed to relieve the pressure. The spinal column was stabilized by fusing the segments from T10 to L2. Despite the spinal fusion, irreversible transverse cord paralysis developed at the T12 level. MR images acquired 8 days after the operation showed diffuse swelling of the spinal cord from the T8 to L1 level with patchy hyperintensity in T2-weighted sequences, consistent with ischemic edema.

Postoperative specimen histopathology revealed a hypervascular osteolytic lesion composed predominantly of spindle cells with numerous osteoclastic giant cells and multiple foci of new bone formation. The tumor was classified as a well-differentiated osteosarcoma with abundant giant cells. There was no evidence of intra- or intercellular edema. The embolization material was dispersed in the precapillary arterioles.

During the next 12 months the patient had a partial recovery of sensation in the lower limbs. The retroperitoneal residual tumor and pulmonary metastases showed partial remission in response to chemotherapy.

Error Analysis and Strategy for Error Prevention

The cord paralysis was caused by the embolization. In the most likely scenario, embolization particles gained access to the radiculomedullary and radiculo-pial arteries arising from the catheterized intercostal and lumbar arteries. The radiculomedullary and radiculo-pial arteries contribute to the blood supply of the spinal cord (**Fig. 7.79**).

Because of their small size and the preferential opacification of tumor vessels, the radiculomedullary and radiculo-pial arteries often are not visible on angiograms taken before the dearterialization of a hypervascular tumor. Once the tumor vessels have been partially occluded, the hemodynamics may change in such a way that the pressure gradient between the intercostal/lumbar arteries and the radiculomedullary/radiculo-pial arteries is higher than the gradient between the intercostal/lumbar arteries and the embolized tumor vessels. When the catheter tip is positioned proximal to the origin of the two radicular arteries, the increasing blood flow toward the spinal canal that occurs during embolization may direct some of the embolic material toward the spinal cord. When the catheter tip is positioned past the origin of the radiculomedullary and radiculo-pial arteries, a similar effect may occur due to reflux.

It has been suggested that this complication can be prevented by performing a provocative lidocaine test (injecting lidocaine through the superselective catheter placement that will be used for embolization) to assess the risk of spinal cord injury. This does not appear promising, however, when we consider the constant pressure and flow changes that occur during the embolization procedure.

In selecting the diameters of the microspheres, the desire to occlude the tumor vessels as completely as possible at the precapillary level should be weighed against the need to protect the spinal cord from ischemia. In the case presented here, the rationale was to use microparticles of the smallest available diameters (40–120 µm range) to reduce the risk of bleeding and its complications while also avoiding the induction of cord ischemia and paralysis. In the literature, it is stated that embolization particles > 150 µm in diameter should be used to reduce the risk of spinal cord injury. This risk cannot be completely eliminated. Finstein et al. (2006) reported one instance of paralysis following the embolization of a giant cell tumor of the same size and location with particles 500–700 µm in diameter.

Sudden compression of the spinal cord by ischemia-induced swelling of the tumor could not have caused the paralysis in this case because histopathology showed no signs of intra- or intercellular edema. Also, because the left pillar of the spinal column had been destroyed, it could not provide a bony fulcrum for mechanical cord compression resulting from an increase in tumor volume.

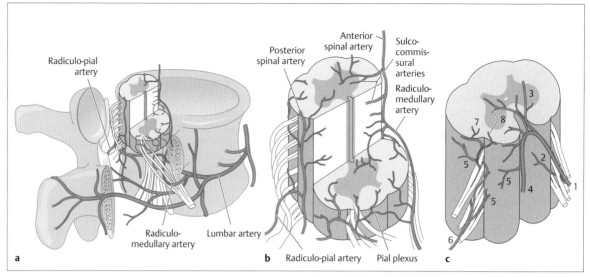

Fig. 7.79 a–c   Blood supply of the spinal cord in the transverse and vertical planes. The spinal cord is supplied in the transverse plane by the radiculomedullary and radiculo-pial arteries, which arise from the lumbar artery. It is supplied in the vertical plane by the anterior spinal artery, which arises from both vertebral arteries, and by the paired posterior spinal arteries, which arise from the inferior cerebellar artery and vertebral artery and are generally distributed to the conus. The transverse and vertical planes of the spinal blood supply have numerous interanastomoses. This particularly applies to the radiculomedullary arteries and anterior spinal artery. Normal variants are common.

a Origin of the radicular artery from the lumbar artery.

b Intraspinal branches of the radiculomedullary artery and radiculo-pial artery. The radiculomedullary artery communicates with the anterior spinal artery and delivers a segmental blood supply to large portions of the anterior spinal cord (gray matter of the anterior horns: motor neurons; white matter: pyramidal tracts and extrapyramidal motor tracts). The radiculo-pial artery makes a segmental contribution to the blood supply of cord areas bordering the spinal pia mater.

c 1 = radiculomedullary artery; 2 = pial vascular plexus; 3 = ascending branch in the anterior cord; 4 = descending branch in the anterior cord; 5 = pial vascular plexus; 6 = radiculo-pial artery; 7 = radial perforating branches of the radiculo-pial artery; 8 = sulcocommissural artery.

References and Further Reading

Berkefeld J, Scale D, Kirchner J, Heinrich T, Kollath J. Hypervascular spinal tumors: influence of the embolization technique on perioperative hemorrhage. AJNR 1999; 20: 757–763

Finstein JL, Chin KR, Alvandi F, Lackman RD. Postembolization paralysis in a man with thoracolumbar giant cell tumor. Clin Orthop Relat Res 2006; 453: 335–340

Lasjaunias P, Berenstein A. Surgical Neuroanagiography. Vol. 3. Functional Vascular Anatomy of the Brain, Spinal Cord and Spine. Berlin: Springer; 1990

Index

Note: images of the most common indexing modalities such as CT and MRI have not been indexed (apart from specialised variations of these techniques such as "diffusion-weighted MRI")